Case-Based
Pathology and
Laboratory Medicine

returned by

k, your l

m

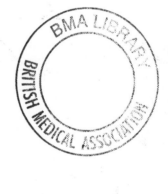

Medicine at a Glance: Core Cases

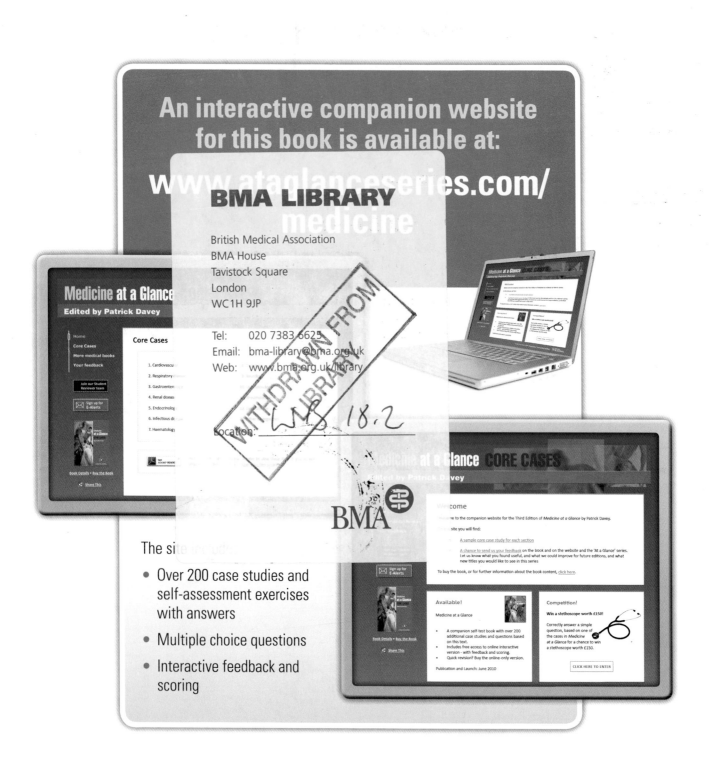

An interactive companion website
for this book is available at:

www.ataglanceseries.com/
medicine

Medicine at a Glance
Edited by Patrick Davey

Home
Core Cases
More medical books
Your feedback

Join our Student
Reviewer team

Sign up for
E-Alerts

Book Details • Buy the Book

Share This

Core Cases

1. Cardiovascu
2. Respiratory
3. Gastroenten
4. Renal diseas
5. Endocrinolog
6. Infectious di
7. Haematolog

Medicine at a Glance **CORE CASES**
Edited by Patrick Davey

Welcome

Welcome to the companion website for the Third Edition of *Medicine at a Glance* by Patrick Davey.

On this site you will find:

A sample core case study for each section

A chance to send us your feedback on the book and on the website and the 'At a Glance' series.
Let us know what you found useful, and what we could improve for future editions, and what
new titles you would like to see in this series

To buy the book, or for further information about the book content, click here.

Sign up for
E-Alerts

Book Details • Share This

Available!

Medicine at a Glance

- A companion self-test book with over 200
  additional case studies and questions based
  on this text.
- Includes free access to online interactive
  version - with feedback and scoring.
- Quick revision? Buy the online-only version.

Publication and Launch: June 2010

Competition!

Win a stethoscope worth £150!

Correctly answer a simple
question, based on one of
the cases in *Medicine
at a Glance* for a chance to win
a stethoscope worth £150.

CLICK HERE TO ENTER

The site includes:

- Over 200 case studies and
  self-assessment exercises
  with answers

- Multiple choice questions

- Interactive feedback and
  scoring

Medicine at a Glance: Core Cases

Edited by

Patrick Davey

Consultant Cardiologist
Northampton General Hospital
Northampton, and
Honorary Senior Lecturer
Department of Cardiovascular Medicine
John Radcliffe Hospital
Oxford

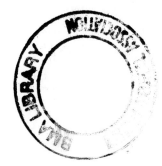

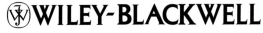

WILEY-BLACKWELL

A John Wiley & Sons, Ltd., Publication

This edition first published 2011, © 2011 by Blackwell Publishing Ltd

Blackwell Publishing was acquired by John Wiley & Sons in February 2007. Blackwell's publishing program has been merged with Wiley's global Scientific, Technical and Medical business to form Wiley-Blackwell.

Registered office: John Wiley & Sons Ltd, The Atrium, Southern Gate, Chichester, West Sussex, PO19 8SQ, UK

Editorial offices: 9600 Garsington Road, Oxford, OX4 2DQ, UK
The Atrium, Southern Gate, Chichester, West Sussex, PO19 8SQ, UK

111 River Street, Hoboken, NJ 07030-5774, USA

For details of our global editorial offices, for customer services and for information about how to apply for permission to reuse the copyright material in this book please see our website at www.wiley.com/wiley-blackwell

Library of Congress Cataloging-in-Publication Data

Medicine at a glance : core cases / edited by Patrick Davey.
      p. ; cm. – (At a glance)
   Companion v. to: Medicine at a glance. 3rd ed. 2010.
   Includes bibliographical references and index.
   ISBN 978-1-4443-3511-8 (alk. paper)
   1. Clinical medicine–Problems, exercises, etc.   2. Clinical medicine–Case studies.
   I. Davey, Patrick.   II. Title: Medicine at a glance.   III. Series: At a glance series (Oxford, England)
   [DNLM: 1. Clinical Medicine–Problems and Exercises.   2. Case Reports–Problems and Exercises.
   WB 18.2 M4893 2010]
   RC58.M478 2010
   616.0076–dc22

                                         2010024528

ISBN 978-1-4443-3511-8

A catalogue record for this book is available from the British Library.

Set in Time New Roman 9/11.5 pt by Toppan Best-set Premedia Limited

Printed and Bound in Singapore by Markono Print Media Pte Ltd

1 2011

Contents

Preface 6
List of Contributors 7
List of Abbreviations 9

1 Cardiovascular: Cases and Questions 13
   Answers 25
2 Respiratory: Cases and Questions 39
   Answers 43
3 Gastroenterology: Cases and Questions 47
   Answers 59
4 Renal: Cases and Questions 71
   Answers 76
5 Endocrinology: Cases and Questions 83
   Answers 88
6 Infectious Disease: Cases and Questions 94
   Answers 107
7 Haematology: Cases and Questions 120
   Answers 130
8 Oncology: Cases and Questions 141
   Answers 146
9 Neurology: Cases and Questions 151
   Answers 158
10 Ophthalmology: Cases and Questions 168
   Answers 172
11 Rheumatology: Cases and Questions 176
   Answers 179
12 Dermatology: Cases and Questions 184
   Answers 190
13 Other Emergencies: Cases and Questions 196
   Answers 206
14 The Acutely Unwell Patient: Cases and Questions 213
   Answers 216

Preface

When studying, it is always important to determine whether or not one has learnt the subject – clearly, this is as true in medicine as any other subject. Different people have very different styles of learning and of testing themselves as to whether they have learnt and understood the subject thoroughly. Some people go on a wing and a prayer, reading and hoping they have retained some information, without testing their knowledge. Some go to the other extreme, reading, shutting the reference book and then writing down that which they have retained. They may do this immediately after reading, or some time later, clearly testing different forms of memory. Yet others, after reading, shut the book, shut their eyes and try to recall mentally their knowledge of the subject. This is often a most enjoyable way of working out what one knows and what one doesn't. Perhaps a down side of this 'shut-eye' mental-testing approach is the degree of mental strength needed to prevent day dreams intruding into working thoughts and distracting us from our studies! Some will discuss the subject with their peers, working out what they know, testing their understanding logically ("if this, then why not this?") and having colleagues help fill in the gaps – this can be a compellingly enjoyable way to learn. In fact, it may be that one of the most important roles of medical student clubs and rooms within medical schools is to encourage this sort of interaction. Perhaps even the most important role of the medical school is to ensure this peer-to-peer bonding, one that allows you to trust colleagues knowledge and judgement sufficiently to ask them questions to which you don't know the answer, sometimes simple questions and sometimes the apparently 'stupid' question, the one everyone has been meaning to ask, the one so obvious you have been frightened to ask, as you feel you should know the answer, but the one in fact which more often than not, is the most pertinent and central question to the problem at hand. This ability to interact with colleagues in this fashion will be, probably, the most important aspect of your competence as a future learner and so as a clinician.

Perhaps in medicine the most potent way of learning and testing knowledge is around a case; students see a patient ('clerk them in') using a fairly rigid and stylized system, synthesize this data into a short presentation, so including all the pertinent positives and negatives, which is then presented to a more senior clinician. The key part of this is not so much the acquisition and presentation of the data, though these are all crucial skills for a competent clinician, rather it is the joy of understanding what the data means, what is the data telling us about the patient and their condition? Does it only mean one illness, and if so why? This seems unlikely, but sometimes is the case. Could there be a differential diagnosis (almost inevitably so)? Why? To understand the data, as well as to collect and present it, one needs a full knowledge of the subject of medicine. There is no doubt that marshalling ones thoughts, rather like the venerable Dr House in the recent successful TV program, as a sleuth and as a detective, can be the most fun way to learn. The data is tested against our knowledge of disease processes, allowing us to reject or accept possible diagnoses. Do all the symptoms fit? Do the investigations support our possible diagnoses? If not, why not? What data needs to fit? What data can be rejected? This allows us to follow one diagnosis or another, reject it, find another, test it and so on. All clinicians are, to a greater or lesser extent, medical detectives in the style of Sherlock Holmes meets Dr House. All this sleuthing can be tremendous fun and is a most potent way to learn and, as importantly, to know that you have learnt and what still needs to be learnt.

Real life cases and real life clinicians, however, may not always be available and another way to learn is the case-based approach from a textbook. This is the aim of this book, to introduce you to a case and then to test your understanding of that case, largely using multiple choice questions and answers. These MCQs are also available on the website accompanying the *Medicine at a Glance* book (www.ataglanceseries.com/medicine). There are different ways to test your knowledge using textbook based MCQs – one could read the question, mentally answer it, then look the answer up. I would suggest, however, that the best way is to read the question and write down the answer you think is right – this way, you commit yourself and so find the truth as to whether you know, or whether you only think you know! Every answer has a detailed explanation of what the answer is and why, and also a suggestion from *Medicine at a Glance* for further reading.

I hope you will enjoy this book and wish you every success in your endeavours. As always, we would be most pleased to have any feedback (medicalstudent@wiley.co.uk).

Patrick Davey

List of Contributors

Laura Benjamin
Wellcome Trust Clinical Research Fellow
London

Chris B. Bunker
Professor of Dermatology & Consultant Dermatologist
Chelsea & Westminster, Royal Marsden Hospitals and
Imperial College School of Medicine
London

Keith Channon
Professor of Cardiovascular Medicine & Honorary Consultant
Cardiologist
Department of Cardiovascular Medicine
University of Oxford
John Radcliffe Hospital
Oxford

Graham Collins
Department of Haematology
John Radcliffe Hospital
Oxford

Ophelia Dadzie
Locum Consultant Dermatopathologist and Dermatologist
St John's Institute of Dermatology
Guy's and St Thomas' NHS Foundation Trust
London

Patrick Davey
Consultant Cardiologist
Northampton General Hospital
Northampton, and
Honorary Senior Lecturer
Department of Cardiovascular Medicine
John Radcliffe Hospital
Oxford

Suzanne Donnelly
Formerly of Department of Rheumatology
St George's Hospital
London

Peggy Frith
Consultant Ophthalmic Physician
The Radcliffe Infirmary
Oxford

Jonathan Gleadle
Lecturer in Nephrology
The Wellcome Trust
Centre for Human Genetics
Oxford

Christopher Hingston
SpR Intensive Care Medicine
University Hospital of Wales
Cardiff

Mark Juniper
Consultant Physician
Great Western Hospital
Swindon

David Keeling
Consultant Haematologist
Oxford Haemophilia Centre
The Churchill Hospital
Oxford

David Lalloo
Reader in Tropical Medicine
Liverpool School of Tropical Medicine
Liverpool

Tim J. Littlewood
Consultant Haematologist
Department of Haematology
John Radcliffe Hospital
Oxford

Andrew McLean-Tooke
Royal Victoria Infirmary
Newcastle-upon-Tyne

Faye Mellington
Specialty Registrar (Ophthalmology)
Oxford Eye Hospital
Oxford

Richard Penson
Director of Clinical Research in Medical Gynecologic Oncology
Massachusetts General Hospital
Boston
USA

Anna Rathmell
Oxford

Jeremy Shearman
Consultant Gastroenterologist
Department of Gastroenterology
Warwick Hospital
Warwick

Gavin Spickett
Consultant in Clinical Immunology, Allergy & General Medicine
Regional Department of Immunology
Royal Victoria Infirmary
Newcastle-Upon-Tyne

David Sprigings
Consultant Cardiologist
Northampton General Hospital
Northampton

Jeremy Steele
Consultant in Medical Oncology
St Bartholomew's Hospital
London

Catherine Stroud
Consultant Immunologist
Royal Victoria Infirmary
Newcastle-Upon-Tyne

Kevin Talbot
MRC Clinician Scientist
Department of Human Anatomy & Genetics, and
Honorary Consultant Neurologist
Department of Clinical Neurology
University of Oxford
The Radcliffe Infirmary
Oxford

Laura Tookman
Academic Clinical Fellow in Oncology
Institute of Cancer
Barts and The London School of Medicine and Dentistry
London

Helen E. Turner
Consultant Endocrinologist
Endocrinology Department
The Radcliffe Infirmary
Oxford

Katherine Whybrew
General Practitioner
Bristol

Matt Wise
Consultant in Intensive Care Medicine
University Hospital of Wales
Cardiff

Paul Wordsworth
Professor of Rheumatology
Nuffield Orthopaedic Centre
Oxford

List of Abbreviations

AAA	abdominal aortic aneurysm		**BMD**	bone marrow density
Ab	antibody		**BMI**	body mass index
ABG	arterial blood gas		**BMZ**	basement membrane zone
ABPA	allergic bronchopulmonary aspergillosis		**BNF**	*British National Formulary*
AC	acromioclavicular		**BOOP**	bronchiolitis obliterans organizing pneumonia
ACE	angiotensin-converting enzyme		**BP**	blood pressure
ACS	acute coronary syndrome		**BRVO**	branch retinal vein occlusion
ACTH	adrenocorticotrophic hormone		**CABG**	coronary artery bypass graft
ADH	antidiuretic hormone		**CAD**	coronary artery disease
ADP	adenosine diphosphate		**CAH**	congenital adrenal hyperplasia
ADPKD	autosomal dominant polycystic kidney disease		**CBD**	common bile duct
AF	atrial fibrillation		**CBT**	cognitive behavioural therapy
AFB	acid-fast bacilli		**CCDC**	consultant in communicable disease control
α-FP	α-fetoprotein		**CCP**	cyclic citrullinated peptide
Ag	antigen		**CCU**	coronary care unit
AIDS	acquired immune deficiency syndrome		**CGD**	chronic granulomatous disease
AIH	autoimmune hepatitis		**CEA**	carcinoembryonic antigen
AIHA	autoimmune haemolytic anaemia		**CF**	cystic fibrosis
AION	anterior ischaemic optic neuropathy		**CFA**	cystic fibrosis alveolitis
ALL	acute lymphoid leukaemia		**CFS**	chronic fatigue syndrome
ALP	alkaline phosphatase		**CFTR**	cystic fibrosis transmembrane conductance regulator
ALT	alanine transaminase		**cGMP**	cyclic guanosine monophosphate
AMA	antimitochondrial antibody		**CHAD**	cold haemagglutinin disease
AML	acute myeloid leukaemia		**CHART**	continuous hyperfractionated accelerated radiotherapy
ANA	antinuclear antibody			
ANCA	antineutrophil cytoplasmic antibody		**CHD**	congenital heart disease
ANF	antinuclear factor		**CIDP**	chronic idiopathic demyelinating polyneuropathy
APC	activated protein C		**CIDP**	chronic inflammatory demyelinating neuropathy
APKD	adult polycystic kidney disease		**CJD**	Creutzfeldt–Jakob disease
APS	antiphospholipid syndrome		**CK**	creatine kinase
APTT	activated partial thromboplastin time		**CLL**	chronic lymphoblastic leukaemia
AR	aortic regurgitation		**CMC**	carpometacarpal
ARDS	adult respiratory distress syndrome		**CML**	chronic myeloid leukaemia
AS	ankylosing spondylitis		**CMV**	cytomegalovirus
ASD	atrial septal defect		**CNS**	central nervous system
ASO	antistreptolysin O		**CO$_2$**	carbon dioxide
AST	aspartate transaminase		**COAD**	chronic obstructive airway disease
α₁-AT	α$_1$-antitrypsin		**COPD**	chronic obstructive pulmonary disease
ATLL	adult T-cell lymphoma/leukaemia		**COX**	cyclo-oxygenase
ATN	acute tubular necrosis		**cP**	centipoise
ATP	adenosine triphosphate		**CPAP**	continuous positive airway pressure
AV	atrioventricular		**CPK**	creatine phosphokinase
AVNRT	atrioventricular nodal re-entrant tachycardia		**CPR**	cardiopulmonary resuscitation
AVRT	atrioventricular re-entrant tachycardia		**CREST**	calcinosis, Raynaud's, oesophagitis, sclerodactyly telangiectasia
AXR	abdominal X-ray			
BAL	bronchoalveolar lavage		**CRH**	corticotrophin-releasing hormone
BBV	blood-borne viruses		**CRP**	C-reactive protein
BCC	basal cell carcinoma		**CRVO**	central retinal vein occlusion
BCE	basal cell epithelioma		**CS**	Churg–Strauss
BCG	bacilli Calmette–Guérin		**CSM**	carotid sinus massage
BCSP	bowel cancer screening programme		**CSF**	cerebrospinal fluid
bd	*bis die* (twice a day)		**CT**	computed tomography
BDZ	benzodiazepine		**CTPA**	computerized tomographic pulmonary angiography
BE	base excess		**CVA**	cerebrovascular accident
BLS	basic life support		**CVID**	common variable immunodeficiency

CVP	central venous pressure	FUO	fever of unknown origin
CWP	coal worker's pneumoconiosis	FVC	forced vital capacity
CXR	chest X-ray	G6PD	glucose-6-phosphate dehydrogenase
CYP	cytochrome P450	GABA	γ-aminobutyric acid
D&V	diarrhoea and vomiting	GBM	glomerular basement membrane
DC	direct current	GCS	Glasgow Coma Score
ddAVP	deamino-D-arginine vasopressin	GFR	glomerular filtration rate
DEXA	dual emission X-ray absorptiometry	GH	growth hormone
DH	dermatitis herpetiformis	GI	gastrointestinal
DHEA	dihydoepiandrosterone	GN	glomerulonephritis
DHF/DSS	dengue haemorrhagic fever/dengue shock syndrome	GnRH	gonadotrophin-releasing hormone
DIC	disseminated intravascular coagulation	GORD	gastro-oesophageal reflux disease
DIF	direct immunofluorecence	GP	general practitioner
DIP	desquamative interstitial pneumonia, distal interphalangeal	GPI	glycosyl-phosphatidylinositol
		γ-GT	γ-glutamyl transferase
DKA	diabetic ketoacidosis	GTN	glyceryl trinitrate
DLB	dementia with Lewy bodies	GU	genitourinary
DM	dermatomyositis, diabetes mellitus	HAART	highly active anti-retroviral therapy
DMARD	disease-modifying antirheumatic drug	HAV	hepatitis A virus
DMSA	[^{99m}Tc] mercaptosuccinic acid	Hb	haemoglobin
DNA	deoxyribonucleic acid	HBsAg	hepatitis B surface antigen
DNAR	'do not attempt resuscitation'	HBV	hepatitis B virus
dsDNA	double-stranded DNA	HCC	hepatocellular carcinoma
DU	duodenal ulcer	hCG	human chorionic gonadotrophin
DVT	deep venous thrombosis	Hct	haematocrit
EAA	extrinsic allergic alveolitis	HCV	hepatitis C virus
EBV	Epstein–Barr virus	HD	Huntington's disease
ECG	electrocardiogram	HDL	high-density lipoprotein
EEG	electroencephalograph	HFE	haemochromatosis gene
EGFR	epidermal growth factor receptor	HHV	human herpes virus
ELISA	enzyme-linked immunosorbent assay	5-HIAA	5-hydroxyindoleacetic acid
EM	electron microscopy	HiB	*Haemophilus influenzae* B
EMA	endomysial antibodies	HIT	heparin-induced thrombocytopenia
EMG	electromyography	HIV	human immunodeficiency virus
EN	erythema nodosum	HLA	human leukocyte antigen
ENT	ear, nose, throat	HMG-CoA	hydroxymethyl-glutaryl coenzyme A
EPAP	expiratory positive airway pressure	HMSN	hereditary motor and sensory neuropathy
ER	endoplasmic reticulum	HNPCC	hereditary non-polyposis colon cancer
ERA	enteric reactive arthritis	HOCM	hypertrophic obstructive cardiomyopathy
ERCP	endoscopic retrograde cholangiopancreatography	HONK	hyperosmolar non-ketotic coma
ESR	erythrocyte sedimentation rate	HPV	human papillomavirus
ESRF	end-stage renal failure	HR	heart rate
ET	essential thrombocythaemia	HRCT	high-resolution computed tomography
EUS	endoscopic ultrasound	HRT	hormone replacement therapy
EVL	endoscopic variceal ligation	HSP	Henoch–Schönlein purpura
FAB	French–American–British classification	HSV	herpes simplex virus
FBC	full blood count	HSV	highly selective vagotomy
FDP	fibrin degradation product	5-HT	5-hydroxytryptamine (serotonin)
FEV$_1$	forced expiratory volume in 1s	HTLV	human T-cell leukaemia virus
FFA	free fatty acid	HUS	haemolytic uraemic syndrome
FFP	fresh frozen plasma	IBD	inflammatory bowel disease
FNAC	fine needle aspiration cytology	IBS	inflammatory bowel syndrome
FOB	faecal occult blood	ICD	implantable cardioverter defibrillator
FPG	fasting plasma glucose	Ig	immunoglobulin
FRC	functional residual capacity	IGF	insulin growth factor
FSGS	focal segmental glomerulosclerosis	IHD	ischaemic heart disease
FSH	follicle-stimulating hormone	IL	interleukin
FTD	frontotemporal dementia	IM	intramuscular
5FU	5-fluorouracil	INR	international normalized ratio

IOP	intraocular pressures		**MUS**	medically unexplained symptom
IPAP	inspiratory positive airway pressure		**MV**	mechanical ventilation
IPPV	intermittent positive pressure ventilation		**MVP**	mitral valve prolapse
IPSS	inferior petrosal sinus sampling		**NaCl**	sodium chloride
ITP	immune thrombocytopenic purpura		**NADPH**	reduced nicotinamide adenine dinucleotide phosphate
ITU	intensive therapy unit			
IV	intravenous		**NG**	nasogastric
IVC	inferior vena cava		**NGU**	non-gonococcal urethritis
IVIG	intravenous immunoglobulin		**NHL**	non-Hodgkin's lymphoma
IVU	intravenous urogram		**NHS**	National Health Service
JVP	jugular venous pressure		**NIV**	non-invasive ventilation
KCl	potassium chloride		**NO**	nitric oxide
KOH	potassium hydroxide		*nocte*	at night
KS	Kaposi's sarcoma		**NPV**	negative pressure ventilation
LA	left artery		**NSAID**	non-steroidal anti-inflammatory drug
LAD	left anterior descending (coronary artery)		**OA**	osteoarthritis
LDH	lactate dehydrogenase		**OCD**	obsessive compulsive disorder
LDL	low-density lipoprotein		**OCP**	oral contraceptive pill
LFT	liver function test		*od*	*omni die* (once a day)
LH	luteinizing hormone		**OGD**	oesophago-gastroduodenoscopy
LMW	low molecular weight		**OGTT**	oral glucose tolerance test
LMWH	low-molecular-weight heparin		**OSA**	obstructive sleep apnoea
LN	lymph nodes		**PAN**	polyarteritis nodosa
LP	lumbar puncture		**PBC**	primary biliary cirrhosis
LSD	lysergic acid diethylamide		**PCI**	percutaneous coronary intervention
LTOT	long-term oxygen therapy		**PCOS**	polycystic ovary syndrome
LUQ	left upper quadrant		**PCP**	phencyclidine, *Pneumocystis carinii* pneumonia
LV	left ventricle, left ventricular		**PCR**	polymerase chain reaction
LVH	left ventricular hypertrophy		**PD**	Parkinson's disease
MAC	*Mycobacterium avium-intracellular* complex		**PDA**	patent ductus arteriosus
MALT	mucosa-associated lymphoid tissue		**PE**	pulmonary embolism
MCA	middle cerebral artery		**PEA**	pulseless electrical activity
MCP	metacarpophalangeal		**PEEP**	positive end-expiratory pressure
M,C&S	microscopy, culture and sensitivity		**PEFR**	peak expiratory flow rate
MCV	mean cell volume		**PEG**	percutaneous endoscopic gastrostomy
MDS	myelodysplastic syndrome		**PEG**	polyethylene glycol
MDT	multidisciplinary team		**PET**	positron emission tomography
ME	myalgic encephalomyelitis		**PION**	posterior ischaemic optic neuropathy
MELAS	mitochondrial encephalopathy, lactic acidosis, stroke-like episodes		**PIP**	proximal interphalangeal
			PM	polymyositis
MEN	multiple endocrine neoplasia		**PML**	progressive multifocal leukoencephalopathy
MET	medical emergency team		**PMR**	polymyalgia rheumatica
MGUS	monoclonal gammopathy of uncertain significance		**PNH**	paroxysmal nocturnal haemoglobinuria
MHC	major histocompatibility complex		**PNS**	peripheral nervous system
MI	myocardial infarction		**PPAR-γ**	peroxisome proliferator-activated receptor γ
MMSE	mini mental state examination		**PPI**	proton pump inhibitor
MND	motor neuron disease		**PR**	per rectum
MODY	maturity-onset diabetes in the young		**PRL**	prolactin
MPS	myocardial perfusion scan		**PRV**	polycythaemia rubra vera
MR	mitral regurgitation		**PS**	psychoactive substance
MRCP	magnetic resonance cholangiopancreatography/ cholangiogram		**PSA**	prostate-specific antigen
			PSC	primary sclerosing cholangitis
MRI	magnetic resonance imaging		**PT**	prothrombin time
MRSA	methicillin-resistant *Staphylococcus aureus*		**PTCA**	percutaneous transluminal coronary angioplasty
MS	multiple sclerosis		**PTH**	parathyroid hormone
MSA	multiple system atrophy		**PUVA**	psoralens and ultraviolet A
MSU	midstream urine		**PV**	polycythaemia vera
MTC	medullary thyroid cancer		**PV**	plasma viscosity
MTP	metatarsophalangeal		**RA**	rheumatoid arthritis, right atrium

RBBB	right bundle branch block	TIA	transient ischaemic attack
RBC	red blood cell	TIBC	total iron-binding capacity
RCC	red cell count	TIMI	thrombolysis in myocardial infarction
RCT	randomised controlled trial	TIPSS	transjugular portosystemic shunt
REM	rapid eye movement	TLC	total lung capacity
RF	rheumatoid factor	TMJ	temporomandibular joint
RNA	ribonucleic acid	TNF	tumour necrosis factor
RP	retinitis pigmentosa	tPA	tissue plasminogen activator
RPGN	rapidly progressive glomerulonephritis	TPN	total parenteral nutrition
RR	respiratory rate	TRUS	transrectal ultrasonography
RUQ	right upper quadrant	TSH	thyroid-stimulating hormone
RV	right ventricle, right ventricular	TT	thrombin time
RVH	right ventricular hypertrophy	TTE	transthoracic echocardiogram
SACD	subacute combined degeneration of the cord	TTP	thrombotic thrombocytopenic purpura
SAH	subarachnoid haemorrhage	TURP	transurethral resection of the prostate
SARA	sexually acquired reactive arthritis	U&Es	urea and electrolytes
SBE	subacute bacterial endocarditis	UC	ulcerative colitis
SBP	spontaneous bacterial peritonitis	UFC	urinary free cortisol
SCC	squamous cell carcinoma	UFH	unfractionated heparin
SCID	severe combined immunodeficiency	UIP	usual interstitial pneumonia
SCLC	small cell lung cancer	URTI	upper respiratory tract infection
SDH	subdural haemorrhage	US	ultrasound
SIADH	syndrome of inappropriate antidiuretic hormone secretion	UTI	urinary tract infection
		UVA	ultraviolet A
SLA	soluble liver antigen	UVB	ultraviolet B
SLE	systemic lupus erythematosus	VC	vital capacity
SMA	smooth muscle actin antibody	VEGF	vascular endothelium growth factor
SOB	shortness of breath	VEP	visual evoked potential
SPB	spontaneous bacterial peritonitis	VF	ventricular fibrillation
SRH	stigmata of recent haemorrhage	VHL	Von Hippel-Landau syndrome
SSRIs	selective serotonin reuptake inhibitors	VIN	vulval intraepithelial neoplasia
STD	sexually transmitted disease	VIP	vasoactive intestinal peptide
STEMI	ST segment elevation myocardial infarction	VLDL	very-low-density lipoprotein
SVC	superior vena cava	$\dot{V}/\dot{Q}$	ventilation/perfusion
SVCO	superior vena cava obstruction	VSD	ventricular septal defect
SVR	sustained viral response	VT	ventricular tachycardia
SVT	supraventricular tachyarrhythmia, supraventricular tachycardia	VWD	von Willebrand's disease
		vWF	von Willebrand's factor
T3	triiodothyronine	VZV	varicella-zoster virus
T4	thyroxine	WCC	white cell count
TB	tuberculosis	WG	Wegener's granulomatosis
tds	*ter die sumendus* (3 times a day)	WHO	World Health Organization
TED	thromboembolic	WoB	work of breathing
TEN	toxic epidermal necrolysis	WPW	Wolff–Parkinson–White
TGF	transforming growth factor		

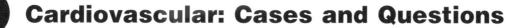

1 Cardiovascular: Cases and Questions

Case 1: A patient with high blood pressure

A 28-year-old woman who has newly registered with her GP has been invited to attend a new patient clinic for a check up. The nurse discovers that her BP is 165/95 mmHg. She says she has rushed to get to the surgery. The value is checked several times over the next few weeks but is persistently elevated. She is otherwise fit and well.

1. *What would you do for this woman next?*
   (a) Offer lifestyle advice including a low-salt diet and increased exercise
   (b) Refer for an echocardiogram to look for left ventricular hypertrophy (LVH)
   (c) Likely 'white coat' hypertension; repeat in 6 months or sooner if symptoms
   (d) 24-hour ambulatory recording

2. *Which of the following are secondary causes of hypertension?*
   (i) *Addison's disease*
   (ii) *Cushing's disease*
   (iii) *Renal disease*
   (iv) *Coarctation of the aorta*
   (v) *NSAIDs*
   (a) All of the above
   (b) i, ii, iii, iv
   (c) ii, iii, iv, v
   (d) ii, iii, v
   (e) ii, iii, iv

3. *What changes on the 12-lead ECG might you expect to see in a patient with chronic hypertension?*
   (a) Bifid P waves
   (b) Prominent S wave in V1 and prominent R in V5/V6
   (c) Right bundle branch block
   (d) ST segment changes throughout the leads

Case 2: A patient with xanthalasma

A 42-year-old non-smoking man is seen by his GP for a routine check up. During the examination the GP notices that the man has xanthalasma around both eyes. Other than being slightly overweight, there is nothing else to note in the history or examination. Blood pressure is 120/80 mmHg. He decides to check the lipid levels:

LDL   4.4 mmol/L
HDL   1.0 mmol/L
Total cholesterol   6.2 mmol/L

1. *How would you initially manage this man's hyperlipidaemia?*
   (a) Do nothing since he has no risk factors for cardiovascular disease
   (b) Commence Simvastatin 20 mg nocte
   (c) Offer lifestyle advice
   (d) Use an alternative lipid-lowering agent, e.g. a fibrate or cholestyramine

2. *Which of the following may cause hyperlipidaemia?*
   (a) Renal failure
   (b) Liver disease
   (c) Hypothyroidism
   (d) Diabetes
   (e) Any of the above

3. *How do the commonly used 'statin' group of drugs work?*
   (a) Decrease absorption of fat from the gastrointestinal tract
   (b) HMG-CoA reductase inhibition (involved in cholesterol synthesis)
   (c) Increase the stimulation of lipoprotein lipase activity
   (d) Bile acid sequestration in the gastrointestinal tract

4. *Which of the following is a well recognized side effect of the statin group of drugs?*
   (a) Lethargy
   (b) Visual disturbance
   (c) Myositis
   (d) Renal failure

Case 3: A patient with severe central chest pain

A 53-year-old man presents to A&E with severe central chest pain radiating through to his scapular. Apparently the pain came on suddenly. He is known to be hypertensive. Examination reveals that he is sweaty, pale and unwell. Although he is in pain he is cooperative and able to answer questions. His BP is 80/40 mmHg. His jugular venous pressure is not raised. There is an early diastolic murmur but his chest is clear. His abdomen is soft. ECG shows sinus rhythm with ECG evidence of left ventricular hypertrophy. There is no ECG evidence of acute myocardial infarction (MI). Chest X-ray film shows a widened mediastinum

1. *What is your provisional diagnosis?*
   (a) Pulmonary embolism
   (b) Myocardial infarction (MI) (non-ST elevation)
   (c) Costochondritis
   (d) Aortic dissection

2. *How will you confirm your suspicions?*
   (a) CT scan
   (b) Lateral chest X-ray
   (c) Transthoracic echocardiography
   (d) Urgent thoracotomy

3. *How will you treat the BP?*
   (a) 1000 mL Hartmann's solution (or Ringer's lactate)
   (b) 500 mL colloid such as gelofusin
   (c) Commence a noradrenaline infusion to aim for BP 120/80 mmHg
   (d) Manage conservatively

Case 4: A patient with dizzy spells and a history of angina

A 68-year-old man who has been having dizzy spells over the last few months is referred to you. He has not lost consciousness but the dizzy spells are becoming more frequent, particularly if he exerts himself. He has a history of angina for which he uses a glyceryl trinitrate (GTN) spray and takes atenolol 50 mg od. He also has hypercholestrolaemia and has had a transurethral resection of his prostate in the past. On examination he has several xanthalasma around the eyes and corneal arcus,

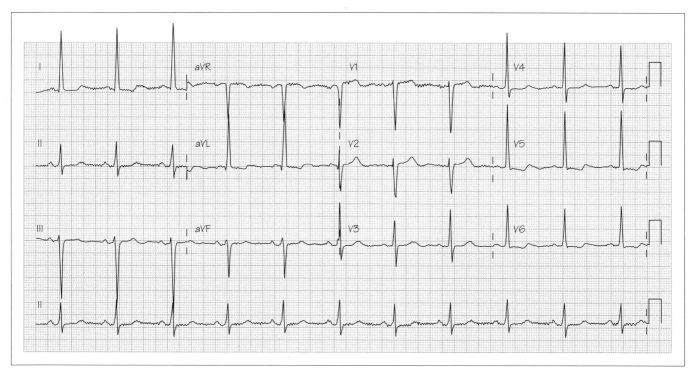

Figure 1.4.1

but no splinter haemorrhages. Neurological examination is normal.

BP is 110/70 mmHg, pulse is slow rising pulse, rate 56 beats/min, sinus rhythm. The apex beat is non-displaced and clearly palpable. He has a systolic murmur which radiates across the praecordium and also to the carotids (Fig. 1.4.1). Chest sounds are clear and chest X-ray appears normal.

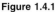

1. *What is the most likely cause of this man's dizziness?*
   (a) Aortic valve stenosis
   (b) Aortic valve regurgitation
   (c) Mitral valve regurgitation
   (d) Micturition syncope
2. *How will you go about investigating this patient further?*
   (a) Exercise stress test
   (b) Coronary angiography
   (c) Transthoracic echocardiogram
   (d) 24-hour ECG
3. *What does the ECG (Fig. 1.4.1) show?*
   (a) Ischaemia in the lateral leads (V4–6)
   (b) Left ventricular hypertrophy (LVH) with a strain pattern
   (c) Right axis deviation
   (d) Normal ECG

Case 5: A woman with sudden shortness of breath and palpitations

A 68-year-old woman is admitted to A&E with sudden increased shortness of breath and palpitations. She is known to have angina and is complaining of chest pain, similar to her usual exertional pain.

Examination reveals that she is clammy and unwell. Her heart rate is 150–170 beats/min, and BP 88/40 mmHg. SpO_2 is 92% with reservoir bag. Her respiratory rate is 22 breaths/min and her chest has fine crepitations throughout. An ECG has been performed (Fig. 1.5.1).

1. *What does the ECG show?*
   (a) Sinus tachycardia
   (b) Atrial fibrillation (AF)
   (c) Atrial flutter
   (d) Wolff–Parkinson–White Syndrome with pre-excitation
2. *How should this tachyarrhythmia be managed acutely?*
   (a) Amiodarone
   (b) Digoxin
   (c) Electrical cardioversion
   (d) Lignocaine
3. *Why has the tachycardia caused the chest pain?*
   (a) It causes a low systolic pressure leading to poor coronary perfusion
   (b) Hyperventilation causes vasoconstriction of the coronary arteries due to low $PaCO_2$
   (c) It causes hypoxia leading to coronary ischaemia
   (d) A short diastolic time leads to poor coronary perfusion
4. *Which of the following electrolytes levels are important to maintain in order to help to maintain sinus rhythm?*
   (a) Sodium, potassium, calcium and magnesium
   (b) Potassium and magnesium
   (c) Calcium and potassium
   (d) Sodium, calcium and potassium

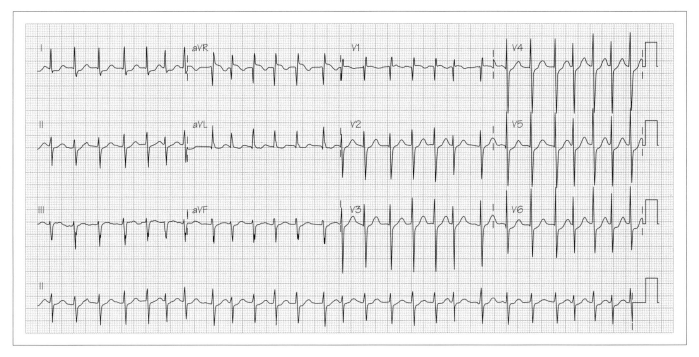

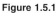

Figure 1.5.1

Case 6: A 72-year-old patient with shortness of breath

A 72-year-old woman has been referred to the chest clinic due to gradually increasing progressive shortness of breath. She is known to suffer with atrial fibrillation and has been treated with digoxin to give rate control. She is also on warfarin.

On examination, she has flushed cheeks and appears well, although is slightly short of breath at rest. She has a low, rumbling murmur heard in mid-diastole and has a tapping apex beat which is undisplaced. A right ventricular (parasternal) heave is noted. Her heart rate is 67 beats/min irregularly irregular, and her jugular venous pressure is elevated at 3 cm. She also has mild oedema of her ankles.

1. *What is the significance of the parasternal heave?*
   (a) Suggests a hyperdynamic circulation
   (b) Probable systemic hypertension
   (c) Probable pulmonary hypertension
   (d) Suggestive of heart failure
2. *What does the clinical examination suggest?*
   (a) Mitral stenosis
   (b) Aortic regurgitation
   (c) Pulmonary regurgitation
   (d) Pulmonary stenosis
3. *What chest X-ray signs are associated with left atrial enlargement?*
   (a) Splayed carina
   (b) Double right heart border
   (c) Bulge in left heart border
   (d) Any of the above

Case 7: A patient in cardiac arrest on the ward

You are called to a cardiac arrest on a medical ward. On arrival cardiopulmonary resuscitation (CPR) has apparently been ongoing

for 4 minutes by nursing staff and the patient is in asystole. There is intravenous access already *in situ*.

1. *What is the first step that you take?*
   (a) Give atropine 3 mg
   (b) Give adrenaline 1 mg
   (c) Check electrode contact and lead selection
   (d) Intubate the patient urgently
2. *With regard to the ECG electrodes what is the correct positioning?*
   (a) Red – left arm; green – right leg; yellow – right arm
   (b) Red – right arm; yellow – left arm; green – left leg
   (c) Red – right arm; yellow – left arm; green – right leg
   (d) It is not important as you are only looking for electrical activity
3. *Asystole is confirmed and CPR continues until an attempt is made to intubate the patient. How long can CPR be interrupted to achieve this?*
   (a) 15 seconds
   (b) 30 seconds
   (c) 45 seconds
   (d) It should not be interrupted under any circumstances
4. *The patient is successfully intubated. What is the correct ratio of compressions to breaths now?*
   (a) 30:2 as before
   (b) 15:2
   (c) 5:1
   (d) Continual compressions at 100 breaths/min and 10 breaths/min

Case 8: A patient in cardiac arrest

A patient is brought by ambulance to A&E. The paramedics have intubated the patient and cardiopulmonary resuscitation is ongoing. They report that the rhythm has been pulseless electrical activity since they arrived at the patient.

1. *Which of the following are reversible causes of pulseless electrical activity (PEA) arrest?*
   (a) Hypomagnesaemia, hypoxia, hypovolaemia, hypothermia
   (b) Toxins, tension pneumothorax, cardiac tamponade, thyroid crisis
   (c) Pulmonary embolism, hyperkalaemia, hypoventilation, hypocalcaemia
   (d) Hypomagnesaemia, pulmonary embolism, hypocalcaemia, hypoxia

2. *Which of the following drugs can be used to treat hyperkalaemia in the arrest situation?*
   (a) Glucagon
   (b) Sodium bicarbonate
   (c) Calcium carbonate
   (d) None of the above

3. *When is atropine 3 mg indicated during the arrest situation?*
   (a) When it is determined that asystole is present
   (b) For both PEA and asystole
   (c) It has benefits in PEA/asystole/VF and VT
   (d) For asystole and PEA provided the rate is <60 beats/min

Case 9: A fit woman with shortness of breath and flu-like symptoms

A 22-year-old woman, who is a keen long distance runner and usually extremely fit and well, has been brought into the A&E department. Since yesterday she has been becoming increasingly short of breath. It is considerably worse today. She had been unwell with a flu-like illness and fever over the last week or so, but had still been able to train until a few days ago. She also has mild central chest discomfort.

On examination she appears distressed, unwell and clearly short of breath. Her respiratory rate is 34 breaths/min, BP 88/50 mmHg, and pulse is 140 beats/min sinus tachycardia. Her temperature is 38.5°C and SpO_2 is 89% with an oxygen reservoir bag and mask. Her jugular venous pressure (JVP) is raised to the ear and there are loud heart sounds including a third heart sound. There is no peripheral oedema. There are widespread fine inspiratory crackles. And the percussion note is resonant. Troponin I is −0.9

1. *What is the most likely cause of her symptoms?*
   (a) Heart failure
   (b) Pulmonary embolus
   (c) Chest infection
   (d) Status asthmaticus

2. *Which of the following would best explain the underlying cause of heart failure?*
   (a) Myocardial infarction
   (b) Congenital heart disease
   (c) Myocarditis
   (d) Pericardial effusion

3. *Which of the following treatment options would you use acutely in her case?*
   (i) *Non-invasive ventilation (CPAP)*
   (ii) *Frusemide*

(iii) *Glyceryl trinitrate (GTN) infusion*
(iv) β-*Blocker*
(v) *Inotropes and vasopressors*
   (a) All of these therapies
   (b) i, ii and v
   (c) i, ii, iii and v
   (d) i, ii and iii

4. *Which of the following are recognized to cause myocarditis?*
   (a) Viruses, bacteria, radiation, drugs, parasite infection
   (b) Viruses, connective tissue disorders, bacteria
   (c) Bacteria, drugs, connective tissue disorders, spirochete infections
   (d) All of the above

Case 10: A patient with shortness of breath and chest tightness

A 58-year-old woman has been brought into A&E complaining of sudden onset of severe shortness of breath and some mild chest tightness whilst eating her breakfast. She has had similar symptoms related to exertion over the past few months, albeit much less severe. These had settled on resting. She has had type 2 diabetes for many years and is now managed with insulin. She smokes 10 cigarettes a day and has a strong family history of ischaemic heart disease.

Examination shows her to be clammy and distressed. She is apyrexial with a BP 90/40 mmHg, pulse 110 beats/min sinus tachycardia. There are no cardiac murmurs but a third heart sound is audible. Her jugular venous pressure (JVP) is raised. The chest sounds rather wheezy. Her respiratory rate is 28 breaths/min, and SpO_2 86% with 4 L/min oxygen.

Her ECG and chest X-ray are shown in Fig. 1.10.1.

1. *What is the most likely cause of this patient's problems?*
   (a) Exacerbation of chronic obstructive pulmonary disease (COPD) or asthma
   (b) Diabetic ketoacidosis
   (c) Myocardial infarction (MI)
   (d) Severe indigestion

2. *What is the most likely cause of the chest X-ray findings?*
   (a) Acute respiratory distress syndrome (ARDS)
   (b) Pulmonary oedema
   (c) Bilateral pneumonia
   (d) Pneumothorax

3. *What is your immediate management?*
   (a) Thrombolysis
   (b) Aspirin 300 mg and clopidogrel 300 mg
   (c) Urgent referral to the cardiology team
   (d) High-flow oxygen

4. *Which of the following are complications of an MI?*
   (a) Arrhythmias
   (b) Mitral valve regurgitation
   (c) Pericarditis
   (d) All of the above
   (e) Only arrhythmias and mitral valve regurgitation

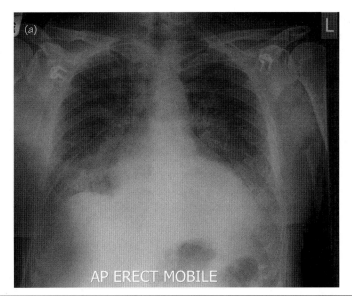

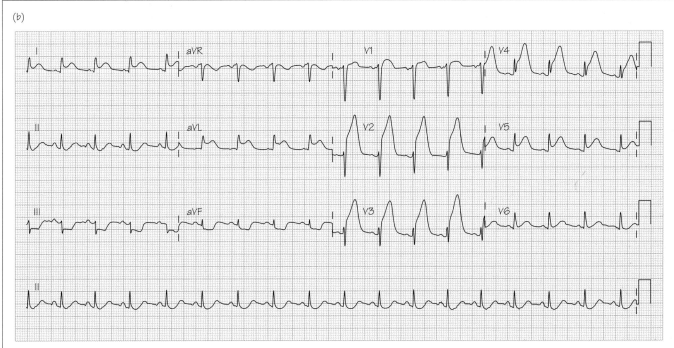

Figure 1.10.1

Case 11: A drug user with a cough and chest pain

A 26-year-old known intravenous drug abuser presents with a long history of cough, pleuritic chest pain and occasional haemoptysis. He also describes night sweats and fevers.

Examination reveals a cachectic man who is pyrexial (temperature of 39.2°C). He has a raised jugular venous pressure and pansystolic murmur, which is loudest over the left sternal edge and accentuated by inspiration. His C-reactive protein (CRP) is 160 mg/L, and his white cell count (WCC) is 18.4×10^9/L. Chest X-ray is normal.

1. *What is the most likely diagnosis to be considered in this patient?*
   (a) Pulmonary tuberculosis
   (b) Chest infection
   (c) Pulmonary embolism
   (d) Infective endocarditis

2. *How many sets of blood cultures should you take in this setting as a minimum?*
   (a) One
   (b) Two
   (c) Three
   (d) Four

3. *What is a mycotic aneurysm?*
   (a) Inflammation and dilatation of a vessel wall caused by septic emboli
   (b) Fungal infection occurring in an aneurysmal dilatation

(c) Fungal infection causing inflammation and dilatation of a vessel wall

(d) Fungal plaque obstructing valvular outflow that is prone to rupture

Case 12: A patient with angina and raised blood pressure

A 67-year-old man who is known to have well controlled angina, albeit well, was recently noted by his GP to be slightly hypertensive despite treatment. He takes bendrofluazide 2.5 mg od, atenolol 50 mg od and ramipril 5 mg bd as well as aspirin 75 mg od. His BP has been found to be 160/95 mmHg on several occasions and it is decided to add further antihypertensive therapy.

1. *Which drug would be appropriate to add to his prescription?*
    (a) Amlodipine (calcium channel inhibitor)
    (b) Hydralazine (nitrate)
    (c) Losartan (an angiotensin II inhibitor)
    (d) Doxazosin (α-antagonist)

2. *What is the likely cause of this man's oedema?*
    (a) Heart failure caused by the calcium channel blocker
    (b) Lymphoedema
    (c) Treatment side effect
    (d) Orthostatic oedema

3. *What is a commonly seen side effect of bendrofluazide?*
    (a) Hyponatraemia
    (b) Paradoxical hypertension
    (c) Hyperkalaemia
    (d) Stevens–Johnson syndrome

Case 13: A pregnant woman with left-sided chest pain

A 36-year-old woman who is 38 weeks pregnant is admitted with a history of some left-sided pleuritic chest pain. This is worse on inspiration. She denies having a fever or cough. She feels more short of breath lately. She usually enjoys good health and her pregnancy has been uneventful.

On examination she is alert and orientated. Her BP is 105/60 mmHg, pulse 95 beats/min, SpO_2 is 95% on room air and respiratory rate is 20 breaths/min. Heart examination reveals a soft systolic murmur over the sternum. Chest sounds are clear but she clearly has pain on deep inspiration. There is no tenderness in her calves.

Arterial blood gas levels are as follows:

pH	7.46
PaO_2	11.8 kPa
$PaCO_2$	4.1 kPa
Base excess	+3
HCO_3^-	20 mmol/L

ECG shows sinus rhythm and borderline left axis deviation.

1. *What is the explanation for the low BP, high respiratory rate and low $PaCO_2$?*
    (a) Probable pulmonary embolism (PE)
    (b) Pleuritic chest pain
    (c) Normal changes in pregnancy
    (d) Mild congenital cardiac defect exacerbated by pregnancy

2. *You decide to request a chest X-ray but the mother is worried it may harm her baby. How do you reassure her? (a) The amount of radiation is similar to a transatlantic flight and unlikely to harm a baby at this stage of development*

(b) The radiation is negligible as you aren't imaging the abdomen

(c) You won't be able to diagnose her problem any other way so she must have it

(d) Decide not to X-ray the chest

3. *The chest radiograph was normal. How would you manage this patient further?*
    (a) Given the normal investigations, reassure her and send her home
    (b) Low molecular weight heparin and further investigation
    (c) Simple analgesics
    (d) Aspirin at an anticoagulant dose

4. *She is sent to the ward but several hours later there is a cardiac arrest call. You arrive to find cardiopulmonary resuscitation (CPR) already in progress and she is in a non-VF/non-VT rhythm. What modifications to the CPR do you make?*
    (a) None, the protocol is standard for everyone
    (b) Position her in the left lateral position and arrange a caesarean
    (c) Give her thrombolysis to break up a probable PE
    (d) Change back to the old 15:2 compression:breath ratio to improve oxygenation of the fetus

Case 14: A patient with calf pain and loss of appetite

A 76-year-old woman was referred to the medical take by her GP with a 2-day history of lower left calf pain and possibly some swelling. Systems questioning reveals that she has been losing weight over the past few months but she attributes this to feeling less hungry and has had some lower abdominal pains due to constipation. She lives independently but states that she lacks energy of late. She has hypertension which is well controlled with bendrofluazide. A diagnosis of osteoarthritis has also been made which affects her hand and knee joints in particular.

Examination reveals that she is cachectic, and there is tenderness in the mid and upper left calf. The left calf is swollen in comparison to the right and there is some increased warmth. Varicosities of both legs are noted. Examination of her cardiovascular and respiratory systems are normal. She has some tenderness on palpation of the left iliac fossa but no masses.

1. *From the following combinations which are the most likely differential diagnoses?*
    (i) *Ruptured Baker's cyst*
    (ii) *Deep venous thrombosis (DVT)*
    (iii) *Varicose veins*
    (iv) *Thrombophlebitis*
    (v) *Cramp*
        (a) i, ii, iii, iv, v
        (b) i, ii, iii, iv
        (c) ii, iii, iv
        (d) ii, iii, iv, v

2. *What is the best way to aid further diagnosis?*
    (a) Urgent X-ray of the left knee
    (b) Check her inflammatory markers (white cell count and C-reactive protein)
    (c) Rheumatology opinion for further advice about possible cyst rupture
    (d) D-dimer and ultrasound left leg

3. *This woman is found to have an extensive DVT which extends into the proximal veins of the leg. What treatment will you initiate?*
   (a) Continue the low molecular weight heparin that you commenced when you suspected a DVT and start warfarin
   (b) Commence thrombolysis to break up the clot
   (c) Change the heparin to warfarin now the DVT is confirmed
   (d) Consider an inferior venal caval (IVC) filter given the large clot

4. *What other treatment or investigation would you consider in this patient's case?*
   (a) Thrombophilia screen
   (b) Rheumatoid factor
   (c) Ultrasound abdomen
   (d) Abdominal X-ray and laxatives

Case 15: A patient with hypertension and chest pain

A 50-year-old smoker with hypertension develops central crushing chest pain radiating to his jaw. He has vomited and he now feels short of breath. He has an ECG performed (Fig. 1.15.1).

1. *What is the diagnosis?*
   (a) Posterior myocardial infarction (MI)
   (b) Inferior myocardial infarction
   (c) Anterior myocardial infarction
   (d) Pericarditis

2. *The patient is given morphine, an anti-emetic and aspirin. He is then taken immediately to the cardiac catheterization laboratory where he undergoes primary coronary angiography and stenting to one of the vessels. Which coronary artery is stented?*
   (a) Right
   (b) Circumflex
   (c) Diagonal
   (d) Left anterior descending (LAD)

3. *The patient returns to the coronary care department where he is now pain free. The ST segment changes on the ECG have resolved with this treatment. He is still breathless and the respiratory rate is recorded as 30 breaths/min with oxygen saturations of 80% on high-flow oxygen via a non-rebreath mask with a reservoir. Crackles are audible throughout the chest on auscultation. The patient is correctly diagnosed as having left ventricular failure (LVF). A chest radiograph confirms pulmonary oedema. Which of the following is indicated?*
   (a) Morphine
   (b) Intravenous nitrate
   (c) Oral frusemide (furosemide)
   (d) Digoxin

4. *The patient is given morphine, 80 mg of intravenous frusemide and glyceryl trinitrate (GTN) at 5 mg/hour. He is in sinus rhythm at 110 beats/min and blood pressure is 100/60 mmHg. He looks grey, clammy and oxygen saturations remain at 80%. Despite being catheterized he has passed little urine in response to the diuretic. Which of the following are indicated to improve his condition?*
   (a) Increase the GTN infusion
   (b) Continuous positive airway pressure (CPAP)
   (c) Angiotensin-converting enzyme (ACE) inhibitor
   (d) Intravenous β-blocker

5. *What are the effects of CPAP?*
   (a) Improves oxygenation
   (b) Gastric distention
   (c) Increased work of breathing
   (d) Reduced venous return
   (e) Reduces left ventricular afterload

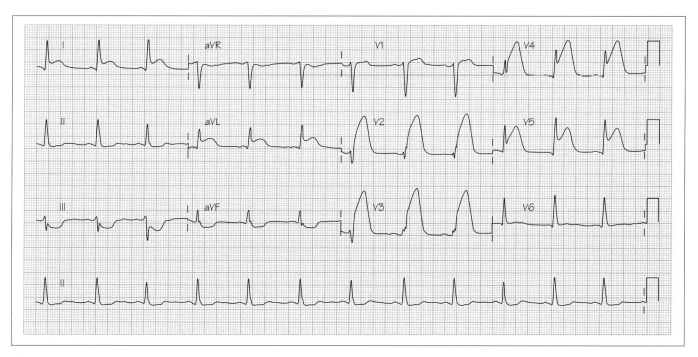

Figure 1.15.1

Case 16: A patient with new onset chest pain

A 48-year-old man is sent by his GP for outpatient evaluation of chest pain. He has noticed chest pains for some 6 weeks. The pain is left sided, described as being 'like toothache', and occurs in episodes lasting about 45-60 mins. He has not identified any clear provoking or relieving factors; his exercise capacity has been unchanged, and he regularly walks the 2 miles to his manual job. He is a smoker of 20 cigarettes a day, he has had 'borderline' hypertension, not treated, for several years, and his total cholesterol is 5.5 mmol/L. There is no family history of premature coronary disease. He drinks 30 units of alcohol per week. Examination shows he is 1.80 m tall, BMI 35, heart rate 70 beats/min, BP 145/90 mmHg, the rest of the exam is normal.

1. *Which syndrome does he have?*
   (a) Non-cardiac chest pain
   (b) Atypical angina
   (c) Typical angina

2. *What is the pre-test probability that he has coronary disease?*
   (a) Low
   (b) Medium
   (c) High

3. *What further investigations should he have?*
   (a) Full blood count
   (b) Resting ECG
   (c) Exercise ECG
   (d) Cholesterol including HDL and LDL subfractions
   (e) Biochemical screen including renal function
   (f) Thyroid function tests
   (g) All of the above

4. *His resting ECG is completely normal. It is therefore likely that:*
   (a) His left ventricular function is normal
   (b) His left ventricular function could be impaired, perhaps severely
   (c) We can tell nothing about his left ventricular function

5. *His exercise stress test shows that he can reach the end of stage IV of the Bruce protocol without symptoms, with heart rate going from 70 to 160 beats/min, his systolic blood pressure from 135 to 180 mmHg. At peak exercise he has 2 mm of planar ST depression inferolaterally. Which of the following statements are true?*
   (a) He has coronary disease
   (b) His prognosis is not good
   (c) He should be offered coronary angiography
   (d) It is unlikely that he has coronary disease

Case 17: Severe chest pain in a man with diabetes

A 58-year-old man with type 2 diabetes is at work when he experiences persistent and severe central chest pain, without any radiation. He hopes that it will go, but it doesn't, and after 1 hour calls 999. He is taken to the local hospital. In A&E, he explains that over the past few weeks he has had three or four similar episodes, each one lasting just a few minutes, none of which have been related to exercise. He does not smoke, is moderately obese, with a BMI of 35, has well treated hypertension, and had a cholesterol of 5 mmol/L about 4 months ago. Other than diabetes, there is no other relevant previous medical history. He is taking metformin, aspirin, and an angiotensin-converting enzyme (ACE) inhibitor. Examination shows him to be obese, in pain, with some mild ten-derness to palpation of the anterior chest wall. He is in sinus rhythm, heart rate 90 beats/min, blood pressure 160/85 mmHg, his jugular venous pressure is not raised, normal heart sounds, no pathological murmurs, clear chest examination. All peripheral pulses are present and undiminished. Abdominal examination was unremarkable. Oxygen saturation is 98% on air. Before the ECG is taken, the diagnosis is considered.

1. *Prior to him developing these symptoms, what is the pre-test probability of coronary disease?*
   (a) Very low
   (b) Low
   (c) Medium
   (d) High

2. *He has mild tenderness to the chest wall. What impact should this have in establishing the diagnosis?*
   (a) None
   (b) It increases the chance of non-cardiac chest pain moderately
   (c) It establishes the diagnosis as being non-cardiac, and musculoskeletal

3. *An ECG is taken (Fig. 1.17.1). What does this show?*
   (a) An anterior wall ST segment elevation myocardial infarction (STEMI)
   (b) No acute changes
   (c) An inferior wall STEMI
   (d) An anterior wall non-STEMI
   (e) Pericarditis

4. *What should be the immediate treatment?*
   (a) Aspirin 300 mg chewed
   (b) Aspirin 300 mg swallowed
   (c) Clopidogrel 300 mg
   (d) Thrombolytic therapy with a fibrin specific thrombolytic
   (e) Percutaneous coronary intervention (PCI) to open the occluded coronary artery, so called primary PCI
   (f) Intravenous opiate

5. *What factors relate to outcome in STEMI?*
   (a) The number of leads showing ST elevation and ST depression
   (b) The age of the patient
   (c) The presence of diabetes
   (d) The BP and presence or absence of heart failure, i.e. the haemodynamic status of the patient
   (e) The method of opening up the occluded coronary artery
   (f) All of the above

6. *The patient progresses well, and discharge home is considered on day 3. However, he mentions that his ankles have started to swell; he is otherwise well, and quite comfortable lying flat in bed. Physical examination now shows that his heart rate is 100 beats/min, BP 100/50 mmHg, jugular venous pressure +10; praecordial examination suggests a thrill, and a loud pansystolic murmur is heard at the base of the left sternal edge. The lungs are dry. What has happened?*
   (a) He has developed an ischaemic ventricular septal defect (VSD)
   (b) He has developed ischaemically mediated acute mitral regurgitation (MR)
   (c) He has developed either a VSD or acute MR
   (d) He has developed pericarditis related to his infarct
   (e) He has developed acute endocarditis from an infected venflon
   (f) He has most likely extended his infarct

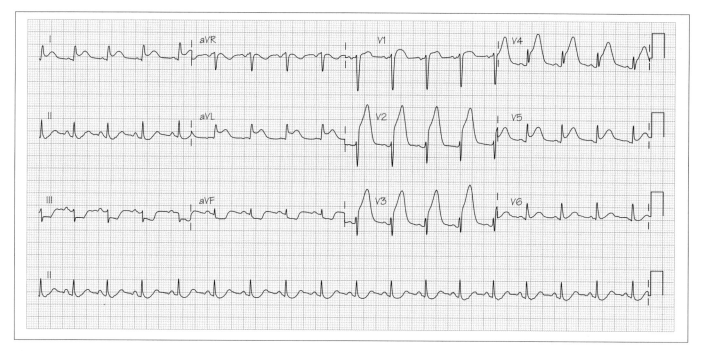

Figure 1.17.1

Case 18: A patient with chronic chest pain

A 48-year-old man presents to hospital with chest pain. The pains started 3 years ago, when he experienced 2 or 3 episodes, each lasting about 10-20 minutes. They were felt retro-sternally, described as being tight, without radiation, of a sort he had never experienced before. They were not effort or respiration related. They were quite severe, and he was admitted to hospital. He is known to have a high, though untreated, cholesterol, high blood pressure and is a smoker. Examination, chest X-ray, full biochemical and haematological screen, and ECGs throughout the 24 hours of his admission were normal and troponin was not raised. His symptoms did not recur during hospitalization and he was discharged home.

1. *What investigations should now be carried out?*
   (a) No more, he has had a full evaluation
   (b) A coronary angiogram
   (c) A CT coronary angiogram
   (d) An exercise stress ECG
   (e) A nuclear myocardial perfusion scan

2. *The patient is treated for hypercholesterolemia with a statin, and hypertension with an angiotensin-converting enzyme (ACE) inhibitor, and remains well for the next 3 years, at which time he then starts to experience similar pains. Again, these occur in episodes lasting about 10-20 minutes; he experiences several episodes over a week, and is admitted following a more prolonged one, lasting 25 minutes. He is fully evaluated within 2 hours of arrival, and examination and initial investigations (including blood count, biochemistry and admission troponin and ECG) are normal. What should happen to the patient next?*

   (a) Discharged home
   (b) Admitted

3. *The patient is admitted. What drugs should he receive?*
   (a) None
   (b) His usual medications (statin and ACE inhibitor) and aspirin, 300 mg chewed then 75 mg a day
   (c) His usual drugs, aspirin, and full dose low molecular weight heparin
   (d) His usual drugs, aspirin and clopidogrel loading with 300 mg, then 75 mg a day
   (e) His usual drugs, aspirin, clopidogrel, and low molecular weight heparin

4. *Sequential ECGs are taken, and his ECG changes to the pattern shown in the figure (Fig. 1.18.1). Where does this ECG suggest the lesion is?*
   (a) In the proximal part of the left anterior descending coronary artery
   (b) In the left main stem
   (c) In the right coronary artery
   (d) In the circumflex coronary artery

5. *His troponin comes back as normal. Clopidogrel and low molecular weight heparin are immediately added to his treatment regime. What should then happen?*
   (a) Coronary angiogram with a view to percutaneous coronary intervention (PCI) with stent insertion if appropriate
   (b) Exercise ECG as his troponin is normal
   (c) CT coronary angiogram
   (d) Mobilization, and provided symptoms settle, early outpatient nuclear myocardial perfusion scan (MPS)

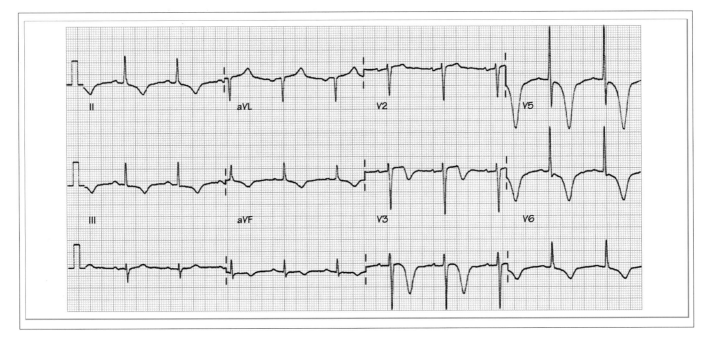

Figure 1.18.1

Case 19: A man with blackouts

A 75-year-old man is sent to see you in the outpatient department with a referral problem of blackout. He is normally fairly fit and well for his age. He has however had blackouts over the past few years, each one being rather similar to the others. He has had 5 or 6 episodes in total. These only occur when he is out of the house, usually when he has been in town, and is standing still looking into a shop window. It may be that he has been in a shop looking at the higher shelves. For a few seconds he will feel slightly light headed with a general feeling of heat. He then falls to the floor; he is unsure as to whether he remembers hitting the floor. There has never been any serious injury. Witnesses describe him as looking pale, a bit sweaty, and being out for only a few seconds. He will be down on the ground for just a few seconds, and then he recovers fully, is completely alert, knows where he is and who he is. He gets up, sits down for a few minutes and is then back to normal. He is otherwise well, has no other major previous medical illness, is treated for high cholesterol with a statin. Physical examination on the couch is normal, blood pressure 145/82 mmHg.

1. *The description of the episodes is best summarized as suggesting?*
   (a) Epilepsy
   (b) A Stokes-Adams attack
   (c) A vasomotor form of syncope
   (d) Hyperventilation
2. *His resting ECG is normal, and a 24-hour ECG, during which he did not have any syncopal episodes, shows 28 ventricular ectopic beats, otherwise unremarkable. An exercise ECG shows no evidence for coronary disease and a cardiac ultrasound is also normal. What is his chance of a cardiac death during follow up?*

   (a) Increased, compared to age matched controls
   (b) The same as age matched controls
   (c) Lower than age matched controls
3. *What investigations should be performed next?*
   (a) None, a watch and wait policy is appropriate
   (b) Coronary angiography
   (c) Cardiac MRI scan
   (d) Prolonged external ECG loop recording
   (e) A tilt table test
   (f) A carotid sinus massage test
4. *He has a tilt table test that is unremarkable; during a carotid sinus massage (CSM) test the following ECG is recorded (Fig. 1.19.1). What is not necessary when performing a CSM test?*
   (a) Auscultation of the neck beforehand to listen for carotid artery bruits
   (b) An ECG machine with a print-out
   (c) A beat-to-beat blood pressure monitor with print out
   (d) A motorized table, so that the CSM can be performed lying down and in the 30-degree head up position.
   (e) Full cardiopulmonary resuscitation equipment
   (f) An infusion of intravenous isoprenaline
   (g) Verbal consent
5. *Given these CSM test results, and the diagnosis of carotid hypersensitivity syndrome, what should be the next step?*
   (a) Watch and wait
   (b) Insertion of a single chamber ventricular pacemaker (a VVI pacemaker)
   (c) Insertion of a single chamber atrial pacemaker (AAI pacemaker)
   (d) Insertion of a dual chamber pacemaker (DDD pacemaker)

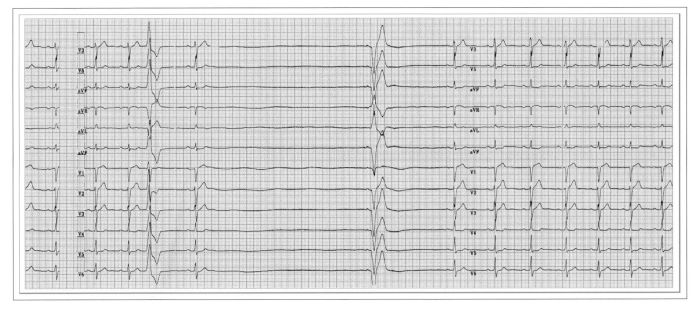

Figure 1.19.1

Case 20: Palpitations in a young woman

A 35-year old woman is seen in outpatients with palpitations. She is normally fit and well, except for these palpitations. She experiences an attack 2 or 3 times a year. They start suddenly, last 20-30 minutes, and stop suddenly 'as if the heart goes back into gear'. They feel fast, and regular. There are no other associated symptoms during the attack, though she does wonder if she passes more urine following an attack. She has never blacked out, or felt like blacking out, during or outside of an attack. They can occur at any time, there are no particular triggers, and she wonders if deep breathing may stop the symptoms. They have been present for 'many years', and she has come to see you really to establish the diagnosis.

1. *What do you think the diagnosis is?*
   (a) Anxiety
   (b) Thyrotoxicosis
   (c) Ectopics, probably ventricular
   (d) Atrioventricular nodal re-entrant tachycardia (AVNRT)
   (e) Atrioventricular re-entrant tachycardia (AVRT)
   (f) Ventricular tachycardia
2. *The physical examination is normal, and a 12 lead ECG is performed (Fig. 1.20.1) What does this show?*

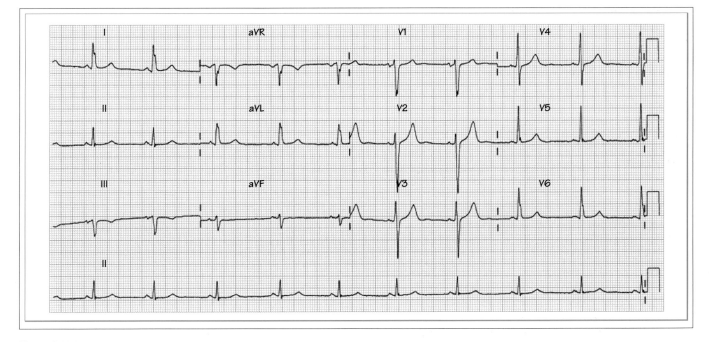

Figure 1.20.1

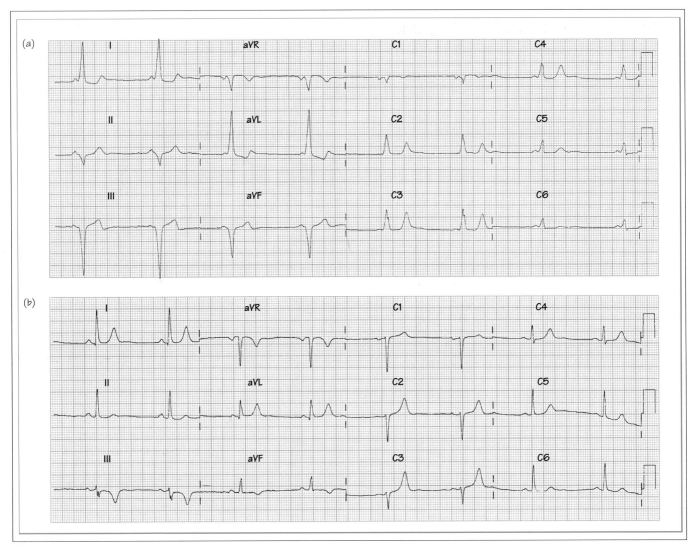

Figure 1.20.2

(a) It is normal
(b) It shows an accessory pathway
(c) Left bundle branch block
(d) It shows an old inferior wall myocardial infarction

3. *What is the next step in establishing the diagnosis?*
  (a) Nothing
  (b) 24-hour ECG
  (c) External 7-day ECG recording
  (d) Cardiac memo device
  (e) Implantable reveal device

4. *She develops sustained palpitations and presents to the local A&E department, where an ECG is taken (Fig. 1.20.2). What does this show?*

(a) Sinus tachycardia
(b) Atrial fibrillation
(c) Supraventricular tachycardia (SVT) due to AVNRT
(d) SVT due to AVRT
(e) Ventricular tachycardia

5. *What treatment should be tried?*
  (a) Neck massage, and if this is not successful, blowing against resistance (valsalva manouvre)
  (b) IV adenosine bolus
  (c) IV verapamil
  (d) IV beta-blocker
  (e) IV amiodarone
  (f) DC cardioversion

Cardiovascular: Answers

Case 1: A patient with high blood pressure

1. (d) 24-hour ambulatory recording

This is a young woman with persistent hypertension. It is less likely that she has primary (essential) hypertension. It may well be 'white coat' hypertension but it is important not to assume this. It should be established if she is indeed persistently hypertensive by means of ambulatory monitoring and if so, to investigate for a secondary cause.

2. (c) ii, iii, iv, v

Addison's disease causes postural hypotension. Other causes include phaeochromocytoma, Conn's disease and other drugs such as the oral contraceptive pill (OCP) and steroids.

3. (b) Prominent S wave in V1 and prominent R in V5/V6

These changes are consistent with LVH. The exact criteria are known as the Sokolow-Lyon criteria. They are S in V1 + R in V5 or V6 (whichever is the larger) ≥ 35 mm or R in a VL ≥ 11 mm. The presence of LVH in hypertension is an independent risk factor of early death.
Further reading: Chapter 79 in Medicine at a Glance.

Case 2: A patient with xanthalasma

1. (c) Offer lifestyle advice

He has a high LDL : HDL ratio. A ratio >4 indicates a high risk for coronary artery disease (CAD). The cholesterol >6.5 mmol/L also doubles his risk of lethal CAD. Despite this, he has no other risk factors for CAD and should be given lifestyle advice regarding diet (especially weight reducing) and exercise and followed up in 3 months. Those with a 10-year cardiovascular disease risk of $\geq 20\%$ stand to benefit from primary prevention. Tables to calculate this can be found in the *British National Formulary* (*BNF*).

2. (e) Any of the above

It is important to determine if this is a primary or secondary hyperlipidaemia. Secondary causes are those listed plus others including excess alcohol, biliary obstruction and certain drugs, e.g. steroids, oestrogens and some antiretroviral drugs. These causes may be excluded by careful clinical examination and by simple blood tests taken when the lipids are checked.

3. (b) HMG-CoA reductase inhibition (involved in cholesterol synthesis)

These are the most widely used group of lipid-lowering drugs. They inhibit HMG-CoA reductase, the rate-limiting enzyme in cholesterol synthesis. They may lower LDL cholesterol by 30% or more but have little effect on triglyceride levels.

4. (c) Myositis

Myositis is a not uncommonly seen side effect of statin therapy. Muscle pain or tenderness should prompt further investigation with a creatinine kinase (CK) level. Stop the statin if the CK is > 10 times the upper normal CK limit. If muscle symptoms are unacceptable, the statin should be stopped even if the CK is normal. Other serious side effects include hepatic damage.
Further reading: Chapter 80.

Case 3: A patient with severe central chest pain

1. (d) Aortic dissection

Aortic dissection is the most likely diagnosis here given the classic onset of symptoms in a known hypertensive patient. The ECG makes an MI very unlikely. The chest X-ray is highly suggestive of a haemo-mediastinum due to aortic rupture.

2. (a) CT scan

A CT scan is likely to be the most accessible in most hospitals. Whilst echocardiography may detect the complications such as haemopericardium and aortic regurgitation, it is not sensitive enough to pick up the area of dissection sufficiently frequently. Transoesophageal may be however, although it is not always widely available and requires sedation in a sick patient.

3. (d) Manage conservatively

The concept of permissive hypotension should apply until the aorta is repaired to prevent further blood loss. Provided the patient is awake (cerebral perfusion) and has a palpable radial pulse (check both in this scenario as BP may be lower in one arm due to aortic dissection) then no further fluid should be given. If needed, he should be resuscitated with blood and clotting products.
Further reading: Chapter 84.

Case 4: A patient with dizzy spells and a history of angina

1. (a) Aortic valve stenosis

Given the symptoms of dizziness and angina together with the clinical findings, it would suggest potentially severe aortic stenosis. Aortic regurgitation gives a wide pulse pressure and a collapsing pulse. The apex beat will be displaced and the murmur does not radiate to the carotids. Aortic stenosis has an ejection systolic murmur and aortic regurgitation a diastolic murmur. Mitral regurgitation gives a pansystolic murmur which may obscure the second heart sound and the apex beat is again displaced.

2. (c) Transthoracic echocardiogram

The least invasive way to assess the severity of the aortic stenosis is to perform a transthoracic echocardiogram in the first instance. Measurement of the pressure gradient across the valve, as well as valve area, can gauge severity. If the aortic stenosis is confirmed to be severe then aortic valve replacement is indicated. He may go on to have coronary angiography to assess his coronary arteries as asymptomatic coronary disease is common in severe aortic stenosis, and any coronary narrowings should be also be bypassed during aortic valve replacement surgery. An exercise stress test is relatively contraindicated, though is sometimes indicated in aortic stenosis of questionable severity, or to determine whether a patient is really asymptomatic.

3. (b) Left ventricular hypertrophy (LVH) with a strain pattern

The complexes are large. There are several criteria for making the diagnosis of LVH (which can also be assessed on echocardiography), none of them perfect. It is, however, important to know at least one method. The Sokolow-Lyon criteria are S in V1 + R in V5 or V6 (whichever is the larger) ≥ 35 mm or R in a VL ≥ 11 mm. There is a left axis deviation. The ischaemic changes appearing in the lateral leads are a 'strain pattern' associated with LVH. LVH can occur in health due to fitness training but occurs pathologically due to hypertrophy of the left ventricular wall. This can be secondary to hypertension, aortic stenosis, aortic insufficiency or cardiomyopathies e.g. hypertrophic obstructive cardiomyopathy (HOCM).
Further reading: Chapter 86.

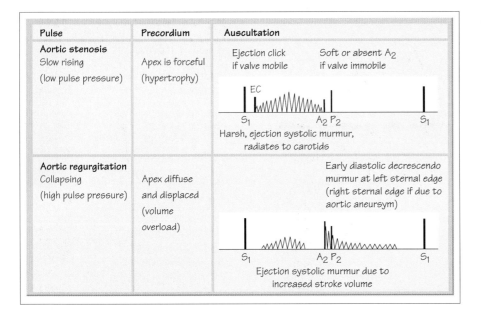

Pulse	Precordium	Auscultation
Aortic stenosis Slow rising (low pulse pressure)	Apex is forceful (hypertrophy)	Ejection click Soft or absent A$_2$ if valve mobile if valve immobile 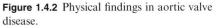 Harsh, ejection systolic murmur, radiates to carotids
Aortic regurgitation Collapsing (high pulse pressure)	Apex diffuse and displaced (volume overload)	Early diastolic decrescendo murmur at left sternal edge (right sternal edge if due to aortic aneursym) Ejection systolic murmur due to increased stroke volume

Figure 1.4.2 Physical findings in aortic valve disease.

Case 5: A woman with sudden shortness of breath and palpitations

1. (b) Atrial fibrillation (AF)

Atrial fibrillation – there are no P waves and the rate of the QRS complexes is irregularly irregular. The baseline shows irregular fibrillatory f waves; the amplitude of these diminished over time, with new AF the wave may be quite large, after several years the f wave may be almost invisible, with the baseline being almost flat. The real clue to the presence of AF is the QRS complexes do not have a regular interval between them, they are irregularly irregular.

2. (c) Electrical cardioversion

This patient is hypotensive and has chest pain. As such an attempt to restore sinus rhythm as soon as possible should be made. Whilst amiodarone may aid the success of electrical cardioversion and a loading of 300 mg can be given intravenously, it should not delay cardioversion, which will require sedation or general anaesthesia by an anaesthetist, depending on her fasting status. If for logistical reasons cardioversion will be delayed by more than a few minutes, then digoxin can be given by slow infusion intravenously. The thromboembolic risk of all patients in AF should always be assessed; this is particularly important when patients are cardioverted as successful restoration of sinus rhythm may well result in the expulsion of any left atrial thrombus into the arterial circulation, most of these thrombi end up in the brain causing a stroke. The risk of left atrial thrombi depends on; duration of AF (traditional teaching suggests that > 48 hours of AF is required for thrombi to form), and the CHADS2 score (1 point each for the presence of congestive heart failure, hypertension, age > 75 years, diabetes, and 2 points for a previous stroke), the higher the score the higher the risk. If AF had been going on for > 48 hours, then the stroke risk of immediate cardioversion must be very carefully considered and balanced against the immediate haemodynamic benefit. This may require careful clinical judgement.

3. (d) A short diastolic time leads to poor coronary perfusion

The left coronary artery fills during diastole (the right coronary during systole). If there is a tachycardia there is less time for this to occur. In patients with structurally normal hearts (no coronary disease, normal left ventricular function) this is rarely sufficient to cause problems. However, in those with coronary disease, this causes myocardial ischaemia which leads to diminished contraction, heart failure and hence shortness of breath and hypoxia. This pathophysiology therefore explains the crucial important of slowing down the heart rate in patients with symptomatic AF. There is an additional mechanism for heart failure in AF, which is the loss of the atrial component of ventricular filling to cardiac output. In those with healthy hearts, atrial systole contributes about 10-15% of ventricular filling and hence cardiac output, whereas in those with stiff hearts (hypertension, the elderly, coronary disease) the atrial contribution to cardiac output is much more, up to 40%; losing this, as occurs in AF, lowers cardiac output, and can lead to heart failure.

4. (b) Potassium and magnesium

Aim to keep the potassium >4 mmol/L. It may be low due to diuretic treatment, which is not uncommon in this patient group. Serum magnesium levels, although not correlating well with total body levels, should be kept within the normal range.

Further reading: Chapter 92.

Case 6: A 72-year-old patient with shortness of breath

1. (c) Probable pulmonary hypertension

It suggests right ventricular enlargement possibly due to pulmonary hypertension. When present, this is a moderately reliable sign of pulmonary hypertension; however, most patients with clinically important pulmonary hypertension do not have this sign, so its absence cannot be relied on to rule pulmonary hypertension out. Rarely it may be that left atrial enlargement has displaced the right ventricle forwards.

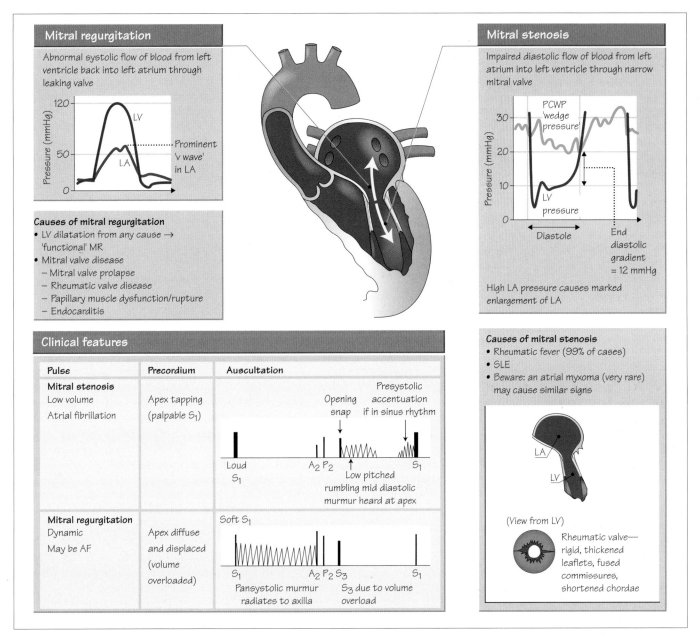

Figure 1.6.1 Clinical features of mitral valve disease.

2. (a) Mitral stenosis

The description of malar flush and clinical findings suggest mitral stenosis with pulmonary hypertension. There is a differential diagnosis of a malar flush, including hypothyroidism, poor cardiac output due to other condition, and outdoor living, hence it is often not that useful a diagnostic sign. The praecordial examination (palpation, auscultation) here are pathognomonic for mitral stenosis

3. (d) Any of the above

All of these signs may be apparent on the chest radiograph. The carina lies directly above the left atrium and may be splayed to >90°. The edge of the enlarged atrium forms the double heart border and the extra bulge is due to an enlarged atrial appendage. Mitral stenosis causes atrial enlargement and eventually pulmonary hypertension as the disease progresses.

Further reading: Chapter 87.

Case 7: A patient in cardiac arrest on the ward

1. (c) Check electrode contact and lead selection

These can be very fraught situations. It is important to reassess the patient yourself to confirm cardiac arrest and adopt an ABC approach. Particularly in the case of asystole it is crucial to check that the ECG electrodes or hands free pads are correctly sited and connected to the machine. Equally important is to ensure that the monitor is reading the correct lead or through the pads and to turn up the ECG gain (size).

2. (b) Red – right arm; yellow – left arm; green – left leg

As an aide memoire, like the traffic lights: Red to Right arm, yeLLow to Left arm, Green to left Groin. The positioning of the leads is important to ensure correct interpretation of the ECG.

3. (b) 30 seconds

Advanced Life Support guidelines suggest that 30 seconds is the longest time permitted at attempting intubation, although ideally there should be no interruption.

4. (d) Continual compressions at 100 breaths/min and 10 breaths/min

Continual chest compressions should now commence. Remember to rotate this duty frequently as it is tiring, particularly in prolonged resuscitation efforts.

Further reading: Chapter 76.

Case 8: A patient in cardiac arrest

1. (c) Pulmonary embolism, hyperkalaemia, hypoventilation, hypocalcaemia

The 4 'H's and 4 'T's. These are: hypoxia, hypovolaemia, hyper- or hypo- kalaemia, hypoglycaemia, hypocalcaemia, acidaemia and other metabolic disorders and hypothermia. The 'T's are tension pneumothorax, tamponade, toxins and thrombosis (coronary and pulmonary).

2. (b) Sodium bicarbonate

Sodium bicarbonate can be used in the acute setting to treat hyperkalaemia. Care must be taken when using concentrated solutions such as 8.4% as extravasation may cause considerable damage. Calcium chloride or gluconate is cardio-protective peri-arrest and will be helpful in the arrest situation. Insulin and dextrose infusions are an alternative.

3. (d) For asystole and PEA provided the rate is <60 beats/min

Atropine 3 mg should be given just once.

Further reading: Chapter 76.

Case 9: A fit woman with shortness of breath and flu-like symptoms

1. (a) Heart failure

The signs taken together suggest heart failure as a cause for her shortness of breath and hypoxia. She has a raised JVP, which may be present in heart failure, pulmonary embolism and (though this is exceptionally unlikely in young patients) acute severe asthma. The third heart sound in a young, fit athlete may not be pathological but otherwise suggests cardiac failure. The clue here is the widespread inspiratory crepitations which would not be present in the other conditions.

2. (c) Myocarditis

The best explanation would probably be a myocarditis secondary to her continued exercise programme with a concurrent viral infection. The ECG also shows widespread ST changes. A pericardial effusion has many similarities with this presentation and may arise secondary to a myocarditis itself. The clearly audible heart sounds go against this, though. Cardiac tamponade is classically described by Beck's triad (muffled heart sounds, a raised JVP and hypotension).

3. (a) All of these therapies

She should be treated with conventional heart failure treatment. This includes diuretics, GTN infusion and non-invasive ventilation. Angiotensin-converting enzyme (ACE) inhibitors and β-blockers are added *when the acute phase has been managed.* GTN is probably best avoided in her case as it will cause vasodilatation and lower her BP further. Inotropes and vasopressors may cause further myocardial damage but in some cases will be necessary. It is a complex case and help from intensive care and cardiology staff will be required. Clearly, after simple blood tests, an ECG and a chest X-ray, the most important investigation is a transthoracic cardiac ultrasound; this will instantly exclude pericardial effusion, and give a good estimate of the severity of the cardiac damage; rarely however does this allow the aetiology of the myocarditis to be diagnosed.

4. (d) All of the above

The causes of myocarditis are extensive, although the most common is a viral aetiology such as coxsackie virus. Other causes include bacterial and spirochete infection, drugs, environmental toxins, connective tissue disorders and even wasp, spider and scorpion stings.

Further reading: Chapter 91.

Case 10: A patient with shortness of breath and chest tightness

1. (c) Myocardial infarction (MI)

She does not present with the classic symptoms of crushing chest pain radiating to the jaw and neck, but this is not always the case. Indeed, a silent MI is recognized in patients with long-standing diabetes, the elderly and postoperative patients. She also has many risk factors for ischaemic heart disease. The sudden onset of the symptoms makes a COPD exacerbation very unlikely.

2. (b) Pulmonary oedema

The chest radiograph demonstrates pulmonary oedema secondary to her MI. The chest X-ray of a patient with ARDS can be impossible to differentiate from pulmonary oedema but occurs due to lung injury in the context of good heart function. The findings in this case clearly point towards heart failure with a raised JVP, third heart sound and 'cardiac' wheeze.

3. (d) High-flow oxygen

All the other options may well be urgent and appropriate but her oxygen saturation is just 86%. It is critically important to quickly optimize the oxygen delivery to the damaged myocardium to prevent further injury. Sitting her upright will also help.

4. (d) All of the above

There are many complications of MI but these include arrhythmias. These may occur at any time but are particularly well recognized firstly at the start of the MI, when ventricular arrhythmias are most common, affect 20-30%, and are the commonest cause of pre-hospital death, and secondly after thrombolysis (reperfusion arrhythmias). Atrial fibrillation is also common. Papillary muscle rupture causes acute mitral valve regurgitation; the typical patient develops severe pulmonary oedema, often treatment refractory so that ventilation is required. The murmur of acute ischaemic mitral regurgitation is often very soft or indeed inaudible, and equally, it is one of the few valve lesions that the transthoracic cardiac ultrasound can substantially underestimate. Accordingly, neither the clinical signs nor the transthoracic echocardiography (TTE) is reliable in diagnosing ischaemic mitral regurgitation. If the diagnosis is under serious consideration, and the TTE fails to confirm the diagnosis, then a trans-oesophageal echo is usually mandatory. Surgery is often required, though is high risk and many patient do not survive acute papillary muscle rupture. Pericarditis (Dressler's syndrome) occurs 2–10 weeks after an MI.

Further reading: Chapter 82.

Case 11: A drug user with a cough and chest pain

1. (d) Infective endocarditis

This patient is a known intravenous drug user and as such is at particular risk of developing endocarditis on the right side of the heart. Although also at risk of tuberculous the murmur makes this less likely and the cause of the murmur should be investigated in the first instance.

2. (c) Three

On suspicion of the diagnosis of endocarditis a minimum of three sets of cultures should be taken. The Duke criteria used to diagnose endocarditis suggest that all of three sets of cultures or a majority of four positive cultures (with only an hour between the first and last set) must be positive to meet one of the major criteria. Three is therefore the minimum. The role of the cardiac ultrasound in diagnosing infective endocarditis is much misunderstood – it should not be used as a screening test in those who are at low probability of endocarditis; low probability is defined as the absence of all of the following criteria: (1) vasculitic/embolic phenomena; (2) central venous access; (3) a recent history of intravenous drug use; (4) presence of a prosthetic valve; and (5) positive blood cultures. The appropriate screening test in low probability patients is 3 sets of blood cultures, provided the patient is antibiotic naïve. Never start antibiotics in a relatively well patient suspected of having endocarditis until you have established the microbiological diagnosis. The cardiac ultrasound is an appropriate test in those with medium or higher chance of endocarditis.

3. (a) Inflammation and dilatation of a vessel wall caused by septic emboli

Septic emboli break off the vegetation on the valve in left-sided endocarditis and may cause either infection of the arterial wall or secondary infection of an existing aneurysm. The name is something of a misnomer, as whilst fungi may cause them, more often they are associated with bacterial infection. The aneurysm may form anywhere in the body.

Further reading: Chapter 91.

Case 12: A patient with angina and raised blood pressure

1. (a) Amlodipine (calcium channel inhibitor)

Amlodipine would be the most appropriate drug to add using the AB/CD principle where A is ACE inhibitor, B is a β–blocker, C is a calcium channel inhibitor and D is diuretics. A drug from either the AB or CD side is chosen, then as escalated a drug from the other selected. He is already on an AB and D drug therefore a calcium channel inhibitor is a good choice. In fact the recommendation is for a calcium channel as first line in those over 55 years.

He is commenced on amlodipine 5 mg od but 2 weeks later returns complaining of swollen ankles. He is otherwise asymptomatic

2. (c) Treatment side effect

Given that there has been no change in the symptomatology it is likely to be a well recognized side effect of the amlodipine that has caused the problem.

3. (a) Hyponatraemia

Electrolyte abnormalities are commonly seen and include hyponatraemia, hypokalaemia and hypomagnesaemia and less commonly, hypercalcaemia.

Further reading: Chapter 79.

Case 13: A pregnant woman with left-sided chest pain

1. (c) Normal changes in pregnancy

Many physiological changes occur during pregnancy that need to be considered when interpreting both physiological parameters and blood test results. Among these are increased minute volume ventilation brought about by a higher respiratory rate which lowers the $PaCO_2$. The murmur is likely to be that of an innocent flow murmur of pregnancy. The ECG finding is also well recognized.

2. (a) The amount of radiation is similar to a transatlantic flight and unlikely to harm a baby at this stage of development

A chest radiograph is an important part of this patient's work up. It may help to exclude other causes of similar symptom groups such as infection, pneumothorax, PE or even fractured ribs if there were a history of trauma.

3. (b) Low molecular weight heparin and further investigation

The incidence of PE ranges between 1 in 1000 to 1 in 3000 deliveries. She is at high risk because of this and her age (risk of PE is doubled in mothers older than 35 years). These are challenging cases and she will need an immediate senior opinion regarding further investigation. Choices between V/Q scanning, CTPA (Computerized Tomographic Pulmonary Angiography) and pulmonary angiography may vary between clinicians because of concerns of radiation exposure. Doppler scans of her legs are not particularly sensitive for deep vein thrombosis (DVT) but if positive are helpful. MRI, although not widely available, is an alternative and is as good as CTPA. While these decisions are being made it is vital she is treated with heparin – indeed, this is perhaps the most important aspect of caring for her, that adequate doses of heparin are given the moment the possibility of pulmonary embolism is considered. There is considerable debate as to what constitutes 'adequate' doses; some protocols specify 5-10,000 units of IV unfractionated heparin immediately, with simultaneous full dose subcutaneous low molecular weight heparin (LMWH). This is because the anticoagulant effect of the IV heparin will be immediate, whereas sub-cut LMWH may take some time to be picked up and start working. Though the anticoagulant action is immediate, the risk of fatal PE will persist for several days following its administration; this is because though heparin will stop new thrombus being made, existing thrombus, for example in the deep calf or pelvic veins, is broken down by the bodies intrinsic fibrinolytic action, and this will take several days or even longer to be completely effective. Clearly while such thrombus is still present, there is always the chance of further PEs and clinical consequences.

4. (b) Position her in the left lateral position and arrange a caesarean

The left lateral position improves venous return to the heart by ensuring the fetus is not compressing the inferior vena cava. If spontaneous circulation has not returned within 5 minutes, emergency caesarean is indicated to improve the mother's circulation, and save the life of the foetus. Thrombolysis in pregnancy is not recommended due to the high risk of placental bed bleeding which may in itself be fatal, unless of course it proves impossible to restore the circulation without thrombolysis, in which case it's use may have to be seriously considered. Case reports demonstrate its occasional successful use in massive PE.

Further reading: Chapter 90.

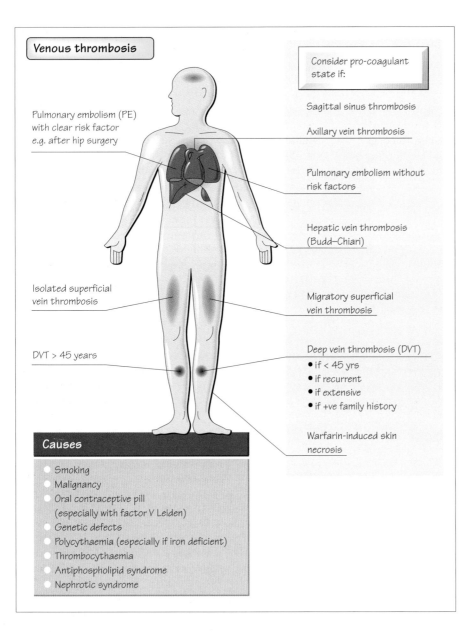

Venous thrombosis

Pulmonary embolism (PE) with clear risk factor e.g. after hip surgery

Isolated superficial vein thrombosis

DVT > 45 years

Consider pro-coagulant state if:

Sagittal sinus thrombosis

Axillary vein thrombosis

Pulmonary embolism without risk factors

Hepatic vein thrombosis (Budd–Chiari)

Migratory superficial vein thrombosis

Deep vein thrombosis (DVT)
- if < 45 yrs
- if recurrent
- if extensive
- if +ve family history

Warfarin-induced skin necrosis

Causes
- Smoking
- Malignancy
- Oral contraceptive pill (especially with factor V Leiden)
- Genetic defects
- Polycythaemia (especially if iron deficient)
- Thrombocythaemia
- Antiphospholipid syndrome
- Nephrotic syndrome

Figure 1.14.1 Clinical features of venous thrombosis.

Case 14: A patient with calf pain and loss of appetite

1. (b) i, ii, iii, iv

A ruptured popliteal cyst (Baker's cyst) is an important differential in any patient with osteoarthritis or rheumatoid arthritis affecting the knee. Fluid escapes into the soft tissue causing pain, swelling and tenderness. It may appear clinically very similar to a DVT. This woman has many potential causes of her calf pain but given the duration of symptoms, swelling and increased warmth, cramp is not one of them.

2. (d) D-dimer and ultrasound left leg

The most important diagnosis to exclude is a DVT of the leg. This has the potential to cause a pulmonary embolism (PE) which may be fatal. Ultrasound is able to detect both a DVT and a Baker's cyst. It is important to recognize that ultrasonography has

a sensitivity as low as 75% for calf DVT. It is much higher for proximal DVT. D-dimer tests (depending on the assay your hospital uses) tend to have a high negative predictive value, so if negative are good at ruling out DVT in low-risk patients. Methods exist to stratify patient risk of having a DVT based on symptoms and signs. Positive D-dimer results may be obtained for many other reasons, including sepsis, malignancy and recent surgery.

3. (a) Continue the low molecular weight heparin that you commenced when you suspected a DVT and start warfarin

Warfarin takes some days to achieve an adequate anticoagulation so it is important to continue the heparin. The evidence for thrombolysis is weak and has high risks associated with it so is not used. An IVC filter may be considered if there are either contraindications to anticoagulation or recurrent PEs despite adequate anticoagulation.

4. (c) Ultrasound abdomen

A worrying feature of this patient's illness is the anorexia, weight loss, fatigue and constipation. She also has abdominal tenderness in the context of a large DVT. Abdominal malignancy should be investigated with ultrasound in the first instance. It is always important to consider if there are any underlying risk factors such as oral contraceptive pill use, immobility, thrombophilia or pregnancy, amongst others.

Further reading: Chapter 185.

Case 15: A patient with hypertension and chest pain

1. (c) Anterior myocardial infarction

The ECG shows ST elevation in the anterior leads.

2. (d) Left anterior descending (LAD)

Anterior myocardial infarctions (MIs) are characterized by disease in the LAD artery. Inferior MI: right artery; posterior MI: right or circumflex arteries; lateral MI: circumflex or diagonal branch of LAD artery.

3. (a) Morphine

(b) Intravenous nitrate

Opiates and intravenous nitrates are used in acute LVF. Loop diuretics are the cornerstone of management but must be given intravenously. Digoxin has no role in acute LVF when the patient is in sinus rhythm.

4. (b) Continuous positive airway pressure (CPAP)

It is difficult to increase the GTN further because of the patient's blood pressure (remember he is normally hypertensive). The hypotension and left ventricular (LV) dysfunction may explain why there has been little response to the diuretic (the patient could be developing an acute kidney injury). Although ACE inhibitors are essential drugs they do not improve acute LVF and reduce blood pressure further. β-Blockers are contraindicated in acute LVF. CPAP is ideally suited to the treatment of pulmonary oedema.

5. (a) Improves oxygenation

(b) Gastric distention

(d) Reduced venous return

(e) Reduces left ventricular afterload

CPAP improves oxygenation by recruiting lung units and improving $\dot{V}/\dot{Q}$ matching. The improvement in lung compliance reduces the work of breathing; this is important because the work of breathing is high in acute LVF and consumes a high proportion of cardiac output. CPAP therefore reduces myocardial oxygen demand whilst at the same time improving oxygen delivery as a result of treating the hypoxia. The positive intrathoracic pressure reduces venous return to the heart (preload) and, importantly, decreases transmural LV systolic pressure, which reduces afterload; both effects can improve myocardial performance.

Further reading: Chapter 85.

Case 16: A patient with new onset chest pain

1. (a) Non-cardiac chest pain

The definition of the different forms of chest pain can be made according to the following scheme:

- Typical angina (definite): (1) substernal chest discomfort with a characteristic quality and duration that is (2) provoked by exertion or emotional stress and (3) relieved by rest or nitroglycerin. Typical pain is a heaviness, tightness, or ache, building up if exercise continues, possibly radiating to the jaw or arm(s), and relieved within 2 minutes by rest
- Atypical angina (probable): meets 2 of the above characteristics
- Non-cardiac chest pain (this is better called non-anginal chest pain, rather than the potentially incorrect non-cardiac chest pain): meets ≤1 of the typical angina characteristics

This man has pain that has an atypical location, is not related to exercise, nor is relieved by rest; by definition, he therefore has non-anginal chest pain.

2. (a) Low

The pre-test probability refers to the likelihood that a patient has an illness before any definitive investigations have been carried out. The pre-test probability for coronary disease can be predicted on the basis of typicality of symptoms, age and sex (see Fig. 1.18.2). Clearly, these odds can be further altered if hypertension, hyperlipidaemia, or other risk factors for coronary disease are present. This data shows that in diagnosing whether coronary disease is the cause of symptoms, it is crucial to know both baseline risk factors as well as the nature of the pain

3. (g) All of the above

Clearly it is crucial to know cholesterol, and hence baseline risk; causes of high cholesterol include hypothyroidism. Renal failure is associated with accelerated coronary disease. Anaemia can provoke anginal symptoms in those with coronary disease. A resting ECG may show evidence of old myocardial infarction. A stress test, while it has many strengths and weaknesses, remains the principle means to diagnose coronary disease and estimate prognosis.

4. (a) His left ventricular function is normal

A completely normal resting ECG is very likely to be associated with normal left ventricular function. Put another way, the vast majority of patients with impaired left ventricular function have some significant abnormality on their resting ECG.

5. (d) It is unlikely that he has coronary disease

Turning the exercise test data into a probabilistic score can be done using the Diamond and Forrester data, some of which is given below (Fig. 1.16.1). This translates the data on age, sex, and exercise test findings into the post-test probability of coronary disease. In essence, the older patients are, the more typical symptoms are, and the greater the ST depression, the more likely there is to be coronary disease. The corollary of this data is that some patients with no ST changes during a stress test have severe coronary disease, and equally some patients with substantial ST depression have no coronary disease. Adding in exercise capacity, and why patients stopped exercising allows a calculation of prognosis (the Duke data).

Further reading: Chapter 64 in ECG at a Glance.

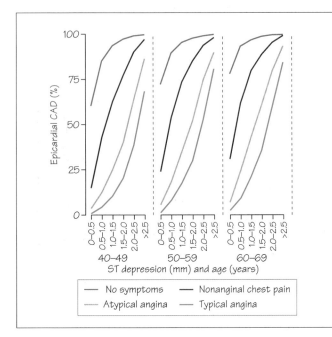

Epicardial CAD (%)

ST depression (mm) and age (years)

40–49   50–59   60–69

— No symptoms   — Nonanginal chest pain
— Atypical angina   — Typical angina

Figure 1.16.1 Diamond and Forrester data.

Case 17: Severe chest pain in a man with diabetes

1. (d) High

He has multiple risk factors for coronary disease, including diabetes, age, sex, treated hypertension, and a cholesterol, which while technically at the upper limit of the population range for the UK, on a world wide basis is very high. The average total cholesterol level in Chinese communities in china is 3.3 mmol/L. Perhaps, though there clearly are assumptions here, the quoted 'normal' UK ranges should be based on what cholesterol should be, i.e. what cholesterol is in peasant communities, rather than on what it actually is in western communities. This would emphasise just how high western cholesterols are, and how unsafe apparently normal cholesterols are in the presence of other major coronary risk factors.

2. (a) None

The findings as reported here are very non-specific. It only establishes the fact that he has chest wall tenderness; if the pain exactly reproduced his symptoms, it would reduce the chance that he had non-cardiac chest pain, but certainly not eliminate them. The clinical factors that increase or decrease the chance that acute chest pain is due to myocardial infarction have been examined.

3. (a) An anterior wall ST segment elevation myocardial infarction (STEMI)

The ECG shows ST elevation in leads I, aVL, V1 through to V5, with ST depression in leads II, III and aVF. The ST elevation is in the anterior leads, and accordingly this is an anterior wall STEMI. It is not pericarditis as the ST elevation is of the wrong pattern, too substantial, and there is inferior lead ST depression. The most sensitive ECG sign of pericarditis is PR interval depression, not seen here.

4. (f) Intravenous opiate

Immediate pain relief is crucial. Clearly the other treatments for STEMI should be given, including aspirin 300 mg chewed (not swallowed, as this takes too long to be absorbed), thrombolytic therapy if speedy primary PCI is not available, otherwise, clopidogrel and immediate primary PCI.

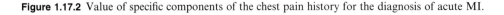

Pain descriptor	Reference	No. of patients	Positive likelihood ratio (95% CI)
Increased likelihood of AMI			
Radiation to right arm or shoulder	29	770	4.7 (1.9–12)
Radiation to both arms or shoulders	14	893	4.1 (2.5–6.5)
Associated with exertion	14	893	2.4 (1.5–3.8)
Radiation to left arm	24	278	2.3 (1.7–3.1)
Associated with diaphoresis	24	8426	2.0 (1.9–2.2)
Associated with nausea or vomiting	24	970	1.9 (1.7–2.3)
Worse than previous angina or similar to previous MI	29	7734	1.8 (1.6–2.0)
Described as pressure	29	11504	1.3 (1.2–1.5)
Decreased likelihood of AMI			
Described as pleuritic	29	8822	0.2 (0.1–0.3)
Described as positional	29	8330	0.3 (0.2–0.5)
Described as sharp	29	1088	0.3 (0.2–0.5)
Reproducible with palpation	29	8822	0.3 (0.2–0.4)
Inframammary locations	31	903	0.8 (0.7–0.9)
Not associated with exertion	14	893	0.8 (0.6–0.9)

Abbreviations: AMI, acute myocardial infarction; CI, confidence interval

Figure 1.17.2 Value of specific components of the chest pain history for the diagnosis of acute MI.

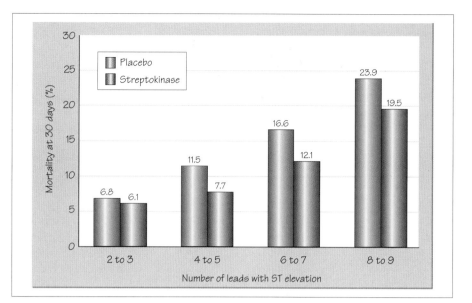

Figure 1.17.3 Relationship between number of leads showing ST elevation and death in STEMI.

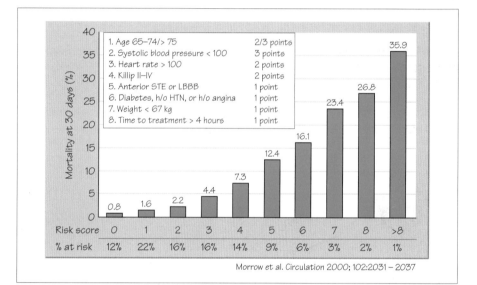

Figure 1.17.4 The outcome for STEMI related to TIMI score.

5. (f) All of the above

The number of leads showing ST segment deviation relates to outcome, as shown in Fig. 1.17.3, where data comes from the GISSI (Gruppo Italiano per lo Studio della Sopravvivenzanell'Infarto miocardico) trial. The effect of the old thrombolytic streptokinase is shown. The haemodynamic status of the patient, as measured by the Killip class, also relates to outcome. Killip class is defined as follows:

- **Killip I** patients with no clinical signs of heart failure
- **Killip II** patients with rales or crackles in the lungs, an S3, and elevated jugular venous pressure
- **Killip III** patients with frank acute pulmonary edema
- **Killip IV** patients in cardiogenic shock or hypotension (measured as systolic blood pressure ≤90 mmHg), and evi-

dence of peripheral vasoconstriction (oliguria, cyanosis or sweating)

The other data also relate to outcome; though there are multiple risk scores for outcome in acute STEMI, a useful one is that produced by the Thrombolysis in Myocardial Infarction (TIMI) study group, and shown in Fig. 1.17.4.

The method and speed of opening up the occluded coronary artery are also critically important in determining outcome; medical therapy with aspirin reduces STEMI mortality overall by about 2%, intravenous thrombolysis by another 2%, with fibrin specific agents, especially in those younger than 65 years, being more effective than streptokinase. Primary PCI reduces mortality by about another 2% overall when compared to thrombolytic therapy. Primary PCI also allows much risk stratification to be done right at the start of the hospital admission, though crucially not all, as a cardiac ultrasound is still needed; if left ventricular function is very depressed, further evaluation may be needed. Duration of hospital stay is also reduced.

It is crucially important to realize that most deaths due to myocardial infarction occur out in the community before medical help is called; of the 20-30% who die during the index event, some 80% die before hospitalization. This clearly means that one of the most important aspects of public health policy is to encourage patients who have symptoms that possibly indicate a heart attack to call for help very early on. In addition, to reduce community mortality the policy of placing large numbers of automatic external defibrillators in public places seems sensible.

6. (a) He has developed an ischaemic ventricular septal defect (VSD)

The time course, symptoms and signs are pathognomonic for an ischaemic VSD. If he only had ankle oedema without a murmur, the likelihood is that the diagnosis would be (mainly right sided) heart failure due to his original infarct. The loud murmur is sited exactly where the murmur from a VSD is sited, at the base of the left sternal edge. Occasionally, the murmur can be difficult to tell apart from that due to MR. However, if he had acute severe, it is highly likely that he would have severe pulmonary oedema due to left heart failure. He would then be quite unable to lie flat, he would sit bolt upright, be very uncomfortable, be very tachypnoiec; lung examination would show extensive inspiratory crepitations. The outlook for ischaemic VSD is still poor; he should be immediately transferred to a surgical centre with good figures for VSD surgery. He may need immediate surgery. In many units, however, the policy , if possible, is to delay surgery for as long as possible, preferably 4-6 weeks, as this allows the boggy oedematous ventricular tissue to heal, such that the stitching of a closure patch is more likely to hold, so greatly reducing surgical mortality and improving outcome. However, many patients suffer a haemodynamic decline before this healing process can be completed, and must be subjected to immediate surgery, with its attendant risks. Some patients are suitable for percutaneous closure using a variety of devices; however, in many there are multiple holes, and satisfactory VSD closure cannot be obtained using the percutaneous route.
Further reading: Chapter 82.

Case 18: A patient with chronic chest pain

1. (d) An exercise stress ECG

An exercise ECG should now be carried out. It would be quite wrong to do nothing in this situation. We are as yet not sure whether his pain has been cardiac, and if so, what his risk of further cardiac events is. Some evaluation is definitely indicated.

An exercise ECG is a simple, cheap, easily available examination that has considerable utility, although there are also major limitations. We already know that the patient is at relatively low risk for further events as he has had normal ECG despite prolonged pain, and was troponin negative, both of these together being moderately predictive for a good future. The exercise ECG can further refine this risk. The exercise ECG is however not that good in this sort of situation in determining whether the pain was cardiac or not.

A coronary angiogram is definitely not indicated in this low risk situation where symptoms have settled. Coronary CT angiography is probably too new to confidently use, and unlikely to be available. An even newer alternative, not yet widely available, would be to consider using CT to obtain a coronary calcium score.

Some units would also consider performing a nuclear myocardial perfusion scan; in this examination a small dose of radioactive technetium is injected during exercise or pharmacological stress, and taken up by viable non-ischaemic cardiac tissue, then imaged using a gamma ray detecting camera. The camera rotates, allowing the different regions of the heart that have and have not taken up the heart to be separately evaluated. The examination is repeated at rest. This allows one to discriminate between normal tissues with a good blood supply (good uptake at rest and stress), normal tissue with a poor blood supply (good image at rest, poor uptake with stress) and infracted tissue (no uptake at rest or with stress). The extent of the abnormalities relates to the risk of further adverse cardiac events.

NICE has issued guidelines for the management of new onset chest pain; they depend on scoring the patient for the pre-test probability of coronary disease, dependent on risk factors and the typicality or otherwise of the chest pain (Fig. 1.18.2). According to this scoring system, our patient had a pre-test probability of coronary artery disease (CAD) of about 40% (atypical angina, as not effort related, and risk factors). NICE then goes on to recommend that:

- If the estimated likelihood of CAD is 61–90%, offer invasive coronary angiography as the first-line diagnostic investigation if appropriate
- If the estimated likelihood of CAD is 30–60%, offer functional imaging as the first-line diagnostic investigation
- If the estimated likelihood of CAD is 10–29%, offer CT calcium scoring as the first-line diagnostic investigation

Our patient has a pre-test probability in the second tertile, which would suggest that according to the guidelines, he should have a functional test, for example, a nuclear myocardial perfusion scan, or a stress echo/MRI. However, provided one is fully conversant with the strengths and limitations of an exercise ECG, many cardiologists would still use this, given its cheapness and widespread availability.

2. (b) Admitted

It would be indefensible to send this man home at this stage. We do not know if he has cardiac chest pain, and we have no real feeling to what his risk is of further adverse events. Low risk patients constitute those in whom symptoms have settled, the ECG is and remains normal, and a properly timed troponin is not raised. In this patient, with bloods taken within 2 hours, it is too early to rely on the troponin measurement (these must be taken 12 hours after pain), and likewise though his admission ECG was normal, this may change. Finally, we do not know if his symptoms have settled.

3. (b) His usual medications (statin and ACE inhibitor) and aspirin, 300 mg chewed then 75 mg a day

The benefit of clopidogrel and low molecular weight heparin relate to risk, and at this stage, though risk is not fully evaluated, his ECG and biomarkers suggest it may be low.

4. (a) In the proximal part of the left anterior descending coronary artery

This ECG shows very widespread T wave inversion, affecting leads I, II, aVL, and V2 to V6. This pattern is very strongly associated with a lesion in the proximal portion of the left anterior

Age (years)	Non-anginal chest pain Men		Women		Atypical angina Men		Women		Typical angina Men		Women	
	Lo	Hi	Lo	Hi	Lo	Hi	Lo	Hi	Lo	Hi	Lo	Hi
35	3	35	1	19	8	59	2	39	30	88	10	78
45	9	47	2	22	21	70	5	43	51	92	20	79
55	23	59	4	25	45	79	10	47	80	95	38	82
65	49	69	9	29	71	86	20	51	93	97	56	84

For men older than 70 with atypical or typical symptoms, assume an estimate > 90%

For women older than 70, assume an estimate of 61–90% EXCEPT women at high risk AND with typical symptoms where a risk of > 90% should be assumed

Values are per cent of people at each mid-decade age with significant coronary artery disease (CAD)[1]

Hi = High risk = diabetes, smoking and hyperlipidaemia (total cholesterol > 6.47 mmol/litre)

Lo = Low risk = none of these three

▨ Represents people with symptoms of non-anginal chest pain, who would not be investigated for stable angina routinely

Note:

These results are likely to overestimate CAD in primary care populations

If there are resting ECG ST-T changes or Q waves, the likelihood of CAD is higher in each cell of the table

Figure 1.18.2 Prevalence of coronary artery disease according to risk factors.

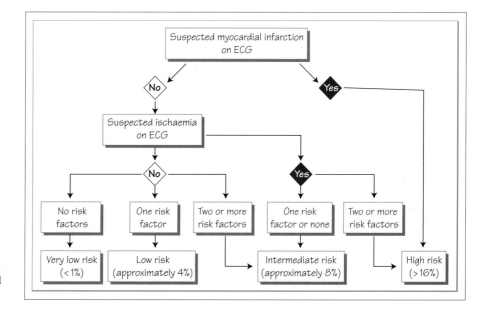

Figure 1.18.3 Annual mortality in suspected MI.

descending (LAD) coronary artery, and as such is termed a 'proximal LAD ECG'. It is also possible that he has a problem in the left main stem, though this is a much rarer diagnosis in this situation. It does not suggest that the acute problem is either in the circumflex or the right coronary artery.

5. (a) Coronary angiogram with a view to percutaneous coronary intervention (PCI) with stent insertion if appropriate

He is at high risk for further adverse events given the ECG changes, so no further risk stratification is needed. Accordingly the exercise ECG and MPS will not be helpful. Indeed, in this situation the exercise ECG could potentially provoke a major anterior infarct. While he still needs his coronary anatomy defining, what he really needs is revascularization. Coronary angiography outlines the coronary anatomy, and so allows the best form of revascularization to be decided. It is highly likely that he has a severe stenosis in the proximal part of the LAD coronary artery, and equally that this can and therefore should be treated by balloon angioplasty and stent insertion. Large randomized trials have shown that early invasive evaluation and revascularization of higher risk patients improves outcome. In this case, a high-grade stenosis was found, and stented successfully. However, a blocked distal right coronary artery was also found, with this artery receiving some collaterals from the left coronary artery; it is highly likely that blocking of this artery was the cause of his pain 3 years ago.

Further reading: Chapter 82.

Case 19: A elderly man with blackouts

1. (c) A vasomotor form of syncope

The description is pathognomonic for this, with stereotyped episodes (i.e. all are similar), warning of the event ('feeling lightheaded'), absence of injury and quick recovery. He is also in the right age range for certain syncopal vasomotor syndromes. The description rules out epilepsy. Stokes-Adams attacks, which are due to a cardiac arrhythmia such as complete heart block or ventricular tachycardia, are random, not location specific, and patients do not experience a warning prior to blacking out. Injury is common, as cerebral blood flow is usually so low during the attack that all protective mechanisms are lost – bilateral black eyes are perhaps their commonest physical sign, and these are frequently seen in patients admitted on the medical take. Stokes-Adams attacks are associated with premature death unless the cause is found and treated; this means that all suspected Stokes-Adams attacks must be fully and urgently evaluated. Hyperventilation is a very rare cause for blackouts, and most commonly affects young women with other manifest forms of psychological illness.

2. (b) The same as age matched controls

The prognosis in syncope depends on the diagnosis; if the diagnosis is vasomotor syncope, then there is no increase in death rate. One could perhaps argue that in this moderately elderly patient, the fact that he has a normal exercise ECG and cardiac ultrasound may actually increase his life expectancy compared to his compatriots, some of whom may have severe coronary disease without realizing it.

The early investigations have some utility in diagnosing the cause of syncope and its danger to the patient; perhaps the most important early investigation is the resting ECG (Fig. 1.19.2). Likewise, occasionally, though not commonly, the 24-hour ECG gives diagnostically useful data. However, the most important aspect of investigation is to try and record an ECG during an event, either one occurring spontaneously, or equally, during some form of provocation test.

3. (f) A carotid sinus massage test

He has had 5 or 6 episodes over the past year or so, it seems unlikely that these will settle spontaneously. There is no evidence either in the history, examination of on simple investigation of structural heart disease, so sophisticated tests looking for structural cardiac abnormalities are not indicated. Prolonged external loop recordings last up to a week; his episodes occur about once every 3 or 4 months, so these devices are unlikely to record an event. His episodes occur while standing, possibly while looking up, so a tilt table test with carotid sinus massage can be used to try and provoke an attack and see what happens to blood pressure and heart rate.

Normal	Interpretation	Further management
Normal	Arrhythmia unlikely, not excluded	If vasomotor syncope likely – tilt-table test; if unlikely, and injury present – Reveal® device
RBBB	Non-specific	Exclude Brugada syndrome (consider ajmaline flecainide challenge)
Long PR interval	Heart block possible; other causes should still be considered	If history of Stokes–Adams attack, permanent pacemaker; if CAD, consider EP study to: (i) measure AH, HV intervals; (ii) to exclude inducible VT; otherwise Reveal® device
Trifasicular block*	Heart block likely	Pacemaker
Q waves	VT related to the scar of the old MI	Ventricular stimulation study or Reveal® device
LVH	Aortic stenosis, hypertrophic cardiomyopathy If hypertensive, VT may underlie syncope	Cardiac ultrasound AVR for aortic stenosis; specialist management for HCM; otherwise Reveal® device
Long QT interval	Polymorphic VT	(i) Exclude relevant drugs; (ii) beta-blockers; (iii) ICD; (iv) family screening

*, Long PR interval + RBBB and L or R axis deviation
AH, atrial – His conduction time; AVR, aortic valve replacement; CAD, coronary artery disease; EP, electrophysiology; HCM, hypertrophic cardiomyopathy; HV, His – ventricular conduction time; ICD, implantable cardioverter defibrillator; LVH, left ventricular hypertrophy; MI, myocardial infarction; RBBB, right bundle branch block; VT, ventricular tachycardia

Figure 1.19.2 The utility of the inter-attack ECG in syncope.

	Vasovagal syncope	Neurocardiogenic syncope	Carotid sinus hypersensitivity	Micturition syncope	Postural hypotension
Age	Usually young	Any age; commoner in middle age	Usually elderly	Usually elderly; only occurs in men	Common in the elderly, people with diabetes
Position when syncope occurs	Upright	Almost always upright; after standing still, e.g. when out shopping	Usually when standing, can occur when sitting	Passing urine, in the middle of the night ± alcohol	Standing – immediately
Preceding symptoms	Modest warning	Presyncope = 'near' syncope = 'as if about to blackout', for 10–30 sec	Often none	Often none	Presyncope very common
Diagnostic test	Usually none required; if intrusive tilt-table test	Tilt-table test • Bradycardic: symptoms with ↓heart rate • Vasodepressor: symptoms with ↓SBP • Mixed	Bradycardia (≥ 3 sec asystole) ±/or hypotension (≥ 50 mmHg fall) on carotid sinus massage, done while lying or standing	History of prostatism	Postural blood pressure

Figure 1.19.3 Forms of vasomotor syncope.

4. (f) An infusion of intravenous isoprenaline

All the other procedures are necessary. Carotis sinus massage is performed by first ausculating the neck arteries for carotid bruit, if present, the risk of stroke is increased marginally, and the utility of the test should be reconsidered. First one and then the other carotid artery are gently massaged, for about 5 seconds, firstly with the patient lying horizontal, then with the table in 30-degree head up position. The definition of a strongly positive carotid sinus massage test is either a fall in systolic blood pressure by ≥50 mmHg with symptoms, or a pause (asystolic) of ≥5 seconds. For the former, a beat-to-beat blood pressure monitor is required; for the latter, it is vital not only to have an ECG machine but also one that can print the rhythm strip. Isoprenaline is sometimes used during a tilt table test to increase the likelihood of a positive result; unfortunately, it also strongly increases the chance of a false positive, and most units rarely use this. It is not used during the carotid sinus massage test.

5. (d) Insertion of a dual chamber pacemaker (DDD pacemaker)

He has had multiple episodes over several years, and they are unlikely to stop spontaneously. If possible therefore effective therapy should be introduced. His CSM shows a prolonged pause with no electrical activity. If an atrial pacemaker were implanted, this would ensure continued atrial activity; however, the vagal tone can be very high during a CSM induced pause, and this may prevent transmission of the electrical impulse from the atria to the ventricles, so that despite the pacemaker induced atrial activity, no ventricular activity results.

A single lead ventricular pacemaker would ensure ventricular activity; however, unless there was coordinated and appropriately timed atrial activity, the atrial component of cardiac output would be lost, and this component may be quite important in maintaining cardiac output and blood pressure in the elderly; indeed, this may be up to 25% of the total cardiac output in the normal elderly, who have quite stiff hearts.

Furthermore, pacemaker syndrome may occur with a VVI pacemaker. In pacemaker syndrome electrical activity from the ventricles retrogradely invades the atrioventricular (AV) nodes and activates the atrial, which then contract at almost exactly the same time as the ventricles. Ventricular contraction increases ventricular pressure and so shuts the AV valves (mitral and tricuspid); this then prevents atrial contraction pushing blood into the ventricles, rather, the atria bulge, and some blood is pushed retrogradely into the lungs and systemic great veins. Stretching of the atria during this ineffective activity results in brain natriuretic peptide release, and activation of various reflexes, both of which act to lower systemic blood pressure. Accordingly, a VVI pacemaker in this situation may prevent bradycardia, but still not prevent hypotension and symptoms.

A DDD pacemaker is indicated to prevent bradycardia and pacemaker syndrome. In patients with pure bradycardic carotid hypersensitivity syndrome, as here, a DDD pacemaker is very good at preventing further symptoms and also the sort of falls that may damage and break bones. In other words, there is some evidence that DDD pacing in this situation may improve outlook. This means that once the diagnosis has been established, treatment should not be delayed.

Further reading: Chapter 62 in ECG at a Glance.

Case 20: Palpitations in a young woman

1. (d) Atrioventricular nodal re-entrant tachycardia (AVNRT)

Clearly, as yet, we know nothing, we do not even have a physical examination or resting 12-lead ECG. However, we know she is young and well, has sudden onset regular palpitations that are fast and regular and of defined duration. This makes it very likely that she has a tachyarrhythmia, not anxiety (palpitations often last for very ill defined time periods, often of many hours). The palpitations are regular, which makes ectopics or atrial fibrillation unlikely. She is young and well, so ventricular tachycardia is highly unlikely. This leaves AVNRT and AVRT; the basis of AVRT is an accessory pathway, and this is a relatively rare phenomena, whereas AVNRT is a very common rhythm abnormality, affecting up to 5% of young women. The symptoms are consistent with AVNRT as are the demographics, so this is the likely diagnosis.

2. (a) It is normal

It is very easy to overinterpret ECGs, particularly in examinations! The computer report, where available, often helps; however, the best guide to what is normal is experience, and you should look at the ECG of all your patients, whether they are 'medical', 'surgical' or something else. Most of their ECGs will be normal, and you will get quite a good feel for the range of normal through this approach.

3. (a) Nothing
   (d) Cardiac memo device

She is extremely unlikely to have a dangerous attack, so implanting a solid state recording device, the reveal device, is not appropriate. If she is not worried by these short relatively infrequent attacks, it would not be unreasonable to do no more, and await events. If, however, she was very keen on a clear cut diagnosis, lending her a cardiomemo device would be appropriate. This is a very simplified external ECG machine, which the patient keeps at their home. During an attack, they apply the device to the left chest wall, and make a simple ECG. The device is good at establishing the diagnosis where attacks last at least a few minutes, and where the events at the onset are not relevant to the diagnosis, i.e. it is not a useful attack in diagnosing the cause of syncope.

The most important advice to give her is that if she were to have a prolonged attack, to immediately go to her GP's surgery, or the local A&E department, for an ECG. She must also be told that when an ECG is taken in this situation, she should request that a copy be given to her; interesting ECGs have a great habit of going missing from patients notes – it is much easier to establish what it showed if the patient can actually produce it for you!

4. (c) SVT due to AVNRT

There is a narrow complex tachycardia (so it cannot be ventricular tachycardia), without P waves visible before each QRS complex (so it is not sinus tachycardia). There is an rSr′ pattern in lead V1 (Fig. 1.20.3); though this may be partial right bundle branch block, if it were also present in the inter-attack sinus rhythm ECG, the second r′ is likely to indicate retrograde passage from a P wave originating in the atrioventricular (AV) node. The diagnosis is clinched when, following treatment, the sinus rhythm ECG no longer showed the r′ deflection.

5. (a) Neck massage, and if this is not successful, blowing against resistance (valsalva manouvre)
   (b) IV adenosine bolus

If (a) is unsuccessful, then (b) should be tried. The patient is well, and it is highly likely that medical therapy will work, so DC cardioversion is unlikely to be needed. Amiodarone is an unpleasant drug to give IV, as it can easily lead to painful phlebitis, and it has a potentially quite toxic side effect profile; many cardiologists feel that it is absolutely contraindicated in this situation for these reasons. Neck massage, and the valsalva manouvre activate the vagal nerve to the heart, and often (in about 50%) break the arrhythmia. If this is not successful, then it is highly likely that a bolus of IV adenosine, provided it is given incrementally, up to a high dose, will do so. Adenosine leads to temporary paralysis of the AV node; this means that all arrhythmias using the AV node will be temporarily stopped. In the case of AVNRT (or AVRT), once the arrhythmia has been stopped, even if only for a brief time period, the sinus node takes over. The old treatment for SVT was either IV verapamil (in a small dose) or IV beta-blocker, though NEVER the two together (which can lead to asystole and death).

Further reading: Chapters 45 and 46 in ECG at a Glance.

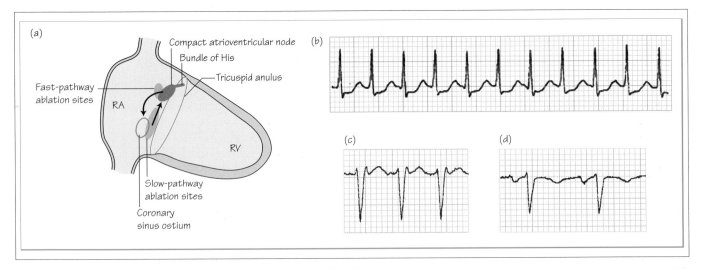

Figure 1.20.3 (a) Atrioventricular nodal re-entrant tachycardia (AVNRT) ablation sites. (b) Atrioventricular nodal re-entrant tachycardia: (b′) rhythm strip; (c) lead V1 showing rSR′ deflection during tachycardia; (d) not present during sinus rhythm.

2 Respiratory: Cases and Questions

Case 1: A patient with sudden-onset breathlessness

A 45-year-old man presents to your clinic. He describes sudden-onset breathlessness waking him from sleep occurring on seven occasions during the last month. When woken he is frightened and unable to breathe. On two occasions he has dialled 999 for an ambulance but has not been admitted to hospital as the paramedics have found no abnormality on arrival at the house.

1. *The patient is a life-long non-smoker, has no significant past medical or family history and is on no regular medication. What is the most likely diagnosis?*
   (a) Acute pulmonary oedema
   (b) Asthma
   (c) Laryngeal spasm
   (d) Hyperventilation syndrome

Case 2: A patient with a recent history of breathlessness

A 65-year-old man presented with breathlessness coming on over several months. There was no history of chest pain, cough or weight loss. He was an ex-smoker and was on no medication. He had just retired from work as a garage mechanic. Physical examination revealed no clubbing or lymphadenopathy. There was stony dullness to percussion with absent breath sounds over the right lower lobe and absent vocal resonance.

1. *What should be done next?*
   (a) Bronchoscopy to identify the cause of the lower lobe collapse
   (b) Needle aspiration of the pleural effusion for cytology
   (c) Plain radiological imaging of the chest
   (d) Sputum cytology

Case 3: A patient admitted with generalized abdominal pain

A 35 year-old woman is admitted with generalized abdominal pain. There is no past medical history. She has been unwell for 1 week and has symptoms of polydipsia and polyuria. She has been given morphine in the emergency department for her pain and is now a little drowsy, but responds to voice by eye opening. Respiratory rate is recorded at 30 breaths/min. Her heart rate is 100 beats/min in sinus rhythm and blood pressure is 100/60 mmHg. She has sweet-smelling breath.

1. *Which bedside test should be performed?*
   (a) Blood sugar
   (b) ECG
   (c) Chest X-ray
   (d) Abdominal X-ray

2. *The blood sugar is 39 mmol/L and the patient is started on intravenous saline and insulin. An arterial blood gas is performed and demonstrates the following:*

pH	7.06
$PaCO_2$	1.3 kPa
PaO_2	23.4 kPa
HCO_3^-	3 mmol/L
Base excess	−27

Which of the following is true?
   (a) The blood gas was performed on air
   (b) There is a respiratory acidosis
   (c) There is a metabolic acidosis
   (d) There is some respiratory compensation

3. *The Na^+ is 146 mmol/L, K^+ 3 mmol/L, Cl^- 110 mmol/L and HCO_3^- 3 mmol/L. What is the anion gap?*
   (a) 8
   (b) 20
   (c) 250
   (d) 36

4. *Which of the following are appropriate?*
   (a) Sodium bicarbonate
   (b) Nasogastric tube
   (c) Insulin and normal saline with potassium supplementation
   (d) Move to a high dependency area

Case 4: An asthmatic patient with dyspnoea and wheeze

A 25-year-old male with long-standing asthma is admitted with 2 days of dyspnoea and wheeze. He has been unable to sleep because of cough and wheeze and his inhalers have run out. On examination he appears dyspnoeic at rest, his respiratory rate is recorded as 28 breaths/min and oxygen saturations on air are 90%. There is reduced but equal expansion of the chest with audible wheeze. There is no evidence of a pneumothorax either clinically or on chest X-ray. The patient is given a nebulizer and put on 60% oxygen. Arterial blood gases are taken as follows:

pH	7.53
PaO_2	11 kPa
$PaCO_2$	3.5 kPa
HCO_3^-	20 mmol/L
SaO_2	96%

1. *Which of the following does the patient have?*
   (a) Acute respiratory acidosis
   (b) Acute respiratory alkalosis
   (c) Acute metabolic acidosis
   (d) Acute metabolic alkalosis

2. *Which of the following is true?*
   (a) The patient is hypoxaemic
   (b) The patient requires intubation
   (c) The oxygen should be reduced as the pH is abnormal
   (d) The patient should be given steroids

3. *What is the approximate A-a gradient?*
   (a) 10
   (b) 25
   (c) 41
   (d) 28

4. *The patient appears more drowsy and no wheeze is audible. A repeat blood gas shows:*

pH	7.22
PaO_2	10.5 kPa
$PaCO_2$	10.1 kPa
HCO_3^-	26 mmol/L
SaO_2	96%

Which of the following may the patient have developed?
  (a) Acute respiratory acidosis
  (b) Acute respiratory alkalosis
  (c) Acute metabolic acidosis
  (d) Acute metabolic alkalosis

Case 5: A patient with fever and dry cough

A 45-year-old man presents to the emergency department with a history of fever and dry cough over 3 days. On the day of presentation he has developed sharp, right-sided chest pain on inspiration. Prior to this he was completely well with no background medical problems. He has never smoked.

On examination he looks flushed but well. His respiratory rate is 20 breaths/min, blood pressure 120/65 mmHg, pulse 100 beats/min and regular, temperature 38.4°C and oxygen saturation 95% breathing room air. A chest X-ray reveals lobar shadowing in the right lower lobe and blood tests reveal a white cell count of 15×10^9/L, C-reactive protein of 50 mg/L, urea of 6.8 mmol/L and creatinine of 104 μmol/L.

1. *How would you treat him?*
  (a) Admit for intravenous fluids and antibiotics and oxygen as required
  (b) Send home on oral antibiotics
  (c) Admit for oral antibiotics, oxygen and observation

Case 6: A patient with persistent cough

A 50-year-old woman presents with a persistent productive cough for several months. The cough occurs in bouts often precipitated by a sore throat. She has never smoked, keeps no pets and has no previous history of chest disease. Physical examination is normal. A chest X-ray and spirometry testing in the outpatient clinic are both normal.

1. *Which of the following statements is true?*
  (a) The physical examination and lung function findings exclude a diagnosis of asthma
  (b) A normal chest X-ray makes a diagnosis of bronchiectasis very unlikely
  (c) A diagnosis of pulmonary fibrosis is effectively excluded
  (d) The absence of signs in the chest makes a diagnosis of sarcoidosis unlikely

Case 7: A patient with a painful shin rash

A 34-year-old woman presents with a painful erythematous rash on the shins. She is on no medication, is previously fit and well with no significant past history. Physical examination is normal other than the rash on the shins, which is healing with bruising. A chest X-ray reveals bilateral hilar lymphadenopathy.

1. *What would you do next?*
  (a) Further investigation including blood tests and CT scan of the chest
  (b) Biopsy of a skin lesion
  (c) Treat with oral corticosteroids
  (d) Treat with anti-inflammatory analgesia

Case 8: A smoker with dyspnoea

An 84-year-old male with a 40 pack year history of smoking is admitted with dyspnoea. He has had a fever with green sputum for the last 5 days. The patient is a little confused and unable to give a coherent history. However, his daughter says that he is normally independent. There is no significant past medical history and he is on no medication. The patient enjoys going out and walks about 5 km each morning before breakfast. He has not done this for the last week. He is never normally breathless.

On examination the patient is disorientated in time and place. He has a fever of 39.2°C, respiratory rate of 32 breaths/min and oxygen saturations of 80%. There is reduced expansion of the right base, where crackles and a pleuritic rub are audible. There is no evidence of wheeze and expiration is not prolonged. His heart rate is 110 beats/min and blood pressure 120/65 mmHg. Routine blood tests show a normal haemoglobin and platelet count. White blood cells are raised at 18.1×10^9/L (90% neutrophils), the urea is raised at 15 mmol/L, but the creatinine is within the normal range.

1. *What is the likely diagnosis?*
  (a) Exacerbation of chronic obstructive pulmonary disease (COPD)
  (b) Community-acquired pneumonia
  (c) Lung cancer
  (d) Empyema

2. *What is the CURB-65 score?*
  (a) 1
  (b) 2
  (c) 3
  (d) 4

3. *How much oxygen should be given to the patient?*
  (a) None
  (b) 24%
  (c) 35%
  (d) High-flow oxygen with a non-rebreath mask with reservoir bag

4. *The patient becomes increasingly drowsy and difficult to rouse; his Glasgow Coma Score (GCS) is documented as 7. An arterial blood gas is performed on high-flow oxygen and is recorded as follows:*

pH   7.25
PaO_2 8 kPa
$PaCO_2$ 8.5 kPa
Base excess −2
HCO_3^- 24 mmol/L
SaO_2 90%
Lactate   1.2 mmol/L

Which of the following is correct?
  (a) Change to 40% oxygen
  (b) Change to 28% oxygen
  (c) Take off oxygen altogether
  (d) The patient needs to be intubated and mechanically ventilated

Case 9: A patient with chronic obstructive pulmonary disease and recent breathlessness

A 64-year-old woman with known chronic obstructive pulmonary disease (COPD) is breathless for 3 days. She is unable to sleep at night and complains of wheeze. She normally uses a salbutamol inhaler and prior to admission to hospital has had to use this more frequently with diminishing effects. In the last year she has been unable to walk more than 200 m without stopping because of dyspnoea. On examinations she is apyrexial. She talks in short sentences. Respiratory rate is 28 breaths/min and she is using her accessory muscles. There is equal expansion of her chest, but wheeze is audible throughout. Examination is otherwise unremarkable. The staff in the emergency department have applied a 28% Venturi mask and performed an arterial blood gas, with the following results:

pH	7.40
PaO_2	12 kPa
$PaCO_2$	5 kPa
HCO_3^-	24 mmol/L
SaO_2	96%
Base excess	−2
Lactate	1.4 mmol/L

1. *Which of the following is true?*
   (a) There is a respiratory acidosis
   (b) There is impaired oxygenation
   (c) The patient is hypoxaemic
   (d) There is a metabolic acidosis

2. *Which of the following treatments are indicated?*
   (a) Salbutamol tablets
   (b) Ipratropium bromide nebulizer
   (c) Oral prednisolone
   (d) Non-invasive ventilation (NIV)

3. *The following day the patient is no better, she remains wheezy with a Glasgow Coma Score (GCS) of 15 and is haemodynamically stable. A repeat arterial blood gas is performed and shows the following:*

pH	7.29
PaO_2	8.9 kPa
$PaCO_2$	7.1 kPa
HCO_3^-	22 mmol/L
SaO_2	93%
Base excess	−1
Lactate	1.0 mmol/L
FIO_2	0.35

Which of the following treatments are essential?
   (a) NIV
   (b) Aggressive physiotherapy
   (c) High-flow oxygen with a non-rebreath mask
   (d) 24% oxygen

4. *Despite institution of NIV the patient deteriorates further and is intubated and mechanically ventilated. Despite intubation the patient is on an inspired oxygen concentration of 80% to maintain SaO_2 >90%. The left side of the chest does not appear to be moving as much as the right. A chest radiograph is performed; what might this show?*
   (a) Pneumothorax
   (b) Endotracheal tube in the right main bronchus
   (c) Pneumonia on left side
   (d) Pulmonary oedema

Case 10: A patient with cough and limb weakness

A 70-year-old male gives a 4-day history of cough with green sputum and fever. He feels short of breath. He has no past medical history. However, on systems review he complains that his limbs feel weak and he has noticed his muscles appear wasted. A chest radiograph shows consolidation of the left lower lobe. Respiratory rate is 28 breaths/min and oxygen saturations 100% on high-flow oxygen via a non-rebreath mask with a reservoir bag. Fasciculation is noticed in the limbs. There is wasting, weakness, brisk reflexes and up-going plantars.

1. *The patient has pneumonia and is started on antibiotics; what other diagnosis does he have?*
   (a) Cerebrovascular accident
   (b) Motor neuron disease (MND)
   (c) Myasthenia gravis
   (d) Duchenne muscular dystrophy

2. *An arterial blood gas is performed on high-flow oxygen with the following results:*

pH	7.29
PaO_2	45 kPa
$PaCO_2$	8.0 kPa
Base excess	−2
HCO_3^-	24 mmol/L
SaO_2	100%
Lactate	1.2 mmol/L

Which of following is best suited to the treatment of this patient?
   (a) Physiotherapy
   (b) Non-invasive ventilation (NIV)
   (c) Continuous positive airway pressure (CPAP)
   (d) Intubation and mechanical ventilation

3. *The patient is moved to a high dependency unit and placed on a BiPapVision (Respironics) ventilator; this is set up in S/T (spontaneous/timed) mode. Inspiratory positive airway pressure (IPAP) is set as 14 cmH₂O and expiratory positive airway pressure (EPAP) at 12 cmH₂O; the back-up rate is set at 10 breaths/min and inspired oxygen at 35%. Respiratory rate is 22/min. The patient has an arterial line inserted and a repeat blood gas performed 30 min later:*

pH	7.29
PaO_2	18 kPa
$PaCO_2$	7.8 kPa
Base excess	−2
HCO_3^-	24 mmol/L
SaO_2	100%

Why have the arterial blood gases not improved?
   (a) This ventilator is ineffective and the patient requires intubation and mechanical ventilation
   (b) IPAP should be increased first
   (c) Both IPAP and EPAP must be increased
   (d) EPAP should be reduced to 4–5 cmH₂O

Case 11: A patient with headache and worsening breathlessness

A 67-year-old woman presents with a history of morning headache and worsening breathlessness over a period of several months. She is sleepy during the day and has had a recent chest infection. She is an ex-smoker with a 30 pack year history. She has recently been started on inhaled bronchodilators with little benefit. She has a history of congenital scoliosis with partial corrective surgery in childhood.

On examination she has a marked scoliosis, basal crackles on the right and is cyanosed and drowsy. Blood gas analysis on air reveals:

pH	7.32
PO_2	7.4 kPa
PCO_2	8.2 kPa
Base excess	8
HCO_3^-	32 mmol/L

1. *What is the likely cause of the blood gas abnormality?*
- (a) Acute exacerbation of chronic obstructive pulmonary disease (COPD)
- (b) Right lower lobe pneumonia
- (c) Scoliosis
- (d) Pulmonary fibrosis

Case 12: Lung function testing in a patient with breathlessness

A 75-year-old retired carpenter presents with gradual-onset breathlessness over several months. He can now walk only 50 m before becoming breathless. He is an ex-smoker of 20 cigarettes per day, having stopped 15 years ago. There is no history of chest pain or wheeze. He takes amlodipine for hypertension. Physical examination reveals a few axillary crackles but no wheeze and his peak flow is reduced at 150 L/min.

1. *What is the significance of the low peak flow rate?*
- (a) It reflects obstructive lung disease due to his smoking
- (b) It cannot be interpreted without further information
- (c) It is likely to be due to respiratory muscle weakness
- (d) It is reduced because the patient is unable to take a deep breath

Case 13: A patient with sleep apnoea

A 45-year-old man presents with a history of loud snoring which disturbs his wife from sleep. She has noticed on several occasions that he appears to hold his breath during the night. There is a background of weight gain of 10 kg over the last 4 years. His body mass index is 32. He is on no medications, has no problems related to sleep and no history of daytime sleepiness.

1. *What would you do next?*
- (a) Reassure him that there is unlikely to be a serious problem
- (b) Advise him on lifestyle measures including weight loss and exercise
- (c) Refer on for a sleep study to look for sleep apnoea

Case 14: A man with gradual-onset breathlessness

A 75-year-old man presents with gradual-onset breathlessness over a period of 18 months. His exercise capacity has reduced from unlimited to 400 m on the flat before becoming breathless. There is no history of chest pain, nocturnal dyspnoea, orthopnoea or ankle swelling. He is an ex-smoker, keeps no pets and worked as a self-employed builder.

On examination he is clubbed. There is no peripheral lymphadenopathy. There are fine bibasal, inspiratory crackles extending into the axillae. Lung function testing reveals an FEV_1 (forced expiratory volume in 1 s) of 1.8 L (62% predicted) and FVC (forced vital capacity) of 1.9 L (50% predicted). A chest X-ray reveals bilateral reticular change.

1. *Which of the following statements is true?*
- (a) The information above is enough to make a diagnosis of pulmonary fibrosis
- (b) A high-resolution chest CT will not add useful prognostic information
- (c) Sequential testing of spirometry will give an accurate measure of disease progression
- (d) Fibrosis in this context is likely to be due to low level exposure to asbestos when working as a builder

Respiratory: Answers

Case 1: A patient with sudden-onset breathlessness

1. (c) Laryngeal spasm

The typical history is of an absolute inability to breathe which is frightening but typically resolves completely over a few minutes. It is often misdiagnosed as asthma. The speed of resolution distinguishes it from asthma and episodes of acute pulmonary oedema.
Further reading: Chapter 19 in Medicine at a Glance.

Case 2: A patient with a recent history of breathlessness

1. (c) Plain radiological imaging of the chest

The most likely diagnosis is pleural effusion. The differential diagnosis based on the clinical signs is an elevated right hemidiaphragm. Radiological confirmation of the effusion is necessary prior to aspiration of fluid, which may be useful for both diagnosis and for relief of breathlessness
Further reading: Chapter 99.

Case 3: A patient admitted with generalized abdominal pain

1. (a) Blood sugar

The patient has the classic presentation of diabetic ketoacidosis.

2. (c) There is a metabolic acidosis

(d) There is some respiratory compensation

The PaO_2 exceeds the partial pressure of oxygen in air and therefore supplemental oxygen must have been given. There is a profound acidosis, but the carbon dioxide is low, the base excess is very negative and there is little bicarbonate. This is a severe metabolic acidosis with an attempt at respiratory compensation, which is only partial because of the severity of the metabolic acidosis.

3. (d) 36

The anion gap is: sum of the cations $(146 + 3)$ – sum of the anions $(110 + 3) = 36 \, mmol/L$. This is due to the ketone bodies, which are present in the breath and give the familiar 'pear drop' breath.

4. (b) Nasogastric tube

(c) Insulin and normal saline with potassium supplementation

(d) Move to a high dependency area

Patients with diabetic ketoacidosis have gastroparesis and are at high risk of aspiration of the gastric contents. If the patient has a reduced Glasgow Coma Score (GCS) more senior help is required, as the patient may have cerebral oedema. Furthermore

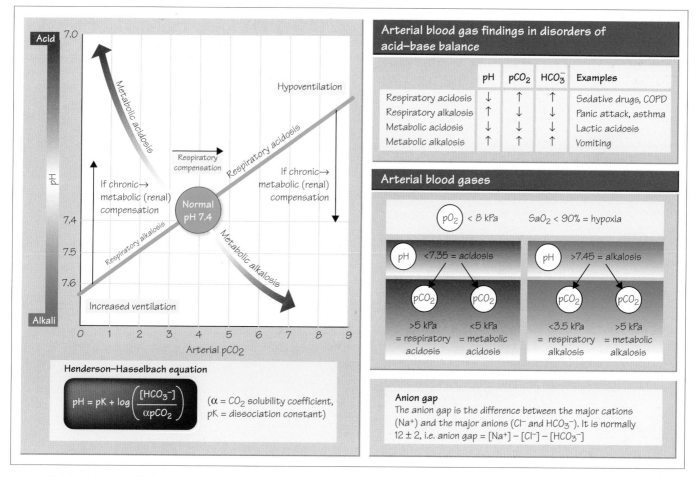

Figure 2.3.1 Blood gas analysis.

insertion of a nasogastric tube in a semiconscious patient may induce vomiting. Bicarbonate therapy is not generally recommended, as it can be deleterious to the patient.

Further reading: Chapter 138.

Case 4: An asthmatic patient with dyspnoea and wheeze

1. (b) Acute respiratory alkalosis

The pH is above 7.45 (alkalosis) and the $PaCO_2$ is low.

2. (d) The patient should be given steroids

The patient has a 'normal' PaO_2, and there are no indications that the patient requires intubation. Reducing oxygen to critically ill patients can precipitate cardiac or respiratory arrest. Steroids will treat the underlying bronchospasm.

3. (c) 41

$$PAO_2 = FIO_2 \text{ (atmospheric pressure} -$$
$$\text{water vapour pressure} - (1.25 \times PaCO_2))$$

$$PAO_2 = 0.6 \, (101 - 6.3) - (1.25 \times 3.5)$$

$$PAO_2 = 56.82 - 4.37 = 52.45$$

$$\text{A-a gradient} = 52.45 - 11 = 41.45$$

Thus although the patient is not hypoxaemic there is a problem with oxygenation.

4. (a) Acute respiratory acidosis

The patient has developed an acute respiratory acidosis because the muscle pump has become exhausted from the increased work of breathing brought about by the airway obstruction (asthma). The patient requires intubation and mechanical ventilation.

Further reading: Chapter 104.

In between attacks	Moderate	Severe	Life threatening
Normal exam Normal lung function tests	PEFR <65% predicted ↓ Admit to hospital	PEFR <50% Pulse rate >110 Respiratory rate >25 Can't complete sentences Wheezy chest Alert → mild confusion	PEFR <33% Bradychardia Exhaustion Can't talk at all Silent chest Confusion → coma
pO2	↓	↓↓	↓↓↓
pCO2	↓	→	↑
pH	Ⓝ or ↑	Ⓝ	↓
			Alert ITU

Figure 2.4.1 Features of asthma.

Case 5: A patient with fever and dry cough

1. (b) Send home on oral antibiotics

The patient has mild pneumonia with no markers of increased severity. He is young and previously fit. A course of oral antibiotics is safe to be administered at home. The case described is most likely to be due to pneumococcal infection as there are typical lobar infiltrates clinically and radiologically. A rapid improvement with penicillin antibiotics is to be expected.

Further reading: Chapter 102.

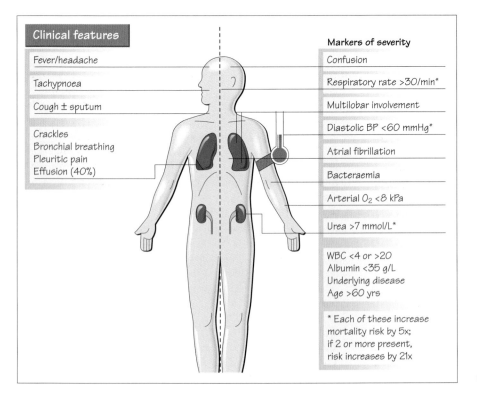

Figure 2.5.1 Clinical features of asthma.

Case 6: A patient with persistent cough

1. (c) A diagnosis of pulmonary fibrosis is effectively excluded

Pulmonary fibrosis is effectively excluded as it presents with a combination of basal crackles (which may be subtle) and a restrictive lung function defect. Asthma can be difficult to diagnose with absence of symptoms, signs and lung function abnormality between attacks. Significant bronchiectasis can be found on CT scanning even with an entirely normal chest X-ray. Sarcoidosis typically causes no abnormality on examination of the chest even in the presence of significant radiological lung infiltrates.

Further reading: Chapter 19.

Case 7: A patient with a painful shin rash

1. (d) Treat with anti-inflammatory analgesia

This patient gives a typical presentation of Lofgren's syndrome, that is to say, acute sarcoidosis, often occuring in younger (<35 years) female patients, typically symptoms include fever, erythema nodosum, arthralgias, and bilateral symmetrical hilar adenopathy. 80% of patients will recover with symptomatic treatment only. Further investigation should be reserved for patients where there is diagnostic doubt, including older patients where a sarcoid reaction to malignancy should be considered.

Further reading: Chapter 108.

Case 8: A smoker with dyspnoea

1. (b) Community-acquired pneumonia

The history and examination findings are consistent with a lobar pneumonia. Despite the history of smoking there is nothing to support a diagnosis of exacerbation of COPD or lung cancer. The latter may be an incidental finding, however. Empyema is a complication of pneumonia.

2. (d) 4

There is confusion, raised urea, a respiratory rate >30 breaths/min and age >65 years. This score is a predictor of mortality as well as a severity score. The score is an acronym for each of the risk factors measured. Each risk factor scores 1 point, for a maximum score of 5: confusion; urea greater than 7 mmol/L (blood urea nitrogen >20 mmol/L); respiratory rate of 30 breaths/min or greater; blood pressure less than 90 systolic or 60 diastolic; age 65 years or older. The risk of death increases as the score increases: 0: 0.7%; 1: 3.2%; 2: 13.0%; 3: 17.0%; 4: 41.5%; 5: 57.0%.

3. (d) High-flow oxygen with a non-rebreath mask with reservoir bag

The patient has pneumonia and is critically ill. An ABCDE approach should be applied and the patient given high-flow oxygen.

4. (d) The patient needs to be intubated and mechanically ventilated

The patient has a failure of oxygenation (he is on high-flow oxygen) and has now developed a respiratory acidosis. His drowsiness is related to the raised carbon dioxide. Reducing the oxygen in a patient who is developing respiratory failure as a consequence of treatment failure will precipitate cardiac arrest. The patient requires mechanical ventilation.

Further reading: Chapter 97.

Case 9: A patient with chronic obstructive pulmonary disease and recent breathlessness

1. (b) There is impaired oxygenation

The pH is normal and therefore there is no acidosis. The patient is not hypoxaemic because the PaO_2 is >8 kPa and SaO_2 is >90%. There is a failure of oxygenation.

$$A\text{-a gradient} = FIO_2 (\text{atmospheric pressure} - \text{water pressure}) - PaO_2 - 1.25(PaCO_2)$$
$$= 0.28(101 - 6.3) - 12 - 1.25 \times 5$$
$$= 26.5 - 12 - 6.25$$
$$= 8.25$$

2. (b) Ipratropium bromide nebulizer

(c) Oral prednisolone

In an exacerbation of COPD, bronchodilators should be given by a nebulizer. The patient does not fit the criteria for NIV.

3. (a) NIV

The patient is developing type II respiratory failure (pH 7.29, $PaCO_2$ 7.1 kPa) and requires assisted ventilation. The patient has adequate oxygenation although this has deteriorated from previously. However, reducing the inspired oxygen from 35 to 24% is likely to make the patient hypoxaemic and may precipitate cardiac arrest.

4. (a) Pneumothorax

(b) Endotracheal tube in the right main bronchus

A pneumothorax may occur as a consequence of overvigorous bagging or high inspiratory pressures. If the endotracheal tube is inserted too far it tends to migrate into the right main bronchus causing collapse of the left lung and poor oxygenation. The step down in oxygenation is related to the intubation and initiation of mechanical ventilation, ruling out answers (c) and (d). The tube is indeed too far in, it is pulled back and oxygenation improves.

Further reading: Chapter 101.

Case 10: A patient with cough and limb weakness

1. (b) Motor neuron disease (MND)

MND presents with wasting and weakness and is characterized by mixed upper and lower motor neuron signs. Duchenne muscular dystrophy presents in childhood. Myasthenia gravis is a disease of the neuromuscular junction, so upper motor neuron signs are absent. It is characterized by proximal muscle weakness, which is fatigueable.

2. (b) Non-invasive ventilation (NIV)

The patient has acute type II respiratory failure and requires a form of ventilation (HCO_3^- is normal, implying this is acute rather than acute on chronic hypercapnia). He is alert, cooperative and haemodynamically stable, and despite the pneumonia he is not difficult to oxygenate and is ideally suited to NIV. His respiratory failure is due to pneumonia in the context of respiratory muscle weakness.

3. (d) EPAP should be reduced to 4–5 cmH_2O

This ventilator is commonly used on high dependency units and is more expensive than the smaller ventilators used for home ventilation. It can deliver inspired oxygen at between 21 and 100%. It has relatively sophisticated monitors and alarms. On many ventilators, including the NIV ventilators, the inspiratory drive is determined by the difference in the IPAP and EPAP, which is only 2 cmH_2O. The IPAP could be increased first but 12 cmH_2O of EPAP is not required because oxygenation is easy to achieve. When EPAP is reduced to 4 cmH_2O, the inspiratory drive is 10 cmH_2O.

Repeat arterial blood gases are now:

pH	7.40
PaO_2	19.8 kPa
$PaCO_2$	5.1 kPa
Base excess	−2
HCO_3^-	24 mmol/L
SaO_2	100%

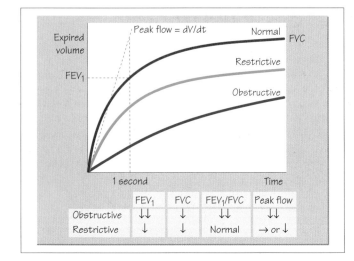

Figure 2.12.1 Spirometry in lung disease.

	FEV$_1$	FVC	FEV$_1$/FVC	Peak flow
Obstructive	↓↓	↓	↓↓	↓↓
Restrictive	↓	↓	Normal	→ or ↓

0 = would never doze or sleep.
1 = slight chance of dozing or sleeping
2 = moderate chance of dozing or sleeping
3 = high chance of dozing or sleeping

Situation	Chance of dozing or sleeping
Sitting and reading	
Watching TV	
Sitting inactive in a public place	
Being a passenger in a motor vehicle for an hour or more	
Lying down in the afternoon	
Sitting and talking to someone	
Sitting quietly after lunch (no alcohol)	
Stopped for a few minutes in traffic while driving	
Total score (add the scores up) (This is your Epworth score)	

Figure 2.13.1 The Epworth score: to assess sleepiness and the probability of sleep apnoea.

With an appropriate EPAP if the patient was still hypercapnic then IPAP could be increased in increments of 2 cmH$_2$O until a normocapnia is achieved.

Other causes of persistent hypercapnia include: inspiratory pressure or tidal volume set too low, back-up respiratory rate too low (if patient is taking few spontaneous breaths), leaks (this is less of a problem with pressure preset ventilators), rebreathing, or patient–ventilator asynchrony (usually related to inappropriate setting of triggering).
Further reading: Chapter 100.

Case 11: A patient with headache and worsening breathlessness

1. (c) Scoliosis

The blood gases reveal a mild compensated respiratory acidosis. The A-a gradient is normal, meaning that the abnormality is due to pure alveolar hypoventilation. This is seen in central and neuromuscular causes of hypoventilation. COPD, pneumonia and pulmonary fibrosis all present with an abnormality of V̇/Q̇ matching, which leads to an increased A-a gradient often combined with hypoventilation in COPD. Basal crackles are common at presentation in patients with previously undiagnosed hypoventilation due to scoliosis.
Further reading: Chapter 97.

Case 12: Lung function testing in a patient with breathlessness

1. (b) It cannot be interpreted without further information

Peak flow measurement is not useful as a diagnostic test. It can be very useful in monitoring changes in lung function in patients with asthma. There is a wide normal range of peak flow and the

test is effort dependent. Patients with restrictive chest diseases may also have a low peak flow rate due to an inability to stretch the expiratory muscles maximally before a rapid expiration.
Further reading: Chapter 95.

Case 13: A patient with sleep apnoea

1. (b) Advise him on lifestyle measures including weight loss and exercise

He also needs reassurance that occasional breathing interruption is common in snorers. The absence of daytime sleepiness suggests he is getting reasonable quality sleep with no respiratory disturbance. The Epworth score is a useful and simple questionnaire to measure sleepiness. The opportunity should be taken to give lifestyle advice.
Further reading: Chapter 96.

Case 14: A man with gradual-onset breathlessness

1. (a) The information given is enough to make a diagnosis of pulmonary fibrosis

CT scanning may add prognostic information if significant ground glass change is present as this can imply steroid-responsive disease. Spirometry will give some information about disease progression but a combination of total lung capacity, alveolar volume, vital capacity, and the transfer factor of the lung for carbon monoxide (TLCO) will give the best measure of progression. Fibrosis due to asbestos (asbestosis) is caused by high-level exposure to asbestos dust. Low-level exposure causes other asbestos complications including pleural plaque formation and mesothelioma.
Further reading: Chapter 109.

3 Gastroenterology: Cases and Questions

Case 1: An ex-smoker with weight loss

A 72-year-old man presents to the clinic with a history of 10 kg weight loss. He is an ex-smoker. His appetite is reduced. He reports fatigue and nausea but no vomiting and has recently developed constipation. On examination he has marked proximal muscle loss and mild dependant oedema. Abdominal examination is normal.

Blood tests showed:

Hb	11.2 g/dL
WCC	7.2×10^9/L
Platelets	450×10^9/L
Na	130 mmol/L
K	4.8 mmol/L
Ca	2.56 mmol/L
Urea	3.4 mmol/L
Creatinine	110 μmol/L

1. *On examination he is noted to have a palpable lymph node in his left supraclavicular fossa. There are no lymph nodes palpable at any other site. This is likely to be due to:*
   (a) Tuberculous lymphadenitis from drinking unpasteurized milk as a child
   (b) Metastasis from a visceral tumour
   (c) Recent infection with Epstein–Barr virus (glandular fever)
2. *What further blood tests would be most useful?*
   (a) Vitamin B_{12} and folic acid
   (b) C-reactive protein (CRP)
   (c) Thyroid function
3. *Prior to referral the patient had already undergone endoscopy and abdominal ultrasound, both of which were normal. Would you request:*
   (a) Chest X-ray
   (b) Repeat endoscopy
   (c) CT headscan

Case 2: A woman with diabetes with weight loss

A 32-year-old female presents with weight loss. She has had insulin-dependant diabetes for 10 years. She has a good appetite but has noticed an increased frequency of pale stools. Her glycaemic control has been poor.

1. *The poor glycaemic control is most likely to be due to:*
   (a) Poor compliance/adherence to treatment
   (b) Insulin resistance
   (c) Malabsorption
2. *The exocrine function of the pancreas is best assessed by:*
   (a) Three-day faecal fat measurement
   (b) A fat provocation ultrasound
   (c) Measurement of pancreatic enzyme activity in faeces
3. *Pancreatic structure would be best assessed by:*
   (a) Ultrasound
   (b) CT
   (c) MRI

Case 3: A man with a history of constipation

A 68-year-old man presents with a 4-month history of constipation. He is having his bowels opened no more than once every week passing an uncomfortably firm stool. On one or two occasions he has experienced bright red rectal bleeding, mainly visible on the toilet paper. He has lost 6 kg in weight. Examination shows him to be dehydrated with dry mucous membranes and a postural blood pressure drop. Examination of the abdomen including digital examination of the rectum is normal. Abdominal X-ray demonstrates constipation but shows no evidence of obstruction. Chest X-ray is normal.

Blood tests showed:

Hb	14.8 g/dL
WCC	6.4×10^9/L
Platelets	272×10^9/L
Plasma viscosity	1.68 cP
Na	135 mmol/L
K	4.5 mmol/L
Corrected Ca	3.24 mmol/L
Urea	18.4 mmol/L
Creatinine	186 μmol/L

1. *In view of the history of bleeding he ought to undergo:*
   (a) Flexible sigmoidoscopy
   (b) Urgent abdominal CT
   (c) Proctoscopy
2. *Further blood test analysis should include:*
   (a) Magnesium levels
   (b) Serum Bence-Jones protein
   (c) Parathyroid hormone (PTH) level
3. *What treatment should he receive?*
   (a) Calcium resonium
   (b) Intravenous fluids
   (c) Phosphate enemas

Case 4: A woman with difficulty defaecating

A 58-year-old woman reports increasing problems with defaecation. She reports that her symptom of bloating is made worse by taking a high-fibre diet and she is only able to defaecate with the use of regular Senna, bought at the local chemist. She has no history of any significant illnesses. She has had three children all by vaginal delivery. The largest child weighed 8 lbs 4 oz and required an episiotomy and forceps. Examination including digital examination of the rectum reveals slightly lax anal tone. Bloods including serum calcium and thyroid are all normal. She has had faecal occult blood (FOB) tests performed by her GP and these were normal also.

1. *What would you advise?*
   (a) CT colonography
   (b) Referral to a dietician
   (c) MRI of the pelvis
2. *To improve her symptomatic control you might advise:*
   (a) Increase in stimulant laxatives
   (b) Attending for regular colonic lavage/hydrotherapy
   (c) Osmotic laxatives
3. *If the patient continues to suffer intolerable symptoms despite initial interventions you might consider referring her for:*
   (a) Psychotherapy
   (b) Anorectal physiology
   (c) Surgery

Case 5: A man with a 6-week history of diarrhoea

A 24-year-old man presents with a 6-week history of diarrhoea after eating out at a restaurant. He is having his bowels opened 8–10 times a day and 2–3 times at night, occasionally witnessing altered blood in his stools. He has had no abdominal pain but has had some soreness in his lower back and gritty eyes. He has lost his appetite and nearly two stone in weight. He has recently given up smoking and in passing mentioned that his cousin has Crohn's disease. He is tachycardic with a pulse of 105 beats/min and febrile with a temperature of 38.7°C. He looks dry and unwell. Abdominal examination reveals some diffuse tenderness in the left iliac fossa.

Blood tests showed:

Hb	8.9 g/dL
WCC	8.6×10^9/L
Platelets	658×10^9/L
Plasma viscosity	2.06 cP
CRP	180 mg/L
Na	138 mmol/L
K	3.2 mmol/L
Urea	11.4 mmol/L
Creatinine	140 μmol/L
Albumin	27 g/L

1. *The best way to manage this patient would be:*
   (a) Urgent colonoscopy
   (b) A course of empirical antibiotics
   (c) Emergency admission to hospital
2. *A plain abdominal X-ray might show:*
   (a) Proximal colonic constipation
   (b) An empty colon
   (c) Wrigler's sign (pneumoperitoneum)
3. *If the patient was no better after 5 days of treatment the following treatment options could be considered:*
   (a) An increased dose of steroid
   (b) Add infliximab
   (c) Colectomy

Case 6: A man with frequent loose stools

An 18-year-old man attends the clinic with a 2-month history of frequent loose stools. He thinks his problem started after attending a rock music festival. His appetite is good but he has lost half a stone in weight. His bowels are open 4–6 times a day but he has not experienced nocturnal diarrhoea. His stools are loose, pale and frequently float, requiring two or more flushes of the toilet. Examination is normal. Bloods are normal. Stool culture is negative.

1. *The clinical presentation is indicative of:*
   (a) Irritable bowel syndrome (IBS)
   (b) Colitis
   (c) Malabsorption
2. *The most likely underlying cause of his symptoms is:*
   (a) Acute pancreatitis
   (b) Crohn's colitis
   (c) Infection
3. *To investigate his problem further would you undertake:*
   (a) An urgent colonoscopy
   (b) Imaging of the small intestine
   (c) Prescribe empirical treatment

Case 7: A man with 'coffee-ground' vomiting

A 78-year-old man is admitted to hospital with 'coffee ground' vomiting. This had become an increasing problem over the previous 6 months. He had been experiencing bloating after meals associated with nausea and vomiting. He had lost 6 kg in weight. On examination it is evident he has lost weight. He has no palpable lymph nodes. Abdominal examination including rectal examination is normal.

Blood tests showed:

Hb	9.2 g/dL
MCV	72 fL
WCC	9.8×10^9/L
Platelets	180×10^9/L
Na	140 mmol/L
K	2.9 mmol/L
Urea	12.4 mmol/L
Creatinine	100 μmol/L

An abdominal X-ray shows dilated loops of small bowel.

1. *'Coffee ground' vomiting is due to:*
   (a) Fresh bleeding into the upper gastrointestinal (GI) tract
   (b) Retching causing abrasion of the gastric mucosa
   (c) The ingestion of too much coffee
2. *The anaemia is due to:*
   (a) Chronic GI blood loss
   (b) An acute GI bleed
   (c) Renal failure
3. *The most likely diagnosis accounting for this clinical presentation is:*
   (a) Caecal cancer
   (b) Gastric cancer
   (c) Rectal cancer

Case 8: A man with vomiting and Crohn's disease

A 24-year-old man presents in the clinic with progressive difficulty with vomiting. Four years previously he had had an ileal resection for Crohn's disease. He has a poor appetite but experiences abdominal pain 15–20 minutes after eating followed by bloating and vomiting. He has lost over a stone in weight and reports mouth ulcers, gritty eyes and low back pain. On examination he looks dry and unwell. His pulse is 110 beats/min and his temperature is 37.5°C. Abdominal examination reveals a diffuse mass in the right iliac fossa. In addition he has tender, raised, red blotches on his shins.

Blood tests showed:

Hb	9.2 g/dL
WCC	12.2×10^9/L
Platelets	650×10^9/L
Plasma viscosity	2.3 cP
Na	135 mmol/L
K	2.7 mmol/L
Urea	4.2 mmol/L
Creatinine	78 μmol/L

1. *The lesions on the shins are most likely to be:*
   (a) Pyoderma gangrenosum
   (b) Dermatitis herpetiformis
   (c) Erythema nodosum

2. *To investigate the nature of his problem he needs:*
   (a) Upper GI endoscopy
   (b) Small bowel imaging
   (c) Colonoscopy
3. *The patient is clinically undernourished. Pending further investigations a dietician could instigate:*
   (a) A liquid diet
   (b) A high-fibre diet
   (c) Total parenteral nutrition

Case 9: An orthopaedic patient who has passed a melaena stool

An 84-year-old man passes a large melaena stool. He is an in-patient on an orthopaedic ward 4 days after repair of a fractured neck of femur. He has a past history of coronary bypass surgery. He normally takes aspirin, atenolol and simvastatin. He has no indigestion or abdominal pain although he has felt nauseated since his surgery. On examination he looks pale and is cool to the touch. His pulse is 110 beats/min and BP is measured at 105/75 mmHg lying and 86/50 mmHg sitting up.

Blood tests showed:

Hb	8.4 g/dL
WCC	4.6×10^9/L
Platelets	230×10^9/L
Na	137 mmol/L
K	6.0 mmol/L
Urea	22.4 mmol/L
Creatinine	130 μmol/L

1. *What is the significance of a postural blood pressure drop?*
   (a) He has had a peri-operative myocardial infarct
   (b) He has had a large GI bleed
   (c) He has autonomic neuropathy
2. *What is the most likely source of his melaena?*
   (a) Diverticular disease
   (b) Duodenal ulcer
   (c) Colon cancer
3. *Prior to undergoing endoscopy the patient should receive:*
   (a) Intravenous fluids
   (b) Gastric lavage
   (c) Intravenous omeprazole

Case 10: A man who has vomited blood

A 54-year-old man is admitted to hospital after vomiting about 500 mL of clotted blood. He has been brought to hospital by ambulance. The crew report that he was found in a collapsed state outside a local off-licence. On examination he is obtunded and smells of alcohol. He has a metabolic flap. He is febrile and tachy-cardic. His pulse is 120 beats/min and his lying BP 100/60 mmHg. He appears to be jaundiced and has palmar erythema and bilateral Dupytren's contractures. Abdominal examination reveals hepat-omegaly and some dullness to percussion in the flanks.

Blood tests showed:

Hb	6.4 g/dL
WCC	14×10^9/L
Platelets	76×10^9/L
PT	36 sec
Na	116 mmol/L
K	3.2 mmol/L
Urea	5.4 mmol/L
Creatinine	90 μmol/L

1. *His clotting is abnormal because:*
   (a) He is taking warfarin
   (b) He is malnourished and deficient in vitamin K
   (c) He has significant liver disease
2. *His bleeding is most likely to be due to:*
   (a) Portal hypertension
   (b) Peptic ulcer
   (c) Gastritis in association with his abnormal clotting
3. *Before his endoscopy you should:*
   (a) Give a vasopressin analogue such as terlipressin
   (b) Withhold antibiotics until there is objective evidence of infection
   (c) Wait until his alcohol withdrawal is complete

Case 11: A man with rectal bleeding

An 82-year-old man is admitted with rectal bleeding. He had felt well earlier in the day. After his evening meal he experienced a sudden urge to have his bowels open with some cramping lower abdominal discomfort. He experienced a single episode of passing clotted blood. During this period he felt quite light-headed. Examination demonstrates a mild tachycardia (pulse 98 beats/min) but a normal lying blood pressure. Abdominal examination reveals no masses, nor areas of localized tenderness. Rectal examination shows some altered blood on the gloved examination finger. Rigid sigmoidoscopy to 15 cm reveals altered blood in the lumen of the bowel only.

Blood tests showed:

Hb	12.2 g/dL
MCV	86 fL
WCC	5.6×10^9/L
Platelets	376×10^9/L
Na	138 mmol/L
K	4.2 mmol/L
Urea	4.2 mmol/L
Creatinine	86 μmol/L
Albumin	40 g/L
Bilirubin	12 μmol/L
ALP	156 U/L
ALT	26 U/L

1. *His blood test results are best explained by:*
   (a) A large bleed with pre-existing polycythaemia
   (b) A long-standing/chronic disease process
   (c) A recent/sudden bleed
2. *The most likely source of the patient's bleeding is:*
   (a) Peptic ulcer
   (b) Colon cancer
   (c) Diverticular change
3. *The best way to investigate this episode of bleeding would be:*
   (a) Urgent abdominal CT scan
   (b) Mesenteric angiography
   (c) Lower GI endoscopy (colonoscopy or flexible sigmoidoscopy)

Case 12: A man with rectal bleeding of increasing frequency

A 72-year-old man is seen in clinic and reports rectal bleeding. This has been occurring intermittently over the previous three to four months but has become more noticeable. Now the bleeding is seen on most episodes of defaecation. The blood is bright red in colour and seen mixed in with the stools. The patient also reports urgency and a sense of incomplete emptying (tenesmus). Examination demonstrates no lymphadenopathy and no palpable abdominal mass. Rectal examination shows some altered blood on the glove.

Blood tests showed:

Hb	9.6 g/dL
WCC	7.3×10^9/L
Platelets	190×10^9/L
Na	140 mmol/L
K	4.2 mmol/L
Urea	4.2 mmol/L
Creatinine	96 μmol/L

Plain X-ray of the abdomen is unremarkable.

1. *The best next investigation would be:*
   (a) Faecal occult blood (FOB) testing
   (b) Flexible sigmoidoscopy
   (c) Colonoscopy
2. *In rectal cancer which investigation provides the best evidence of distal metastatic disease?*
   (a) Abdominal ultrasound
   (b) CT
   (c) Pelvic MRI
3. *Tumour markers that may be of use in monitoring patients after bowel cancer treatment include:*
   (a) Carcinoembryonic antigen (CEA)
   (b) α-fetoprotein (α-FP)
   (c) Carbohydrate antigenic determinant (CA) 19.9

Case 13: A man with difficulty in swallowing

A 65-year-old man presents with a 2-week history of progressive difficulty in swallowing. This is worse with meat and solid foods and he has had to vomit to clear obstruction on occasions. He has lost 6 kg in weight over the last 4–6 weeks. Examination demonstrates evidence of weight loss but is otherwise unremarkable.

Blood tests showed:

Hb	10.5 g/dL
WCC	6.9×10^9/L
Platelets	276×10^9/L
Na	136 mmol/L
K	3.6 mmol/L
Urea	8.9 mmol/L
Creatinine	120 μmol/L

Chest X-ray is normal.

1. *The best next investigation would be:*
   (a) Barium swallow
   (b) CT, chest and abdominal
   (c) Endoscopy
2. *Which is the more common type of oesophageal cancer?*
   (a) Squamous carcinoma
   (b) Adenocarcinoma
   (c) Lymphoma
3. *Which is the most useful investigation for determining the role for surgery?*
   (a) Endoscopy
   (b) CT
   (c) Endoscopic ultrasound

Case 14: A man with heartburn and painful swallowing

A 38-year-old man attends the outpatient department describing heartburn. He experiences a retrosternal burning discomfort on a daily basis. His appetite is good and he admits to having gained 12 kg over the preceding 2 years. He denies dysphagia but does have painful swallowing (odynophagia) and effortless regurgitation. He has tried over the counter antacids with some benefit but his symptoms are getting worse. His paternal uncle recently died from oesophageal cancer. Examination is normal.

1. *This patient would benefit most from:*
   (a) Trial of treatment with a proton pump inhibitor (PPI)
   (b) Endoscopy
   (c) *H. pylori* eradication
2. *If the patient was to undergo endoscopy what would be the most likely finding?*
   (a) Normal
   (b) Reflux oesophagitis
   (c) Barrett's oesophagus
3. *The main risk from taking long-term PPIs is:*
   (a) Malabsorption
   (b) Rash
   (c) Food poisoning

Case 15: A patient with sudden-onset upper abdominal pain

A 48-year-old woman presents with severe upper abdominal pain. This was of sudden onset after eating a meal out at a restaurant. It is situated in the epigastrium and right upper quadrant (RUQ). The pain is coming in waves (i.e. colicky) causing intense nausea, sweating and retching. She has had one or two previous episodes like this but none quite as intense or as prolonged.

On examination the patient is obviously in pain with a tachycardia of 110 beats/min. Her BP is 130/85 mmHg and her temperature is 37.3°C. Abdominal examination reveals marked right upper quadrant tenderness. There is no palpable organomegaly and no masses.

Blood tests showed:

Hb	13.6 g/dL
WCC	12.2×10^9/L
Platelets	168×10^9/L
Plasma viscosity	1.56 cP
Na	140 mmol/L
K	4.2 mmol/L
Urea	3.8 mmol/L
Creatinine	89 μmol/L
Albumin	42 g/L
Bilirubin	12 μmol/L
ALP	150 U/L
AST	24 U/L

1. *The best next investigation would be:*
   (a) Endoscopy
   (b) Ultrasound
   (c) CT
2. *Her immediate treatment should include:*
   (a) High doses of opioid painkillers
   (b) Emergency cholecystectomy
   (c) Conservative management

3. *The treatment option of greatest proven benefit in reducing the risk of complications from gallstones is:*
(a) Cholecystectomy
(b) Low-fat diet
(c) Ursodeoxycholic acid

Case 16: A patient with worsening upper abdominal pain

A 78-year-old woman presents to hospital as an emergency with upper abdominal pain. This had been occurring on and off over the preceding months but has been getting worse. On admission she is febrile with a temperature of 39°C. Her pulse is 110 beats/min, and her BP is 100/70 mmHg She has jaundice but no other signs of liver disease. Abdominal examination reveals some diffuse upper abdominal tenderness but no masses.

Blood tests showed:

Hb	12.5 g/dL
WCC	15.7×10^9/L
Platelets	172×10^9/L
Na	137 mmol/L
K	3.9 mmol/L
Urea	8.4 mmol/L
Creatinine	120 μmol/L
Albumin	30 g/L
Bilirubin	140 μmol/L
ALP	450 U/L
AST	110 U/L

1. *Which clinical term best describes this patient's presentation?*
(a) Cholangitis
(b) Cholecystitis
(c) Choledocolithiasis
2. *What other investigations might be needed urgently?*
(a) Ultrasound
(b) Antimitochondrial antibody
(c) Hepatitis A serology
3. *The most suitable definitive treatment for this presentation would be:*
(a) Extra-corporeal shock wave lithotripsy
(b) Open cholecystectomy and bile duct exploration
(c) Endoscopic retrograde cholangiopancreatography (ERCP)

Case 17: A heavy drinker with jaundice

A 45-year-old man is admitted with jaundice. He admits to being a very heavy drinker, consuming a bottle of spirits a day. His only previous admission to hospital was following a road traffic accident a number of years ago. He has had a number of visits to A&E for minor injuries and falls. He is unemployed having lost his job as a labourer due to drink-related problems. He is separated from his wife and two young children. He takes no regular prescription medications.

On examination he is drowsy and smells ketotic. He has a fever of 38.5°C. He is quite deeply jaundiced and has palmar erythema and scattered spider naevi. Abdominal examination reveals marked hepatomegaly and some flank percussion dullness consistent with ascites.

Blood tests showed:

Hb	10.8 g/dL
MCV	110 fL
WCC	15.2×10^9/L
Platelets	98×10^9/L
PT	20 sec
Na	122 mmol/L
K	3.2 mmol/L
Urea	1.7 mmol/L
Creatinine	98 μmol/L
Albumin	22 g/L
Bilirubin	328 μmol/L
ALP	340 U/L
AST	450 U/L

1. *Why do patients with liver disease develop spider naevi and palmar erythema?*
(a) High pressure in capillary vessels associated with portal hypertension
(b) An excess of endogenous oestrogen hormones
(c) A direct toxic effect of alcohol on small capillaries
2. *Immediate treatment should include:*
(a) Broad-spectrum antibiotics
(b) Fresh frozen plasma to correct the abnormal clotting
(c) Intravenous omeprazole to reduce the risk of gastrointestinal bleeding
3. *If the patient becomes agitated and more confused one should consider:*
(a) Sedation with a long-acting benzodiazepine
(b) CT headscan
(c) Transfer to the intensive care unit for ventilation
4. *Once the patient's condition has been stabilized other treatment options that might be considered on this same admission might include:*
(a) Liver transplant
(b) Renal dialysis
(c) Steroids

Case 18: A patient with lower abdominal pain, diarrhoea and weight loss

An 84-year-old man is referred with a month's history of lower abdominal pain, diarrhoea and weight loss. His appetite has been poor and he has lost a stone in weight. More latterly he has developed fever and dysuria. Prior to this time he has been well. He had a transureathral resection for benign prostatic hypertrophy 2 years before. He had had a barium enema performed 10 years earlier for symptomatic constipation. This had shown diverticular change only.

On examination he looks unwell with a fever of 38.4°C and a tachycardia. He looks dry although he is peripherally vasodilated with a bounding pulse and low blood pressure. Abdominal examination demonstrates a large tender mass in the left iliac fossa. This mass is dull to percussion and hot to the touch.

Blood tests showed:

Hb	11.8 g/dL
WCC	14.5×10^9/L
Platelets	305×10^9/L
Na	140 mmol/L

K	4.2 mmol/L
Urea	8.7 mmol/L
Creatinine	120 µmol/L
Urine dipstick	protein ++, blood +, nitrites ++

Plain abdominal film shows an unremarkable gas pattern. There is no evidence of pnemoperitoneum.

1. *This mass would be best investigated by:*
   (a) CT
   (b) Ultrasound
   (c) Flexible sigmoidscopy
2. *The early management of the patient might include:*
   (a) Emergency surgery
   (b) Fluid resuscitation and systemic antibiotics
   (c) Colonic stenting
3. *The most likely cause of this mass is:*
   (a) Caecal cancer
   (b) Diverticulitis
   (c) Kidney tumour
4. *The definitive treatment of this mass is likely to be:*
   (a) Conservative management with laxatives and antibiotics
   (b) Emergency surgery (Hartman's procedure)
   (c) Interval sigmoid resection

Case 19: A patient with abdominal distension

A 62-year-old man is admitted with abdominal distension. He admits to having been unwell for the previous 12 months experiencing fatigue, weight loss and difficulty sleeping. He had had previous surgery for peptic ulcer disease 20 years ago but since then had not been a regular attender at his GP practice. He gave up work as a pub landlord 7 years ago.

On examination he appears to have lost proximal muscle mass. He has palmar erythema and 2–3 spider naevi over his chest but no other peripheral signs of chronic liver disease. He is in atrial fibrillation. Abdominal examination demonstrates gross ascites and possible splenomegaly. He has mild pitting oedema of the ankles.

Blood tests showed:

Hb	12.2 g/dL
WCC	5.6×10^9/L
Platelets	98×10^9/L
PT	18 sec
Na	125 mmol/L
K	3.2 mmol/L
Urea	1.4 mmol/L
Creatinine	98 µmol/L
Albumin	23 g/L
Bilirubin	65 µmol/L
ALP	140 U/L
AST	38 U/L

1. *The clinical detection of organomegaly in the presence of ascites might be helped by:*
   (a) Dipping
   (b) Auscultation
   (c) Percussion
2. *The patient's wife explains to you that she has become concerned that her husband might have cancer causing his problem. Which single test gives you the best evidence that the ascites is not primarily a malignant problem?*

   (a) Ascitic protein
   (b) Abdominal ultrasound
   (c) Ascitic cytology
3. *After his initial evaluation it is decided to treat his ascites by total abdominal paracentesis. What measures need to be undertaken to support this intervention?*
   (a) Pre-treatment with high-dose diuretics
   (b) High-salt diet
   (c) Infusion of human albumin solution
4. *Several months later the patient returns to the out-patient clinic and despite reasonable doses of diuretics he is still accumulating ascites and requiring admission to the ward for paracentesis every 2 weeks. What other treatment options could be considered?*
   (a) Perito-venous (Leveen) shunt
   (b) A transjugular intrahepatic portosystemic shunt (TIPSS)
   (c) Lieno-renal shunt

Case 20: A patient with large-volume ascites

An 83-year-old woman is seen in the out-patient clinic with large-volume ascites. She feels otherwise well although has experienced fatigue over recent weeks. She had previously undergone a trans-vaginal hysterectomy for prolapse. She takes aspirin, simvastatin and alendronate.

On examination she looks well. She has no palpable lymphaden-opathy and no peripheral signs of chronic liver disease. On abdominal examination she has gross ascites but no detectable organomegaly or masses.

Blood tests showed:

Hb	11.3 g/dL
WCC	8.4×10^9/L
Platelets	256×10^9/L
Na	137 mmol/L
K	4.2 mmol/L
Urea	11.2 mmol/L
Creatinine	110 µmol/L
Albumin	32 g/L
Bilirubin	12 µmol/L
ALP	136 U/L
AST	14 U/L

An ascitic tap reveals a protein content of 28 g/dL.

1. *The best form of imaging to consider in this case would be:*
   (a) MRI
   (b) Ultrasound
   (c) CT scan
2. *Which tumour marker might be useful in the initial assessment?*
   (a) CA19-9
   (b) CA125
   (c) CA
3. *The best initial treatment of the ascites would be:*
   (a) Diuretics
   (b) TIPSS
   (c) Therapeutic paracentesis

Case 21: A patient with bloody diarrhoea

A 34-year-old woman is admitted to hospital with 72 hours of severe bloody diarrhoea. She had been fit and well the previous week but had taken ill 24 hours after dining out with friends at a local restaurant. No one else in the party was affected. Initially she felt nauseated and then developed frequent loose stools associated with severe, cramping lower abdominal pain. She has been having her bowels open every hour and was up in the night 5 or 6 times. She has no significant past medical history but takes the oral contraceptive pill and uses proton pump inhibitors (PPIs) on an as-needed basis for reflux symptoms. Her mother has ulcerative colitis.

On examination she looks unwell. She is febrile with a temperature of 39.2°C. She has dry mucous membranes and is tachycardic with a pulse of 110 beats/min. She is hypotensive with a BP of 80 mmHg systolic and feels light headed when sitting up.

Blood tests showed:

Hb	13.8 g/dL
WCC	22.1 × 10⁹/L
Platelets	198 × 10⁹/L
Na	145 mmol/L
K	2.7 mmol/L
Urea	11.4 mmol/L
Creatinine	130 µmol/L

Plain abdominal X-ray shows an empty colon with marked mucosal oedema and thumb-printing.

1. *The most likely cause of this presentation is:*
   (a) Food poisoning
   (b) Ulcerative colitis
   (c) Acute pancreatitis
2. *Initial investigations should include:*
   (a) Blood cultures
   (b) Flexible sigmoidoscopy
   (c) Campylobacter serology
3. *First-line treatment should be with:*
   (a) Probiotics
   (b) Intravenous fluid resuscitation
   (c) Anti-diarrhoeal agents (e.g. loperamide)
4. *During the recovery period after this illness the patient might be advised to eat:*
   (a) More chocolate
   (b) Less tea and coffee
   (c) More milk

Case 22: A patient with community-acquired pneumonia and diarrhoea

You are asked to see an 87-year-old woman on the medical ward. She had been admitted to hospital 10 days previously with a community-acquired pneumonia and has been receiving broad-spectrum oral antibiotics. In the last 24 hours she has developed anorexia and diarrhoea. She had reported no gut symptoms on admission to the hospital. On examination she looks dry with reduced skin turgor and has a mild tachycardia (pulse 100 beats/min). Her temperature is recorded at 37.4°C. Abdominal examination reveals some mild lower abdominal tenderness.

Blood tests showed:

Hb	12.2 g/dL
WCC	16.4 × 10⁹/L
Platelets	180 × 10⁹/L
Na	149 mmol/L

K	3.0 mmol/L
Urea	10.4 mmol/L
Creatinine	220 µmol/L

1. *The most likely cause of her diarrhoea is:*
   (a) *Campylobacter jejuni*
   (b) Antibiotic-associated diarrhoea
   (c) Ulcerative colitis
2. *Diagnostic tests to consider would include:*
   (a) Stool microscopy
   (b) Abdominal CT scan
   (c) Assay for *C. difficile* toxin
3. *Principles of treatment should include:*
   (a) Give antibiotics for the diarrhoea
   (b) Consider different antibiotics for the chest infection
   (c) Keep the patient 'nil by mouth' until the diarrhoea has stopped

Case 23: A patient with reflux and increasing heartburn

A 52-year-old man is referred back to the gastroenterology clinic. He was diagnosed as having reflux on the basis of an endoscopy performed 10 years previously. Since that time he has been taking omeprazole 20 mg daily. Over the last year he has had increasing problems with heartburn and belching (northerly wind) and has been using over the counter antacids. He has gained 12 kg in weight over the last 18 months and claims to be under a lot of stress going through a difficult divorce. He is otherwise physically well. He was recently started on a calcium antagonist for hypertension and a statin for hypercholesterolaemia.

On examination he weighs 94 kg (BMI 34). Examination is otherwise unremarkable. His blood tests were normal.

He recently underwent a repeat endoscopy. He remembers belching and retching a lot during the procedure which he chose to have done under local anaesthetic spray only. He was told that the examination was 'unremarkable'.

1. *What is the source of belching?*
   (a) Fermentation of gastric contents associated with slow gastric emptying
   (b) Air swallowing
   (c) Carbon dioxide caused from *Helicobacter pylori* splitting urea
2. *Given that the patient is getting symptoms despite omeprazole (a proton pump inhibitor; PPI) they should consider:*
   (a) Increasing the dose (or frequency) of the PPI
   (b) Switching to an H2 receptor antagonist (e.g. ranitidine)
   (c) Using regular antacids
3. *The patient asks about being considered for surgery. What operations could be considered?*
   (a) Nissen's fundoplication
   (b) Highly selective vagotomy (HSV)
   (c) Ramstead's pyloroplasty

Case 24: A patient with Barrett's oesophagus

A 65-year-old man attends the clinic for discussion regarding his diagnosis of Barrett's oesophagus. This was first identified 10 years previously and since that time he has been attending for surveillance endoscopies every 1–3 years (depending on the integrity of the recall system at the local hospital and his own memory). He takes 20 mg of omeprazole daily and experiences no heartburn. His last endoscopy was performed 6 months ago and this revealed 6 cm of Barrett's. Biopsies taken at that time showed columnar metaplasia (with intestinal metaplasia) but no dysplasia. His elder brother has just been diagnosed with prostate cancer but he has no other family history of cancer. He has just retired and admits that the Barrett's issue worries him.

1. *He has read several articles in the press and wishes to clarify the varying claims:*
   (a) Patients with Barrett's oesophagus are at high risk of developing cancer
   (b) Treatment with photodynamic therapy might reduce the risk of cancer
   (c) Adenocarcinoma of the distal oesophagus is increasing in incidence
2. *He is keen to manage his risk more pro-actively. Which of the following actions will significantly reduce his risk of oesophageal cancer?*
   (a) Stopping drinking alcohol
   (b) Taking a double dose of omeprazole (40 mg per day instead of 20 mg)
   (c) Increasing his frequency of surveillance endoscopy to every 6 months
3. *The patient wishes to consider having anti-reflux surgery. If this were to be successful could he expect:*
   (a) To be able to stop using omeprazole
   (b) No symptoms at all
   (c) To no longer need endoscopic surveillance

Case 25: A patient with a 6-month history of indigestion

A 35-year-old man presents with a 6-month history of indigestion. His discomfort is situated above the umbilicus and is present most days. He has noticed that it is worse with spicy and rich foods. On occasions the discomfort has made him vomit. He is a smoker.

1. *Which is the best non-invasive diagnostic test for* Helicobacter pylori?
   (a) Blood culture
   (b) Analysis of stool
   (c) Lactulose breath test
2. *If* Helicobacter *testing was positive should the patient:*
   (a) Have an endoscopy to determine whether or not he has an ulcer
   (b) Have a course of antibiotics
   (c) Continue to use antacid medication on an as-needed basis
3. *If the patient then returns with ongoing symptoms should he:*
   (a) Undergo endoscopy
   (b) Have a barium swallow
   (c) Have a 4-week trial of treatment with a PPI

Case 26: A patient with indigestion and nausea

A 78-year-old man is referred with a 6-week history of indigestion. This is present every day and situated above the umbilicus. Associated with this discomfort he has felt nauseated and has lost 4 kg in weight. In 1974 he had undergone surgery for peptic ulcer disease. Examination reveals some evidence of weight loss. Abdominal examination shows a midline upper abdominal scar but no masses and no organomegaly.

Blood tests showed:

Hb	11.7 g/dL
WCC	4.3×10^9/L
Platelets	379×10^9/L
Na	136 mmol/L
K	4.2 mmol/L
Urea	6.7 mmol/L
Creatinine	130 µmol/L

1. *On the basis of the history he should be advised to:*
   (a) Undergo urgent endoscopy
   (b) Have a trial of a proton pump inhibitor (PPI)
   (c) Have a *Helicobacter* breath test
2. *Pending specific investigations he could try and control his symptoms with:*
   (a) Antacids
   (b) Centrally acting anti-emetics
   (c) Eating small meals
3. *If he was eventually found to have developed a gastric cancer this would be best treated by:*
   (a) Total gastrectomy
   (b) Radiotherapy
   (c) Chemotherapy

Case 27: A man with abnormal liver blood tests

A 37-year-old man is referred for an opinion regarding abnormal liver blood tests. These were identified as part of a routine 'screening' health check arranged by his employer. He has no symptoms. His weight has gone up by 12 kg over the previous 5 years since having a family. He drinks alcohol no more than twice a week. He is on no regular prescribed medications and has no family history of liver disease.

On examination he looks fit and well. He weighs 120 kg (BMI 34). He has no peripheral signs of chronic liver disease and abdominal examination is normal.

Blood tests showed:

Hb	14.5 g/dL
WCC	6.7×10^9/L
Platelets	276×10^9/L
PT	11 sec
Glucose	5.6 mmol/L
Na	142 mmol/L
K	4.3 mmol/L
Urea	4.7 mmol/L
Creatinine	100 µmol/L
Albumin	41 g/L
Bilirubin	14 µmol/L
ALP	150 U/L
AST	110 U/L

Ultrasound showed increased reflectivity of liver parenchyma with increased prominence of portal tracts. There was no focal liver lesion. His bile duct, kidneys and spleen were normal. His pancreas was obscured by overlying bowel gas.

1. *The ultrasound report is consistent with which pathology?*
   (a) Haemochromatosis
   (b) Cirrhosis
   (c) Fatty liver
2. *The patient has read about haemochromatosis in the* Daily Mail. *What blood tests would screen for this condition?*

(a) Fasting transferring saturation
(b) Zinc protoporphyrin
(c) HFE mutation analysis

3. *Which hepatitis viruses should he be tested for?*
    (a) Hepatitis C
    (b) Hepatitis A
    (c) Hepatitis E

4. *What advice would you give the patient pending his investigation results?*
    (a) To use condoms
    (b) To lose weight
    (c) To take milk thistle

Case 28: A woman with abnormal liver blood tests

A 54-year-old woman is referred for investigation of abnormal liver blood tests. The tests were initially performed by the GP prior to the patient being started on statins. A recent cholesterol was elevated at 7.6 mmol/L. The patient has no symptoms other than mild fatigue. She drinks alcohol no more than 2–3 times a month. She has previously had gynaecological interventions following atypical smear tests but has had no admissions to hospital. She takes bendroflumethiazide and fluoxetine on prescription and evening primrose oil. Her mother had thyrotoxicosis and her maternal aunt had diabetes.

On examination she looks well. She weighs 87 kg (BMI 34). She has mild xanthelasmata under both her eyes. Her BP is 120/70 mmHg and there are no signs of chronic liver disease. Abdominal examination is normal.

Blood tests showed:

Hb	13.4 g/dL
WCC	6.4×10^9/L
Platelets	306×10^9/L
PT	12 sec
TSH	0.4
Na	138 mmol/L
K	3.5 mmol/L
Urea	4.3 mmol/L
Creatinine	110 μmol/L
Albumin	38 g/L
Bilirubin	2 μmol/L
ALP	275 U/L
AST	24 U/L
γ-GT	350 U/L
Cholesterol	7.6 mmol/L

Abdominal ultrasound is normal.

1. *The raised gamma glutamyl transferase (γ-GT) implies:*
    (a) That the patient is drinking more alcohol than she claims
    (b) That she has significant liver disease
    (c) That the raised alkaline phosphatase (ALP) is of liver origin

2. *Which blood test will determine whether or not this patient has primary biliary cirrhosis (PBC)?*
    (a) Antinuclear antibody (ANA)
    (b) Smooth muscle actin antibody (SMA)
    (c) Anti-mitochondrial antibody (AMA)

3. *If PBC is suspected the patient needs:*
    (a) A liver biopsy
    (b) Treatment with immunosuppressants
    (c) Information leaflets on the nature of the condition

Case 29: A patient with epigastric pain and vomiting

A 64-year-old woman is admitted to hospital with severe epigastric pain and vomiting. The pain was of sudden onset coming on an hour after eating. The pain radiates through to her back and had only just improved with intravenous morphine given in the casualty department. She is hypertensive on treatment with an ACE inhibitor and a thiazide diuretic. She had been investigated previously 2 years ago for abdominal pain.

On examination she is in obvious pain. Her temperature is 38.2°C. She is tachycardic with a pulse of 120 beats/min and a BP of 90/60 mmHg. She is tachypnoeic with a respiratory rate of 25 breaths/min. Abdominal examination reveals marked tenderness in the upper abdomen associated with guarding.

Blood tests showed:

Hb	11.4 g/dL
WCC	22.4×10^9/L
Platelets	110×10^9/L
CRP	250 mg/L
Glucose	9.8 mmol/L
Arterial pH	7.30
PO_2	7.4 kPa
PCO_2	3.2 kPa
HCO_3	19 mmol/L
Na	38 mmol/L
K	5.6 mmol/L
Corrected Ca	1.95 mmol/L
Urea	12.4 mmol/L
Creatinine	120 μmol/L
Albumin	32 g/L
Bilirubin	35 μmol/L
ALP	146 U/L
AST	120 U/L
Amylase	3560 U/L

Chest X-ray is normal.

1. *What further tests are necessary to confirm a diagnosis of acute pancreatitis?*
    (a) Abdominal ultrasound
    (b) ERCP (endoscopic retrograde cholangiopancreatography)
    (c) None

2. *Which of the test results are most significant with regard to her prognosis?*
    (a) $pO_2 < 8$ kPa
    (b) Amylase >3000 U/L
    (c) WCC $>12 \times 10^9$/L

3. *Which of the following investigations are necessary?*
    (a) Ultrasound on the day of admission
    (b) ERCP after 5 days
    (c) CT on day 2

4. *If gallstones are confirmed as the cause of a severe pancreatitis the best management is:*
    (a) Life-long low-fat diet
    (b) ERCP and endoscopic sphincterotomy
    (c) Cholecystectomy

Case 30: A patient with epigastric pain and weight loss

A 58-year-old man presents on the medical admissions ward with a 3-month history of epigastric pain and 12 kg in weight loss. He had previously been a very heavy drinker but had cut back recently due to his pain and vomiting. He has experienced diarrhoea, passing a pale and offensive stool 4–5 times a day. He has had marked thirst and nocturia.

On examination he looks dehydrated and unwell. His pulse is 100 beats/min, and his BP 110/60 mmHg. He smells ketotic. Abdominal examination demonstrates upper abdominal tenderness but no palpable mass, no organomegaly and no ascites.

Blood tests showed:

Hb	11.2 g/dL
MCV	105 fL
WCC	14.8×10^9/L
Platelets	380×10^9/L
Glucose	22.3 mmol/L
Na	128 mmol/L
K	3.1 mmol/L
Urea	22.4 mmol/L
Creatinine	110 µmol/L
Albumin	28 g/L
Bilirubin	12 µmol/L
ALP	170 U/L
AST	46 U/L
Amylase	45 U/L

Urine dipstick showed:

Ketones ++

Blood –

Protein –

1. *His 'diarrhoea' is most probably due to:*
   (a) Continued alcohol consumption
   (b) Fat malabsorption
   (c) Lactose intolerance
2. *Typical CT features of chronic pancreatitis include:*
   (a) Pancreatic oedema
   (b) Pancreatic glandular calcification
   (c) Pancreas divisum
3. *Once his condition has been stabilized he will need treatment with:*
   (a) Oral hypoglycaemic agents
   (b) Pancreatic enzyme supplements
   (c) Probiotics

Case 31: A patient with severe abdominal pain

An 85-year-old man is admitted with severe abdominal pain. This was of sudden onset, starting at 7.30 in the evening. The pain is situated above the umbilicus radiating through to the back. It is colicky in nature and associated with vomiting and rigors.

On examination he looks unwell. He is dry and has a fever of 39°C. His pulse is 115 beats/min, and BP is 80/40 mmHg. He is jaundiced. Abdominal examination reveals upper abdominal tenderness but no palpable masses or organomegaly.

Blood tests showed:

Hb	12.5 g/dL
WCC	22.4×10^9/L
Platelets	235×10^9/L
PT	11.9 sec
Na	138 mmol/L
K	4.8 mmol/L
Urea	12.8 mmol/L
Creatinine	150 µmol/L
Albumin	30 g/L
Bilirubin	140 µmol/L
ALP	350 U/L
ALT	95 U/L

1. *The combination of abdominal pain, fever and jaundice is known as:*
   (a) Charcot's triad
   (b) Saint's triad
   (c) Murphy's sign
2. *The most important feature to look for with an abdominal ultrasound would be:*
   (a) Gallbladder stones
   (b) Dilated bile ducts
   (c) Pancreatic oedema/pancreatitis
3. *After initial resuscitation with fluids and antibiotics the patient would best be treated with:*
   (a) Laparoscopic cholecystectomy
   (b) Open cholecystectomy and bile duct exploration
   (c) Endoscopic retrograde cholangiopancreatography (ERCP)

Case 32: A man with acute pancreatitis

A 52-year-old lawyer attends the clinic following a recent discharge from hospital. He had just suffered a second episode of acute pancreatitis. He is teetotal and has no other significant past medical history. During his admission it was noted that his liver blood tests were mildly abnormal but an abdominal ultrasound showed a normal calibre bile duct and 2–3 small stones in an otherwise healthy looking gallbladder.

Blood tests showed:

Hb	14.5 g/dL
WCC	6.4×10^9/L
Platelets	186×10^9/L
Na	135 mmol/L
K	4.2 mmol/L
Urea	3.8 mmol/L
Albumin	42 g/L
Bilirubin	14 µmol/L
ALP	180 U/L
AST	46 U/L

1. *He wishes to avoid having a further attack of pancreatitis. The best investigation for him to have at this stage would be:*
   (a) A further ultrasound now that his pancreatitis has settled
   (b) A CT scan
   (c) MRI
2. *To reduce his risk of further problems he should consider:*
   (a) A low-fat diet
   (b) Ursodeoxycholic acid to dissolve his stones
   (c) Cod liver oil
3. *If further imaging is unremarkable he would be best advised to:*
   (a) Continue conservative management indefinitely
   (b) Have an elective cholecystectomy
   (c) Consider having an emergency cholecystectomy if he has a further episode of pancreatitis

Case 33: A former drug user on a methadone programme

A 28-year-old man is referred to the clinic by the local drug action team. He is now established on a methadone programme and has not used intravenous drugs for 6 months. He has never been jaundiced nor had any admissions to hospital. He has requested screening for blood-borne viruses (BBV).

Blood tests showed:

Hb	13.4 g/dL
WCC	4.2×10^9/L
Platelets	320×10^9/L
Na	142 mmol/L
K	4.5 mmol/L
Urea	4.2 mmol/L
Creatinine	110 µmol/L
Albumin	38 g/L
Bilirubin	14 µmol/L
ALP	110 U/L
ALT	22 U/L
HBsAg	–ve
HCV Ab	+ve
HIV Ab	–ve

1. *From the results gained already he can be told:*
   (a) That he does not have hepatitis B
   (b) That does not have a significant liver problem
   (c) That he has hepatitis C virus (HCV)
2. *Chronic HCV infection is treated with:*
   (a) α-Interferon
   (b) Lamivudine
   (c) Adefovir
3. *The duration of antiviral treatment is:*
   (a) Determined by the viral genotype
   (b) 6 weeks
   (c) Indefinite
4. *During treatment the patient should be advised to:*
   (a) Take milk thistle
   (b) Exercise regularly
   (c) Abstain from alcohol

Case 34: A jaundiced woman with profound fatigue

A 42-year-old woman presents to the ward with a recent onset of jaundice. She has not been well for 4–6 weeks with profound fatigue and aching joints and muscles. Over the last week she has been noted by her family to have jaundice. She has lost three-quarters of a stone in weight and has been off her food. She has no significant past medical history other hypothyroidism. She takes thyroxine 100 µg and the oral contraceptive pill. Her mother also had thyroid disease and diabetes. Her father has haemochromatosis.

On examination she looks tired and unwell. She is obviously jaundiced. She is haemodynamically stable and afebrile. She has bilateral palmar erythema and a few spider naevi on her upper chest. Abdominal examination is unremarkable.

Blood tests showed:

Hb	12.1 g/dL
WCC	7.8×10^9/L
Platelets	98×10^9/L
PT	16 sec
Na	32 mmol/L
K	4.2 mmol/L
Urea	2.8 mmol/L
Creatinine	110 µmol/L
Albumin	27 g/L
Bilirubin	140 µmol/L
ALP	115 U/L

ALT	320 U/L
Fe	12 µg/dL
Ferritin	72 ng/mL
HBsAg	–ve
HCV Ab	–ve
HAV IgM	–ve
IgG	30 g/dL
IgA	3.4 g/dL
IgM	2.4 g/dL
TIBC	68 µg/dL

1. *The clinical presentation is most in keeping with a diagnosis of:*
   (a) Autoimmune hepatitis
   (b) Primary biliary cirrhosis
   (c) Haemochromatosis
2. *The autoantibody most likely to support the working diagnosis would be:*
   (a) Antinuclear antibody(ANA)
   (b) Anti-mitochondrial antibody
   (c) Anti-neutrophil cytoplasmic antibody
3. *The patient has an abdominal ultrasound that demonstrates a small amount of ascites and a mildly enlarged spleen. There is no focal liver abnormality and no biliary dilatation. The next investigation should be:*
   (a) Liver biopsy
   (b) Abdominal CT
   (c) Endoscopic ultrasound
4. *Once the diagnosis has been consolidated/confirmed:*
   (a) An expectant policy needs to be followed
   (b) Steroids need to be avoided
   (c) Steroids need to be started

Case 35: A man with no symptoms whose brother has haemochromatosis

A 48-year-old man is referred to the clinic. He is of Irish descent. His elder brother has emigrated to Australia and has recently been identified as having haemochromatosis. The patient has no symptoms and is on no medications. He has no significant past medical history. His father died of heart disease in his 70s. His mother is alive, in her late 60s and has arthritis. He has a younger sister who is alive and well.

Examination is unremarkable.

Blood tests showed:

Hb	15.2 g/dL
WCC	4.2×10^9/L
Platelets	420×10^9/L
Na	138 mmol/L
K	4.6 mmol/L
Urea	4.5 mmol/L
Creatinine	100 µmol/L
Albumin	42 g/L
Bilirubin	12 µmol/L
ALP	110 U/L
ALT	25 U/L
Fe	42 µg/dL
Ferritin	570 ng/mL

1. *The patient has heard about haemochromatosis from his brother and from having read about the condition on the internet. From the evidence presented to you, you can say that:*
   (a) It is unlikely that he has haemochromatosis
   (b) He definitely has haemochromatosis
   (c) He is likely to have haemochromatosis

2. *The patient asks to be tested for* HFE *mutations. The most common genotype associated with haemochromatosis is:*
(a) HH/CC
(b) HD/CY
(c) HH/YY

3. *His genetic testing supports the diagnosis of haemochromatosis. In view of this he should:*
(a) Start venesection treatment
(b) Be discharged and told to return to clinic if and when he develops symptoms
(c) Have a liver biopsy

4. *The patient has two children aged 16 and 18 years and wishes for them to be tested for haemochromatsosis. This could be done by:*
(a) Testing them for HFE mutations
(b) Measuring their iron indices
(c) Waiting until they develop symptoms

Case 36: A woman who drinks heavily and has had a seizure

A 34-year-old woman is admitted to your ward following a seizure. She admits to being a heavy drinker, consuming at least 2 litres of strong cider daily. She has been trying to cut down her alcohol intake because of persistent nausea and vomiting. Her only previous admissions to hospital were due to a head injury and an impulsive overdose. She takes no regular prescribed medications but admits to smoking tobacco and cannabis socially and previously to having used ecstasy. She has never used intravenous drugs.

On examination she is tremulous and sweaty. She is orientated and cooperative. She has a tachycardia with a pulse of 120 beats/min and has a hyperdynamic circulation with a bounding high volume pulse and relative hypotension (systolic BP 80 mmHg). She is jaundiced and febrile with a temperature of 38°C. Abdominal examination reveals some RUQ (right upper quadrant) tenderness and moderate hepatomegaly. She has no detectable spleen nor large volume ascites.

Blood tests showed:

Hb	9.4 g/dL
WCC	16.4×10^9/L
Platelets	78×10^9/L
PT	20 sec
Na	118 mmol/L
K	2.3 mmol/L
Urea	1.6 mmol/L
Creatinine	98 μmol/L
Albumin	24 g/L
Bilirubin	240 μmol/L
ALP	265 U/L
ALT	358 U/L

On ultrasound her liver is enlarged with an irregular outline and heterogeneous echopattern. There is mild splenomegaly (12 cm) and small volume ascites. Reverse flow is noted in portal vein on Doppler.

1. *She feels like she is 'having the DTs' (experiencing withdrawal). Which of the following should you give her?*
(a) Intravenous vitamins
(b) Oral chlordiazepoxide
(c) Intramuscular haloperidol

2. *Spontaneous bacterial peritonitis (SBP) can be determined by:*
(a) Positive blood cultures
(b) Abdominal tenderness
(c) An ascitic tap

3. *If after 5 days the patient is deteriorating despite broad-spectrum antibiotics and all the cultures are negative, the other treatment to consider is:*
(a) Steroids
(b) Liver transplant
(c) Haemofiltration

Case 37: A man with dysphagia and weight loss

An 88-year-old man presents to your hospital with 6 weeks of progressive dysphagia to solids. He has lost 9 kg in weight. He has ischaemic heart disease having previously had coronary artery by-pass surgery and currently uses GTN spray in anticipation of angina before walking to his corner shop for the morning newspaper. He no longer smokes. He lives with his wife who has cognitive impairment. Their only daughter now lives in Australia.

On examination he looks emaciated and dehydrated. He has no palpable lymphadenopathy. Abdominal examination reveals a small but palpable aortic aneurysm but is otherwise unremarkable.

An open-access endoscopy has demonstrated the patient to have a malignant oesophageal stricture at 25 cm from the incisors. The stricture precluded completion of the examination and a biopsy taken at the time of the procedure has shown squamous carcinoma.

1. *His further management should include:*
(a) Discussion of his case at an upper gastrointestinal cancer multidisciplinary team meeting (MDT)
(b) Endoscopic ultrasound (EUS)
(c) CT of chest and abdomen

2. *In order to address his symptoms and his poor nutrition it would be reasonable to consider:*
(a) Total parenteral nutrition (TPN)
(b) Sip feeds
(c) Percutaneous endoscopic gastrostomy (PEG)

3. *To relieve his dysphagia the best treatment option would be:*
(a) Placement of an oesophageal stent
(b) Chemotherapy
(c) Radiotherapy

Gastroenterology: Answers

Case 1: An ex-smoker with weight loss

1. (b) Metastasis from a visceral tumour

Virchow's node should always be actively sought in any patient where there is any suspicion of underlying malignancy. A Virchow's node is an enlarged supraclavicular lymph node on the left side, where the lymphatic drainage from much of the abdomen comes up via the lymphatic duct and enters the venous system via the subclavian vein. There are many causes of Virchow's node, including; metastatic intra-abdominal malignancy (Virchow spotted the node in himself, the presenting feature of his gastric cancer), breast cancer (rare), and occasionally infection or lymphoma.

2. (c) Thyroid function

Thyrotoxicosis should be excluded in all patients with weight loss. Neither CRP nor vitamins levels are likely to add to this patient's assessment.

3. (a) Chest X-ray

Chest X-ray is mandatory in all cases of weight loss and may be forgotten if the patient has any gut/abdominal symptoms.

Further reading: Chapter 23 in Medicine at a Glance.

Case 2: A woman with diabetes with weight loss

1. (c) Malabsorption

Even if the patient adheres to the prescribed insulin regime, glycaemic control can be upset by malabsorption. Clearly if this patient had not had pale frequent stools, one of the hallmarks of malabsorption, then the most likely cause of her poor glycaemic control would be poor compliance.

2. (c) Measurement of pancreatic enzyme activity in faeces

Although quantifying faecal fats used to be the standard test for exocrine function, this can now be reliably determined with measurement of faecal elastase or chymotrypsin activity. Fat provocation ultrasound is used in some circumstances to determine gallbladder function.

3. (b) CT

CT is useful for documenting the presence of pancreatic glandular calcification and cyst formation in chronic pancreatitis. It can also estimate glandular size and in most circumstances rule out a significant mass lesion.

Further reading: Chapter 124.

Case 3: A man with a history of constipation

1. (a) Flexible sigmoidoscopy

Although these blood tests show some renal impairment (raised urea and creatinine), the most important abnormality is the high calcium, which is at least moderately elevated. Clearly, the cause of this needs urgent evaluation, and as part of this, it is good and safe practice to consider investigation of any reported rectal bleeding. Proctoscopy and rigid sigmoidoscopy are procedures that can safely be performed in the clinic or on the ward although in an unprepared bowel views might be limited and only the last 15 cm of the rectum can be clearly seen. Even if one identifies haemorrhoids it is imperative to exclude a more significant source of the bleeding proximal to the rectum and a carefully performed flexible sigmoidoscopy after suitable bowel preparation would be desirable. An abdominal CT is not imperative at this stage. Malignant hypercalcaemia is a rare occurrence with intra-abdominal cancers being associated more frequently with squamous cancers (i.e. skin, bronchus, cervix).

2. (c) Parathyroid hormone (PTH) level

The patient has significant hypercalcaemia; though there are many possible causes, the most common two causes are primary hyperparathyroidism and disseminated malignancy. In distinguishing these two apart, PTH level is very useful: a normal or elevated PTH level is diagnostic of primary hyperparathyroidism, whereas a suppressed PTH suggests disseminated malignancy. Magnesium levels may be informative in investigating *hypo*calcaemia. Myeloma is a possible alternative diagnosis, although the normal plasma viscosity would be somewhat against this. Bence -Jones protein is detected in *urine* and not in serum.

3. (b) Intravenous fluids

In addition to having significant hypercalcaemia he is clinically and biochemically dehydrated and should receive intravenous saline before receiving an *intravenous* bisphosphonate. In assessing dehydration, one should always *be certain* to measure postural blood pressure, as clinical assessment of the dryness of mucus membranes, or the lack of turgor in the skin is a very insensitive clinical means of assessing fluid status.

Further reading: Chapter 24.

Case 4: A woman with difficulty defaecating

1. (a) CT colonography

Although the history is suggestive of a pelvic floor problem, it is necessary to exclude a mechanical cause for the patient's symptoms. Colonoscopy can be technically challenging in patients with constipation as the colon is frequently long and convoluted. Although one might consider a barium enema, modern CT imaging with bowel preparation and colonic insufflation gives a very good structural evaluation of the colon.

2. (c) Osmotic laxatives

Osmotic agents such as milk of magnesia or polyethylene glycol (PEG) preparations are very safe in the long-term management of chronic constipation. Stimulant laxatives such as Senna will often exacerbate pain and are of limited benefit. Colonic lavage is not risk free and leads to short-term symptom relief only.

3. (b) Anorectal physiology

The history is consistent with pelvic floor dysynergia consequent on pelvic trauma during childbirth. If the patient's symptoms are not manageable with medical interventions then anorectal physiology with a biofeedback programme might be necessary. Surgery may have to be considered in very exceptional circumstances.

Further reading: Chapter 24.

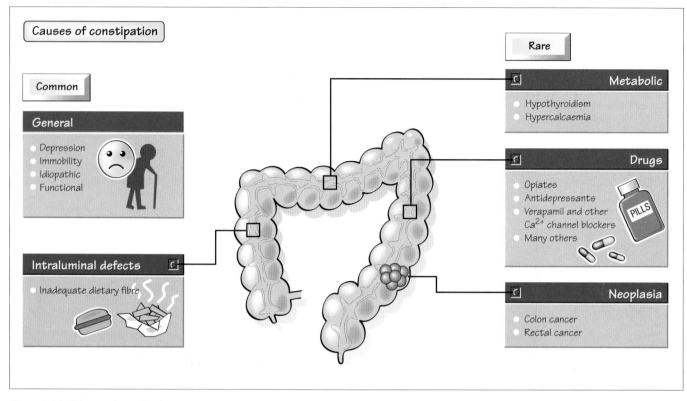

Figure 3.4.1 Causes of constipation.

Case 5: A man with a 6-week history of diarrhoea

1. (c) Emergency admission to hospital

This presentation satisfies the Truelove–Witts criteria for severe acute colitis and regardless of the underlying cause, this man needs urgent medical care with admission to the gastroenterology ward, intravenous fluids and intravenous steroids. A stool culture should be sent as part of his assessment and antibiotics might be considered. A colonoscopy would not be undertaken at this stage, a sigmoidoscopy (either rigid or flexible) together with a plain abdominal X-ray should be sufficient to guide treatment.

2. (b) An empty colon

The presentation with weight loss and raised inflammatory markers is typical of an extensive colitis and the colon is likely to be empty. The X-ray might show evidence of mucosal oedema (i.e. 'thumb-printing') and dilatation. Wrigler's sign (air outlining the

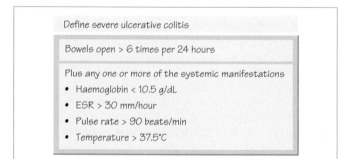

Define severe ulcerative colitis

Bowels open > 6 times per 24 hours

Plus any one or more of the systemic manifestations
- Haemoglobin < 10.5 g/dL
- ESR > 30 mm/hour
- Pulse rate > 90 beats/min
- Temperature > 37.5°C

Figure 3.5.1 Truelove and Witt's criteria for diagnosing severe ulcerative colitis.

wall of the bowel) is indicative of perforation. Proximal constipation might be seen in patients presenting with proctitis.

3. (c) Colectomy

Failure to respond to medical therapy should always prompt consideration of surgery. A pan-proctocolectomy would be undertaken and in most circumstances the patient would be left with a temporary ileostomy. Restorative ileoanal pouch surgery might then be offered once the patient has recovered. Infliximab is licensed for severe Crohn's disease and for mild to moderate ulcerative colitis, but its role in severe colitis has yet to be defined.
Further reading: Chapter 123.

Case 6: A man with frequent loose stools

1. (a) Irritable bowel syndrome (IBS)

(c) Malabsorption

Weight loss despite preservation of appetite is typical of malabsorption. It is unwise to assume that symptoms are purely functional (i.e. IBS) when the patient reports significant weight loss. Although the patient reports frequent loose stools the description is of steatorrhoea and not typical 'colonic' diarrhoea, which is more likely to be watery and possibly bloody.

2. (c) Infection

Although the presentation has quite a long history the most likely diagnosis is Giardiasis. This protozoa colonizes the small intestine and can lead to significant malabsorption. It is commonly acquired from contaminated water supplies. Small bowel Crohn's disease can present with small bowel malabsorption but would typically be associated with pain (i.e. subacute intestinal obstruction). Chronic pancreatitis can present with malabsorption but acute pancreatitis most commonly presents with pain.

3. (c) Prescribe empirical treatment

In cases of suspected *Giardia* one can send a 'hot' stool sample for microscopy but the diagnostic yield is often low. The infection can be determined by biopsy of the duodenum undertaken at gastroscopy or by culture of duodenal aspirates, but in many instances the infection is cleared adequately with a single dose of Tinidazole (2 g). Imaging of the small intestine is rarely useful in the absence of symptoms of intestinal obstruction.
Further reading: Chapter 25.

Case 7: A man with 'coffee-ground' vomiting

1. (b) Retching causing abrasion of the gastric mucosa

Any cause of protracted vomiting is likely to result in 'coffee grounds'.

2. (a) Chronic GI blood loss

A microcytic anaemia is characteristic of iron deficiency. Acute blood loss or renal failure will more commonly result in a normocytic, normochromic anaemia. A microcytic anaemia does not exclude acute blood loss, such as may occasionally lead to severe cardiovascular disturbance.

3. (a) Caecal cancer

Caecal cancer will commonly present with iron deficiency and subacute *small-bowel* obstruction. Conversely, rectal cancer will present with overt rectal bleeding – possibly with features of large-bowel obstruction. Gastric cancer will usually cause anaemia with feelings of early satiety (feeling full after meals) and foregut (i.e. upper abdominal) bloating.
Further reading: Chapter 131.

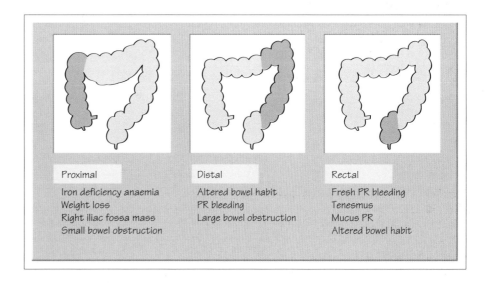

Figure 3.7.1 Features of colonic carcinoma.

Proximal	Distal	Rectal
Iron deficiency anaemia	Altered bowel habit	Fresh PR bleeding
Weight loss	PR bleeding	Tenesmus
Right iliac fossa mass	Large bowel obstruction	Mucus PR
Small bowel obstruction		Altered bowel habit

Case 8: A man with vomiting and Crohn's disease

1. (c) Erythema nodosum

The description is of classic erythema nodosum which is associated with Crohn's disease: other causes include drug reactions, streptococcal sore throat, sarcoidosis, mycobacterial infections, and in addition viral illnesses. It is sometimes idiopathic. Pyoderma gangrenosum usually presents as largely painless ulcers. Dermatitis herpetiformis is an itchy blistering rash associated with coeliac disease.

2. (b) Small bowel imaging

The presentation is typical of subacute intestinal obstruction and is most likely to be secondary to recurrent Crohn's disease at the anastomosis resulting from his previous surgery. Although one might consider endoscopy to investigate vomiting or colonoscopy to directly visualize the anastomosis he is best served by formal imaging of the small intestine. This could be by contrast radiography (enteroclysis) or by MRI (enterography or enteroclysis). Magnetic resonance imaging has the advantage of defining extraluminal disease (fistulae, abscesses) and would probably be the investigation of choice.

3. (a) A liquid diet

The patient's symptoms are in part exacerbated by subacute obstruction as undigested food is forced through a relative narrowing in the gut. A high-fibre diet would make his symptoms worse rather than better, but a low residue or even a liquid diet will lead to some improvement. An *elemental* diet is a balanced liquid diet in which the 'protein' element is in the form of amino acids. A *polymeric* diet is one in which 'protein' is delivered in the form of peptides. Each can be taken in the form of 'sip feeds' (i.e. taken orally) or delivered by naso-enteral tube (e.g. an NG feeding tube). Total parenteral nutrition would only be considered in exceptional circumstances.
Further reading: Chapter 127.

Case 9: An orthopaedic patient who has passed a melaena stool

1. (b) He has had a large GI bleed

Postural hypotension is a very important physical sign in patients with gastrointestinal bleeding and should be sought and documented in all cases. This man has clearly had a significant GI bleed from the history, though the clues from the laboratory investigations pointing to a large GI bleed are anaemia, and the urea being raised in the setting of a nearly normal creatinine. This high urea is partly due to intravascular volume depletion (pre-renal renal failure), but also to the large protein load in the GI tract (blood) that is being digested and absorbed. A history of syncope or postural dizziness should similarly alert clinicians to a significant bleed. Very rarely GI bleeds present to A&E only with symptoms of brief syncope; put another way, all patients who present to casualty with syncope, and in whom there is no obvious alternative explanation should have postural blood pressures performed, a rectal examination (for melaena), and bloods including full blood count (especially for haemoglobin) and biochemistry screen (particularly for urea).

2. (b) Duodenal ulcer

The presentation is one of an *upper* gastrointestinal bleed and the disproportionate rise in urea over creatinine is typical of blood in the proximal gut. Although there is no prior history of indigestion a peptic ulcer is the most likely cause. Diverticular disease can cause acute *lower* GI bleeding but this will usually present with identifiable blood per rectum (i.e. haematochezia).

3. (a) Intravenous fluids

An emergency endoscopy should be considered but only after appropriate fluid resuscitation. This could initially be undertaken with saline or colloidal fluids such as gelofusine. Transfusion requirements need to be carefully judged to maintain a haematocrit of 0.3. The rationale behind giving an intravenous proton pump inhibitor is that in raising the intragastric pH one is likely to facilitate stabilization of any formed blood clot. Some evidence has been published to suggest early/blind treatment with intravenous omeprazole but the benefit is probably greater in patients with a proven peptic ulcer with identifiable stigmata of recent haemorrhage (i.e. after endoscopy). Gastric lavage has no established role.
Further reading: Chapter 27.

Case 10: A man who has vomited blood

1. (c) He has significant liver disease

Prothrombin time (PT) is an essential parameter of liver *function*. The normal PT is 12-15 seconds, the patients here has a PT of 36 seconds, so his INR is 3.0. Prothrombin time measures the action of factors II, V, VII, X and fibrinogen. Warfarin therapy, malaborption (of vitamin K), and liver disease can all prolong the PT, as does increased consumption of clotting factors, such as occurs with disseminated intra-vascular coagulation, where the activated partial thromboplastin time is prolonged, fibrinogen levels are low, and fibrin degradation products raised. These tests were not reported here, they should be carried out, though the clinical context is highly suggestive of a prolonged PT due to liver disease. Although he might be malnourished it is unlikely that his clotting would improve with the administration of vitamin K. If correction of his clotting is clinically indicated he should be given fresh frozen plasma. His platelet count may be low due to alcohol induced bone marrow depression (consistent with his low haemoglobin), hypersplenism (splenic enlargement secondary to cirrhosis induced portal hypertension).

2. (a) Portal hypertension

The most likely source of his bleeding is oesophageal varices secondary to cirrhosis with portal hypertension. For this reason he should undergo emergency endoscopy – preferably within six hours of his admission. If varices are identified these should be treated by endoscopic variceal ligation (EVL or 'banding').

3. (a) Give a vasopressin analogue such as terlipressin

Vasopressin analogues such as terlipressin reduce portal pressures and have been demonstrated to be effective in portal hypertensive bleeding. They work in a way that is complementary to endoscopic therapy and will also reduce bleeding from 'ectopic' varices that lie further down the gut beyond the reach of endoscopy. Terlipressin may also provide a protective effect against hepato-renal syndrome. Blind antibiotic therapy has been demonstrated to improve outcomes in portal hypertensive bleeding and has led to a theory that many cases of bleeding are associated with (or even precipitated by) episodic portal pyaemia causing transient rises in portal pressures.
Further reading: Chapter 128.

Case 11: A man with rectal bleeding

1. (c) A recent/sudden bleed

Although there appears to be little if any evidence of anaemia on the blood tests the haemoglobin might be disproportionately high due to vaso-constriction and 'haemo-concentration'. Features of a chronic disease process might include microcytosis (indicating iron deficiency), thrombocytosis (suggesting chronic inflammation) or hypoalbuminaenia.

2. (c) Diverticular change

Diverticular change may commonly present with sudden lower GI bleeding. Diverticulae form at areas of localized weakness in the muscular layer of the colon where the blood vessels penetrate through to the submucosa. The exact precipitant of bleeding episodes is unknown but usually the bleeding is unheralded and short lived. Colon cancers can present with rectal bleeding but usually this is of lower volume over a longer period of time, culminating in iron deficiency.

3. (c) Lower GI endoscopy (colonoscopy or flexible sigmoidoscopy)

On the whole bleeding is best investigated by 'endoscopy'. Ideally one would manage the patient conservatively and then undertake flexible sigmoidoscopy or colonoscopy with appropriate bowel preparation. If bleeding is particularly severe or ongoing direct mesenteric angiography or even laparotomy with 'on-table' colonscopy might be considered to identify the site of bleeding.
Further reading: Chapter 120.

Case 12: A man with rectal bleeding of increasing frequency

1. (b) Flexible sigmoidoscopy

Testing for *occult* bleeding is completely inappropriate in the context of *overt* rectal bleeding. Colonoscopy could be undertaken but this is unnecessary and moreover patients with possible colonic malignancy might experience bowel obstruction with the bowel preparation necessary for a total colonic examination. A rigid sigmoidoscopy will examine the last 15–20 cm of the colon whereas flexible sigmoidoscopy is the examination of choice allowing examination of the colon distal to the splenic flexure.

2. (b) CT

Ultrasound might identify liver metastases but is of less use for identifying lymph node or pulmonary deposits. MRI is useful for assessing local pelvic invasion but CT of chest, abdomen and pelvis provides the best investigation for metastatic disease. This approach might be refined by the development and greater access to CT PET (positron emission tomography).

3. (a) Carcinoembryonic antigen (CEA)

CEA may be elevated in up to 65% of patients with colon cancer, but this depends very much on the extent of the disease, those with limited (and thus resectable) disease often having only minor or no rises (Fig.3.12.1). For this reason, it has only limited utility in establishing a diagnosis but may be of use in monitoring response to treatments such as chemotherapy and in screening for metastatic disease during follow-up. CA19.9 is a marker of pancreatic/biliary malignancy. aFP is elevated in hepatocellular carcinoma and some germ cell/testicular tumours.

Further reading: Chapter 131.

Stage of colon cancer	% raised CEA
I	4
II	25
III	44
IV	65

Figure 3.12.1 Staging of colonic cancer.

Case 13: A man with difficulty in swallowing

1. (c) Endoscopy

Although barium swallow might delineate an oesophageal stricture endoscopy has greater sensitivity and specificity. Biopsies can be taken of suspicious appearances and if appropriate, strictures might be dilated or even stented.

2. (b) Adenocarcinoma

Although in the past squamous cancer of the mid-oesophagus was very common, with the reduction of cigarette smoking the incidence has fallen. This has been superceded by adenocarcinoma of the distal oesophagus/gastric cardia.

3. (b) CT

Endoscopy is useful for establishing diagnosis but provides little 'staging' information. Although endoscopic ultrasound might be crucial for early-stage cancers, the majority of upper GI cancers are already advanced at the point of presentation and CT of chest and abdomen is usually required to determine whether or not surgery might be performed.

Further reading: Chapter 130.

Case 14: A man with heartburn and painful swallowing

1. (a) Trial of treatment with a proton pump inhibitor (PPI)

It could be argued that testing and treating for *H. pylori* might achieve symptom relief but the history is very typical of gastro-oesophageal reflux and he is likely to get a good response to acid suppression. There is no immediate indication for endoscopy.

2. (a) Normal

From the symptom description it is most likely that the role of endoscopy would be to provide qualified reassurance.

3. (c) Food poisoning

Many people's perception is that gastric acid has a critical role in digestion but the main theoretical risk of long-term acid suppression is an increased risk of food poisoning. Though this is generally important, there is one area where this knowledge is critically important, that is, in the avoidance of hospital acquired GI infection. Currently there is an epidemic of *Clostridium difficile* associated diarrhoea in UK hospitals. Whilst there are many risk factors for this, including increasing age, antibiotic use (particularly cephalosporins), co-morbidity, a critical factor in promoting spread of the toxogenic *C. difficile* species is ease of entry to a patients GI tract, and this is promoted by PPIs. In other words, there should be a high threshold in prescribing PPIs to elderly patients admitted acutely to general hospitals. Evidence is accumulating that osteopenia might also be a long-term risk, although the mechanism behind this is not clear.

Further reading: Chapter 118.

Case 15: A patient with sudden-onset upper abdominal pain

1. (b) Ultrasound

The history is typical of biliary colic and an ultrasound should either show gallstones and/or evidence of gallbladder inflammation (thickened gallbladder wall). Other important aspects of the ultrasound report would be whether or not there is evidence of bile duct dilatation (suggestive of stones in the common bile duct) or evidence of a focal liver abnormality (such as a liver abscess).

2. (c) Conservative management

Analgesics may well be necessary but biliary pain is relatively resistant to opioids and morphine in particular can exacerbate bile duct spasm. Surgery might be considered but where possible this will be deferred and undertaken as an 'interval' intervention.

3. (a) Cholecystectomy

A low-fat diet will reduce the incidence of pain by reducing the likelihood of gallbladder contraction. Ursodeoxycholic acid had been developed in the hope that this synthetic and very soluble bile salt might lead to the chemical dissolution of gallstones. Unfortunately it does not achieve this in the majority of symptomatic stones as they are already calcified by the time they present. Cholecystectomy not only removes the existing stones but also reduces the risk of bile stasis, reducing the risk of further stones forming.

Further reading: Chapter 126.

Case 16: A patient with worsening upper abdominal pain

1. (a) Cholangitis

She might have gallstones in the common bile duct (choledocolithiasis) but the combination of pain, fever and jaundice is definitive of infection in the biliary tree or cholangitis (Charcot's triad). Cholecystitis refers to inflammation/infection in the gallbladder, not the bile ducts.

2. (a) Ultrasound

An ultrasound scan is necessary to confirm the presence of stones and to demonstrate dilatation of the bile ducts. It is also necessary to exclude liver abscess.

3. (c) Endoscopic retrograde cholangiopancreatography (ERCP)

Lithotripsy is not useful in dealing with bile duct or gallbladder stones. Open surgery used to be the treatment of choice but this has now been replaced with ERCP at which the bile duct can be

cut open (sphincterotomy) and the stones extracted with an endoscopic basket or balloon.
Further reading: Chapter 126.

Case 17: A heavy drinker with jaundice

1. (b) An excess of endogenous oestrogen hormones

Spider naevi, palmar erythema, gynaecomastia, loss of body hair and testicular atrophy are all due to an excess in circulating levels of endogenous oestrogens. They are often described together as the 'oestrogenic signs of chronic liver disease'.

2. (a) Broad-spectrum antibiotics

Although the presentation is consistent with an acute alcoholic hepatitis it can be difficult to clinically distinguish this from an infection leading to a decompensation of chronic liver disease. Blood and urine cultures should be taken in addition to a diagnostic tap of the ascites looking for spontaneous bacterial peritonitis (SBP). Antibiotic treatment should not be delayed. Omeprazole will not alter the risk of bleeding and the effect of fresh frozen plasma on the coagulopathy would only be short lived.

3. (b) CT headscan

With a history of falls and abnormal clotting the patient is at risk of having a sub-dural haemorrhage. Transfer to intensive care would be considered after a diagnosis has been established. Long-acting benzodiazepines are cleared poorly in liver failure. If any sedation is necessary short-acting drugs such as chlordiazepoxide are preferable.

4. (c) Steroids

Systemic corticosteroids have been demonstrated to be of benefit in selected patients with acute alcoholic hepatitis. Once infection has been excluded the patient should be scored according to validated criteria (discriminant function or Maddrey score; Glasgow Alcoholic Hepatitis Score) before steroids are considered. Patients with acute alcoholic hepatitis fare badly with transplantation regardless of the ethical issues. Renal replacement therapy such as haemofiltration might be used in exceptional circumstances but where possible renal dysfunction will be treated with a combination of terlipressin and human albumin solution.
Further reading: Chapter 128.

Case 18: A patient with lower abdominal pain, diarrhoea and weight loss

1. (a) CT

CT would be the investigation of choice for this mass. Ultrasound is good for primary problems of the urinary tract but not as useful for deeper abdominal masses and lesions associated primarily with the gut. Although it is reasonable on the basis of the clinical presentation to think that the mass arises from the sigmoid colon, a flexible sigmoidoscopy will give no information regarding extra-luminal disease and could be a very high-risk intervention.

2. (b) Fluid resuscitation and systemic antibiotics

The patient is clinically dehydrated and septic. There are no features of bowel obstruction and therefore stenting would not be appropriate. If surgery was ultimately necessary this would be best deferred until the patient is better and the diagnosis consolidated.

3. (b) Diverticulitis

A diverticular mass will often present with localized tenderness and urinary symptoms sometimes with more overt clinical evidence of a colovesical fistula (pneumaturia, air in the bladder on CT). It may be difficult to distinguish from a cancer of the sigmoid colon.

4. (c) Interval sigmoid resection

The definitive treatment would be an operation performed at an interval with the intention of resecting the diseased bowel, taking down any fistulae and aiming for a primary anastomosis. A Hartman's procedure involves the creation of an end colostomy leaving the distal bowel in situ, usually as a mucous fistula. It is only really a temporary intervention.
Further reading: Chapter 120.

Case 19: A patient with abdominal distension

1. (a) Dipping

'Dipping' is a specific technique useful for eliciting hepatomegaly and/or splenomegaly in the presence of ascites. It involves a sort of push with the hand into the abdomen followed by a second

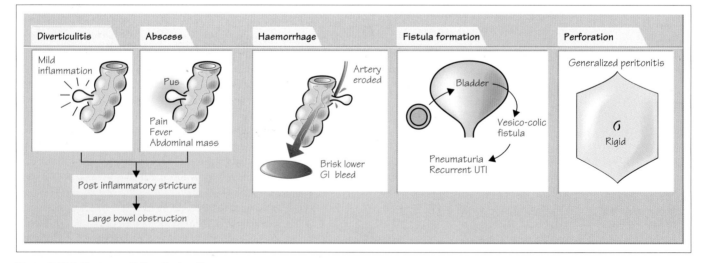

Figure 3.18.1 Features of diverticular disease.

movement whereupon the enlarged organ pushes back towards the abdominal wall.

2. (a) Ascitic protein

An ascitic protein content of less than 10 g/L is typical of a transudate and characteristic of ascites from chronic liver disease. Ultrasound images may be sub-optimal in the presence of large-volume ascites and imaging is often best deferred until after the ascites has been treated. Ascitic fluid cytology can be very difficult to interpret and a negative cytology report should not deflect from a diagnosis of malignancy if there are other features of concern.

3. (c) Infusion of human albumin solution

The major risk of undertaking high-volume paracentesis is post-paracentesis circulatory dysfunction and hepatorenal failure. This risk can be reduced by the infusion of plasma expanders and human albumin solution has been proven to provide the greatest protection. Diuretic treatment will increase the risk of renal failure and although the patient might have mild hyponatraemia, this is largely dilutional and patients should be advised to take a 'no added salt' diet.

4. (c) Lieno-renal shunt

A TIPSS is a stent that is placed as an interventional radiological procedure. It establishes direct communication between the portal vein and the hepatic vein through the liver. This has been demonstrated to control ascites in selected patients.

Further reading: Chapter 33.

Case 20: A patient with large-volume ascites

1. (b) Ultrasound

The presentation is very suspicious for ovarian cancer and transvaginal ultrasound by an experienced gynaecological ultrasonographer would provide the best evaluation of the ovaries.

2. (b) CA125

Although tumour markers are best used for the monitoring of response to treatment and detection of disease relapse, a very elevated CA125 in the presence of exudative ascites (with or without an ovarian mass on imaging) would be strongly suggestive of ovarian cancer. CA19-9 is a marker of pancreatic and bile duct cancer. CA 15.3 and 27.29 are raised in breast cancer.

3. (c) Therapeutic paracentesis

Good symptom relief can be obtained by paracentesis. Malignant ascites responds less well to diuretic therapy.

Further reading: Chapter 33.

Case 21: A patient with bloody diarrhoea

1. (a) Food poisoning

The short history and sudden onset of symptoms very much favour an infective cause for the problem and the history is typical for infection with *Campylobacter jejuni* infection. The fact that no other members of the party were affected is not unusual.

2. (a) Blood cultures

Blood cultures should be taken in addition to stool cultures. Serology for campylobacter is not universally available. The sigmoidoscopic appearances of ulcerative colitis and severe campylobacter colitis are virtually indistinguishable.

3. (b) Intravenous fluid resuscitation

Intravenous fluid rehydration is often all that is necessary, although antibiotics might be considered in the light of a positive culture and if progress after the first 24 hours is slow. Probiotics might help symptoms during the recovery phase but there is no randomized controlled trial (RCT) data to support this. Antidiarrhoeal agents are contraindicated as they are likely to prolong the course of the illness and have been associated with a greater risk of toxic dilatation of the colon.

4. (b) Less tea and coffee

After a severe episode of food poisoning patients are frequently left with recurrent symptoms of pain and altered bowel frequency (post-infective irritable bowel syndrome). Patients are recommended to reduce their consumption of gut stimulants such as coffee, tea, chocolate and alcohol. Similarly patients are often advised to limit their intake of dairy products (mainly milk and cream) in case they might have a temporary lactose intolerance.

Further reading: Chapter 117.

Case 22: A patient with community-acquired pneumonia and diarrhoea

1. (b) Antibiotic-associated diarrhoea

The presentation is typical of a colitis secondary to *Clostridium difficile*. Campylobacter could cause an illness such as this but is typically more florid with bloody diarrhoea. *Clostridium difficile* associated diarrhoea is a major problem in many hospitals. The toxogenic strain is spread by the faeco-oral route of transmission; small number of the bacteria in the normal gut do not result in symptoms, but when bacterial overgrowth occurs when normal gut bacteria are suppressed with antibiotics, the bacteria secretes toxins, including an enteropathic one (toxin A), a cytotoxin (toxin B), and other toxins. These result in a pseudomembranous colitis, and an offensively smelling diarrhoea; the illness can be quite persistent, results in very long hospital admissions (on average, prolonging hospital stay by 20 days), has a significant mortality (up to 10-20%) and is very unpleasant both for patients and relatives. Patients, if they survive, are very debilitated afterwards and may require prolonged rehabilitation. The organism is relatively resistant to antibiotics, requiresprolonged treatment and recurs in up to 10-20% of cases within 20 days after initially apparently successful treatment. Clearly, it is crucially important to take all steps to avoid this infection, including avoiding PPIs in those at risk, avoiding antibiotics, or if this is not possible, avoiding those with the highest risk of provoking *Clostridium difficile* diarrhoea, and, critically, meticulous isolation of patients with the condition, and meticulous approach to all aspects of nosocomial infection transmission, particularly hand hygiene.

2. (c) Assay for *C. difficile* toxin

The *C. difficile* toxin should be tested at the earliest opportunity. The diagnosis of *C. difficile* colitis has implications not only for the patient but also for other patients being nursed on that ward. If the diagnosis is suspected, the patient should be effectively barrier nursed and everyone in contact with the patient (including visiting relatives) should be informed of the potential diagnosis and reminded of the principles of basic hand hygiene. The spores of *C. difficile* are highly transmissible and are resistant to commonly used alcohol gels – hands should be washed thoroughly with soap and water.

3. (a) Give antibiotics for the diarrhoea

If possible any existing on-going broad-spectrum antibiotics should be stopped and far from starving the patient, one should consider nutritional support with either sip-feed supplements or even enteral nutrition delivered via a nasogastric tube. If *C. difficile* is confirmed or strongly suspected it should be actively treated with metronidazole or oral/enteral vancomycin.

Further reading: Chapter 25.

Case 23: A patient with reflux and increasing heartburn

1. (b) Air swallowing

Subconscious air swallowing is the cause of belching. It is often useful to explain this to patients in some detail as the symptom can be very distressing at times.

2. (a) Increasing the dose (or frequency) of the PPI

Although many patients gain good control of reflux symptoms with a standard dose of a generic PPI, some patients require a higher dose to achieve optimal acid suppression and some patients ultimately need to be maintained on a specific branded (i.e. more expensive) agent. Ultimately the patient should be maintained on the lowest dose of the cheapest agent *sufficient to control the symptoms* (NICE guidance 1999). H2 antagonists have a lower potency with respect to acid suppression and probably have a greater range of reported side effects. Antacids taken at the same time as PPIs inhibit PPI absorption.

3. (a) Nissen's fundoplication

Nissen's fundoplication (usually performed laparoscopically) is the operation of choice. Ramstead's pyloroplasty is a procedure performed for neonatal pyloric stenosis. HSV was a procedure performed for recurrent/resistant duodenal ulcers in the days before the characterization of *Helicobacter pylori*.

Further reading: Chapter 118.

Case 24: A patient with Barrett's oesophagus

1. (c) Adenocarcinoma of the distal oesophagus is increasing in incidence

The incidence of most intestinal cancers is static or falling. However the incidence of adenocarcinoma of the distal oesophagus is rising. Barrett's oesophagus is a risk factor for developing cancer but the risk is in the order of 0.5% per year. Photodynamic therapy has been tried in Barrett's but most commonly in patients identified with severe dysplasia who are otherwise not fit for oesophagectomy.

2. (a) Stopping drinking alcohol

Excess alcohol consumption is associated with an increased risk of gastrointestinal cancers. The effect of differing doses of proton pump inhibitors (PPIs) is unknown but at present there is no hard clinical evidence to recommend a dose beyond that which controls heartburn/indigestion. The benefits of endoscopy surveillance are unproven. Currently the recommendation is for this to be performed every 2–3 years in patients deemed suitable for surveillance. Patients are always encouraged to report interval symptoms (i.e. heartburn, dysphagia, etc.).

3. (a) To be able to stop using omeprazole

The expectation of anti-reflux surgery would be that symptoms of reflux would be managed without the need for PPIs. In the immediate period after surgery some patients will experience dysphagia and 'gas-bloat' (aka 'trapped wind'). Most of these symptoms settle in time. Whether or not successful anti-reflux surgery reduces the risk of Barrett's is unproven and if it has been deemed appropriate for the patient to undergo surveillance this decision should not be altered by even clinically successful surgery.

Further reading: Chapter 118.

Case 25: A patient with a 6-month history of indigestion

1. (b) Analysis of stool

The blood test commonly relied upon for the diagnosis of *Helicobacter* is measurement of *Helicobacter*-specific IgG – this provides evidence of previous exposure to the bacteria. Helicobacter infection can be determined by a breath test but this relies upon the use of ^{14}C labelled urea which is split by the bacterial urease enzyme leading to the exhalation of ^{14}C labelled CO_2. Detection of *Helicobacter* antigens in stool has now become a routine diagnostic test for the infection.

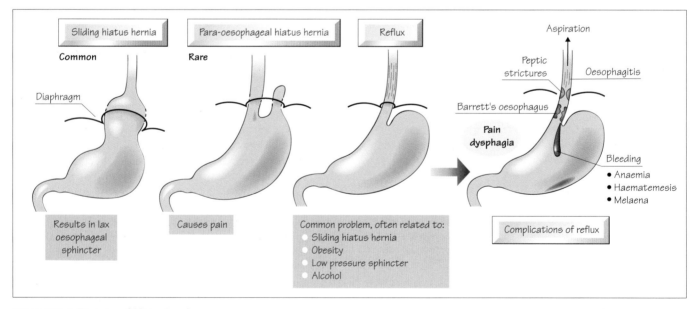

Figure 3.23.1 Features of hiatus hernia.

2. (b) Have a course of antibiotics

If *Helicobacter* is identified in a patient with 'dyspepsia' he should be offered eradication therapy with a combination of two antibiotics (including clarithromycin) and a high-dose proton pump inhibitor (PPI). Proof of eradication should be confirmed with a urease breath test.

3. (c) Have a 4-week trial of treatment with a PPI

In a significant number of patients the underlying cause for their indigestion symptoms is reflux. The NICE guidelines for the management of dyspepsia in primary advise trial of a PPI prior to any assessment by endoscopy.

Further reading: Chapter 119.

Case 26: A patient with indigestion and nausea

1. (a) Undergo urgent endoscopy

Dyspepsia with weight loss, anaemia and/or history of previous gastric surgery is an indication for urgent endoscopy. The reason being that there is a significant chance that he may have a malignancy, such as gastric cancer. The risk factors for gastric cancer include:

- Pernicious anaemia
- Vagotomy
- Partial gastrectomy–the most likely surgery for our patient
- Dietary factors; including low fruit diet, high intake of preserved food, high alcohol consumption, smoking
- *H. pylori* infection doubles the risk, and the risk is even higher with cagA positive *Helicobacter pylori*.
- Obesity increases the risk about two-fold.

2. (c) Eating small meals

It is most likely that his ulcer surgery constituted a partial gastrectomy and by removing the gastric antrum it is likely that he produces less gastric acid. However, he will have a small residual stomach and would be advised to take small but frequent meals.

3. (a) Total gastrectomy

Most gastrointestinal cancers, if found prior to the development of distal metastases, are best treated with surgery. Most gastrointestinal cancers are adenocarcinoma and have very limited response to radiotherapy. The role of chemotherapy for most gut tumours is restricted to either adjuvant regimes or palliation.

Further reading: Chapter 130.

Case 27: A man with abnormal liver blood tests

1. (c) Fatty liver

A 'bright' liver on ultrasound is typical of fatty change. There were no particular features of chronic liver disease in the report (such as irregular liver outline, patchy echogenicity, splenomegaly). Ultrasound signal does not alter significantly in iron overload although this can be identified on CT and/or MRI.

2. (a) Fasting transferring saturation

Haemochromatosis is defined as primary iron overload and measurements of iron excess such as a raised transferrin saturation and/or a raised ferritin are the best diagnostic tests. HFE mutation analysis is useful for cascade screening for haemochromatosis (i.e. identifying other affected family members). Zinc protoporphyrin is elevated in iron deficiency but not of use in assessing iron overload.

3. (a) Hepatitis C

Although he has no declared risk factors for hepatitis C up to 10% of infected patients have an apparently idiopathic infection. Hepatitis C is potentially curable with combination antiviral treatment and if undetected carries an increased risk of cirrhosis and primary liver cancer. Depending on where in the world the patient was born and brought up it would also be worth screening for hepatitis B. Hepatitis A and Hepatitis E each cause acute liver inflammation but neither is associated with chronic liver disease.

4. (b) To lose weight

Fatty liver is associated with centripetal obesity and if he were to lose weight it is likely that his liver enzyme abnormalities might well resolve. Moreover he will reduce his future risk of hypertension, diabetes and vascular disease. There is insufficient evidence to advise him at this stage of changing his sexual practices. Milk thistle is promoted in health food shops as being beneficial in liver diseases. There is no clinical evidence to support this.

Further reading: Chapter 122.

Case 28: A woman with abnormal liver blood tests

1. (c) That the raised alkaline phosphatase (ALP) is of liver origin

γ-GT is useful in confirming that a raised alkaline phosphatase is of liver and not bony origin. It is not a reliable indicator of alcohol consumption.

2. (c) Anti-mitochondrial antibody (AMA)

Anti-mitochondrial antibody (and in particular the M2 isoform) is typical of PBC. Many patients are now diagnosed with this autoimmune condition at an asymptomatic phase. ANA and SMA are associated with autoimmune hepatitis (AIH).

3. (c) Information leaflets on the nature of the condition

PBC is a chronic disease, often with many years before the development of symptoms or physical signs. It is imperative that the patient is provided with information regarding the condition and its usual natural history. A biopsy is no longer considered mandatory although would be considered if there were atypical features of her illness. Immunosuppressants are of no proven benefit in PBC. Treatment is more commonly with the synthetic bile acid ursodeoxycholic acid.

Further reading: Chapter 127.

Case 29: A patient with epigastric pain and vomiting

1. (c) None

In the context of the clinical history a three-fold elevation of serum amylase is diagnostic of acute pancreatitis. However, had there been doubt about the diagnoses, for example, due to there being a non-diagnostic rise in amylase, then it would be crucial to consider other diagnoses, for example, ruptured abdominal aortic aneurysm (AAA). In most centres, AAA are best diagnosed with abdominal CT rather than abdominal ultrasound examination.

2. (a) $pO_2 < 8\,kPa$

Hypoxia is a poor prognostic sign and implies intrapulmonary shunting and may herald adult respiratory distress syndrome (ARDS).

3. (a) Ultrasound on the day of admission

Urgent ultrasound is indicated to look for gallbladder stones and/or evidence of common bile duct dilatation. In severe gallstone pancreatitis ERCP might be indicated but this is best

Assessment of severity of pancreatitis	
White cell count	> 15 x 10⁹/L
Urea	> 16 mmol/L
Calcium	< 2.0 mmol/L
Albumin	< 32 g/L
Glucose	> 10 mmol/L
PO₂	< 8 kPa
Aspartate transaminase	> 200 U/L
Lactate dehydrogenase	> 600 U/L
C-reactive protein	> 150 mg/L

Figure 3.29.1 Markers of severe pancreatitis.

performed within the first 24–48 hours. CT is best undertaken between 7–10 days and should if possible be contrast enhanced to determine the extent of pancreatic necrosis.

4. (c) Cholecystectomy

Cholecystectomy should be performed early after a severe gallstone pancreatitis and preferably on the same admission. ERCP and endoscopic sphincterotomy may be considered in patients deemed unfit for gallbladder surgery. Pancreatitis is a risk of ERCP.
Further reading: Chapter 125.

Case 30: A patient with epigastric pain and weight loss

1. (b) Fat malabsorption

He presents with features of steatorrhoea and is likely to have exocrine pancreatic insufficiency due to a deficiency of lytic enzymes secreted from the pancreas.

2. (b) Pancreatic glandular calcification

Calcification is a typical feature of chronic pancreatic disease and may even be seen on plain abdominal X-ray. Oedema of the pancreas is more typical in acute pancreatitis. Pancreas divisum is an embryological fault resulting from failure of fusion of the ventral and dorsal pancreatic buds.

3. (b) Pancreatic enzyme supplements

He has features of exocrine pancreatic insufficiency and is likely to need pancreatic supplements long term. Although he might ultimately manage with oral diabetic agents his presentation with weight loss and ketosis implies that he should be treated with insulin in the first instance.
Further reading: Chapter 125.

Case 31: A patient with severe abdominal pain

1. (a) Charcot's triad

The combination of pain, jaundice and fever is known as Charcot's triad and is typical of cholangitis. Murphy's sign is right upper quadrant tenderness exacerbated by inspiration and is a feature of cholecystitis. Saint's triad is the association of gallstones, hiatal hernia and diverticular change.

2. (b) Dilated bile ducts

The presence of gallbladder stones would not be unusual in an 85 year old and would not necessarily change your immediate approach to management. The presence of a dilated biliary system would be supportive of obstruction even if a stone was not visible within the common bile. The sensitivity of ultrasound is less for abnormalities deep within the abdomen such as at the lower end of the bile duct and the pancreas.

3. (c) Endoscopic retrograde cholangiopancreatography (ERCP)

ERCP would be the treatment of choice and even if cholecystectomy were to be considered, this would have to be deferred until the biliary obstruction had been addressed.
Further reading: Chapter 126.

Case 32: A man with acute pancreatitis

1. (c) MRI

A magnetic resonance cholangiogram (MRCP) would determine whether or not he had any stones or debris within the distal common bile duct. Endoscopic ultrasound would be an alternative option.

2. (a) A low-fat diet

A low-fat diet might give him some short-term relief. Fat stimulates gallbladder and bile duct contraction through the secretion of cholecystokinin. This might typically reduce gallstone symptoms. No drug treatment or dietary intervention will lead to gallstone dissolution.

3. (b) Have an elective cholecystectomy

He should undergo any intervention that would significantly reduce his risk of a further attack and provided he has no residual stones in his bile duct he would be well advised to have his gallbladder removed.
Further reading: Chapter 126.

Case 33: A former drug user on a methadone programme

1. (a) That he does not have hepatitis B

Hepatitis B surface antigen remains the most widely used marker of chronic HBV infection. Although he has antibodies to HCV, 10–15% of individuals exposed to HCV generate a sufficient immune response to clear the virus. He should be tested with an HCV PCR (polymerase chain reaction) which measures viral RNA and is the only way to determine chronic infection. If he has HCV he could still have significant liver fibrosis despite normal liver transaminases.

2. (a) α-Interferon

α-Interferon in combination with ribavirin has the potential to achieve a 'sustained viral response' (SVR) or 'cure' in up to two-thirds of patients. Lamivudine and adefovir are licensed for the treatment of HBV.

3. (a) Determined by the viral genotype

Combination treatment regimes are tailored to the viral genotype. Genotype 1 is most resistant to antiviral therapy and requires 48 weeks of treatment. Most non-1 genotypes (i.e. type 2 and 3) are adequately treated with 24 weeks of treatment and it is hoped that in time even shorter treatment regimes may be facilitated by more intensive monitoring of viral load and the development of newer antiviral drugs.

4. (c) Abstain from alcohol

Alcohol is a co-factor for most forms of liver injury and reduced viral response rates are likely if patients drink heavily during treatment. It is good advice for the patient to exercise regularly, although this is unlikely to have any specific influence on his treatment outcome. Milk thistle is of no proven benefit although many patients with liver disease take it.

Further reading: Chapter 127.

Case 34: A jaundiced woman with profound fatigue

1. (a) Autoimmune hepatitis

A subacute presentation of an inflammatory hepatitis with evidence of immune activation would support a working diagnosis of autoimmune hepatitis. Primary biliary cirrhosis is a chronic cholestatic liver disease. Haemochromatosis rarely presents with jaundice and would be effectively excluded by the normal iron indices.

2. (a) Antinuclear antibody(ANA)

Antinuclear antibody is most frequently associated with autoimmune hepatitis. Anti-neutrophil cytoplasmic antibody is associated with primary sclerosing cholangitis and anti-mitochondrial antibody defines primary biliary cirrhosis.

3. (a) Liver biopsy

Although a transthoracic liver biopsy is contraindicated (coagulopathy, ascites), histology is essential for the patient's management and a biopsy should be performed via the transjugular route.

4. (c) Steroids need to be started

Even if on the biopsy the patient has an established cirrhosis autoimmune hepatitis is very sensitive to steroids and these should be started without delay. Primary biliary cirrhosis is the autoimmune condition of the liver in which steroids are not used.

Further reading: Chapter 127.

Case 35: A man with no symptoms whose brother has haemochromatosis

1. (c) He is likely to have haemochromatosis

Provided the iron indices were performed in the fasting state, the tests demonstrate iron overload (raised ferritin and transferring saturation >90%). There is no evidence of end organ injury.

2. (c) HH/YY

Homozygosity for C282Y is strongly associated with haemochromatosis. Compound heterozygosity (one copy of C282Y and one copy of H63D or HD/CY) does increase the risk of iron loading but is not strongly associated with classical haemochromatosis.

3. (a) Start venesection treatment

The key to improving the prognosis in haemochromatosis is early detection and treatment. Although in the past the diagnosis relied on the demonstration of excess liver iron, it is now recognized that in C282Y homozygotes without abnormal liver enzymes or hepatomegaly and with a ferritin of less than 1000, the risk of them having significant liver fibrosis is low.

4. (a) Testing them for HFE mutations

In a pedigree in which the genotype of the proband is known, cascade screening is possible using mutation analysis. This approach is likely to identify individuals 'at risk' of iron loading. Advice regarding future monitoring can then be tailored to the individual.

Further reading: Chapter 129.

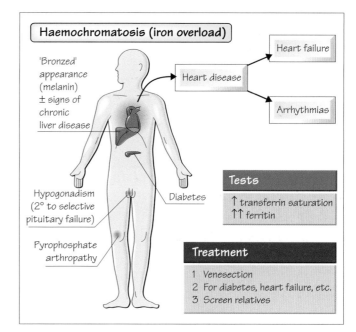

Figure 3.35.1 Features of haemochromatosis.

Case 36: A woman who drinks heavily and has had a seizure

1. (b) Oral chlordiazepoxide

She needs sedation to prevent another seizure or development of acute confusion. This is best given orally and titrated to the clinical response. Intravenous vitamins are an important element in her early treatment but will not alter her risk of seizures. Intramuscular injections should be avoided inpatients with coagulopathy and major tranquilizers such as haloperidol if anything lower patients' seizure threshold and make fits more likely.

2. (c) An ascitic tap

A high-protein ascitic fluid with >250 nucleated cells per ml is diagnostic of SBP. Patients should not have antibiotics withheld pending positive culture results.

3. (a) Steroids

Steroids are proven to benefit *selected* patients with acute alcoholic hepatitis. The benefit is limited to those with very severe inflammatory disease (discriminant function >32, Glasgow alcoholic hepatitis score >9). Patients with acute alcoholic hepatitis fare very badly with transplantation. MARS (molecular adsorbents recirculating system) therapy, a form of artificial liver, may be beneficial as a temporizing treatment in patients with fulminant liver failure but has no proven role in acute alcoholic hepatitis.

Further reading: Chapter 129.

Case 37: A man with dysphagia and weight loss

1. (a) Discussion of his case at an upper gastrointestinal cancer multidisciplinary team meeting (MDT)

EUS is of limited benefit in patients with circumferential and stenosing cancers. Likewise the benefit of traditional 'staging' investigation in a patient who is unlikely to be a good

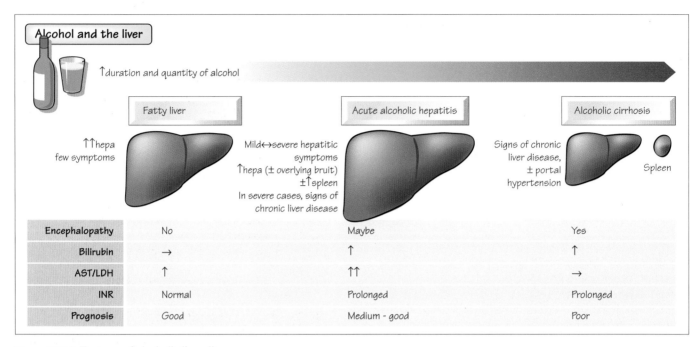

Figure 3.36.1 Features of alcoholic liver disease.

	Fatty liver	Acute alcoholic hepatitis	Alcoholic cirrhosis
Encephalopathy	No	Maybe	Yes
Bilirubin	→	↑	↑
AST/LDH	↑	↑↑	→
INR	Normal	Prolonged	Prolonged
Prognosis	Good	Medium - good	Poor

surgical candidate is low. His case should be discussed in an MDT meeting.

2. (b) Sip feeds

A high-calorie liquid diet should be advised pending a definitive treatment plan. Although TPN might benefit some patients pending surgery for upper GI cancer, the benefits do not outweigh the risks in patients in whom surgery is not deemed appropriate. Malignant dysphagia is not a good indication for PEG feeding.

3. (a) Placement of an oesophageal stent

Chemotherapy is unlikely to help his symptoms and although squamous cancers of the oesophagus may respond to radiotherapy, dysphagia might get worse due to tumour oedema or get no better due to scarring. A self-expanding metal stent can be placed either endoscopically or radiologically. This does not return the patients swallowing to normal but does give good relief of dysphagia.
Further reading: Chapter 130.

4 Renal: Cases and Questions

Case 1: A patient with polyuria

A 65-year-old man is getting up at night three times to pass urine, feels thirsty and is passing a lot of urine during the day.

1. *What blood tests should be requested, with what possible diagnosis in mind?*
   (a) Glucose for diabetes insipidus
   (b) Calcium for hypocalcaemia
   (c) Urea/creatinine for chronic renal failure
   (d) Plasma osmolality for syndrome of inappropriate antidiuretic hormone secretion (SIADH)

Case 2: A patient with oliguria

An 80-year-old man has only passed 100 mL of urine since an operation for a perforated duodenal ulcer 18 hours ago. You insert a urethral catheter but no urine is produced.

1. *Which of the following medications or procedures could have adversely affected renal function?*
   (a) Gentamicin
   (b) A contrast-enhanced CT scan 3 days ago
   (c) Ibuprofen
   (d) Lisinopril
   (e) All of the above
2. *Which of the following are suggestive of hypovolaemia?*
   (a) A rise in pulse rate from 80 beats/min lying to 120 beats/min standing
   (b) A central venous pressure of +20 mmHg
   (c) A jugular venous pressure of +9 cm above the sternal angle at 45 degrees
   (d) Pulmonary oedema on a chest X-ray

Case 3: A patient with dysuria

A 23-year-old woman is known to have a solitary right kidney and has become unwell with a fever (39°C), rigors and pain in her back and right loin. Her sister has had previous episodes of renal calculi. Urine microscopy shows >100 000 white cells/mL.

1. *What tests should be arranged urgently?*
   (a) Urine microscopy for casts
   (b) MRI of her back
   (c) 24-hour urinary calcium
   (d) Blood and urine cultures

Case 4: A patient with haematuria

A 40-year-old woman presents to A&E with a 3-day history of passing blood-stained urine. She has no pain or dysuria but is starting to feel nauseous. Her serum creatinine is 500 µmol/L.

1. *What features would suggest glomerulonephritis as a cause of her presentation?*
   (a) Urinary white cells
   (b) Negative urine dipstick for proteinuria
   (c) Hyaline casts
   (d) Coughing up blood (haemoptysis)

Case 5: A patient with diabetes and anaemia

An 82-year-old woman is referred with a creatinine of 322 µmol/L. She has had diabetes mellitus and hypertension for 20 years. Her urine contains 5 g of protein in 24 h, her serum albumin is 23 g/L and she has swelling of her legs. Her haemoglobin is 8.7 g/dL.

1. *Her glomerular filtration rate (GFR) is likely to be which of the following?*
   (a) >100 mL/min
   (b) <10 mL/min
   (c) 10–30 mL/min
   (d) 30–60 mL/min
2. *The measurement of creatinine clearance requires knowledge of which of the following?*
   (a) Urine protein
   (b) Serum creatinine, urine creatinine and 24-hour urine volume
   (c) Serum creatinine, serum albumin and 24-hour urine volume
   (d) Weight, age, serum creatinine, urine creatinine and 24-hour urine volume
3. *The patient is most likely to be suffering from which condition?*
   (a) Nephrotic syndrome
   (b) Nephritic syndrome
   (c) Congestive cardiac failure
   (d) Hypertensive nephropathy
4. *What is her anaemia likely to be due to?*
   (a) Iron deficiency
   (b) Diabetes mellitus
   (c) Deficient erythropoietin production
   (d) α_1-Hydroxylated vitamin D deficiency

Case 6: A patient with hyperkalaemia

A 41-year-old woman is unwell and presents to A&E. She has a 12-year history of hypertension and is on multiple medications. Blood tests show advanced renal failure with a creatinine of 789 µmol/L and a potassium of 7.2 mmol/L.

1. *Which of the following urgent treatments should be instituted?*
   (a) Frusemide (furosemide) infusion and dopamine
   (b) Intravenous calcium gluconate, intravenous glucose and insulin
   (c) Intravenous saline infusion
   (d) β-Blockers and calcium infusion
2. *The ECG signs of hyperkalaemia include which of the following?*
   (a) J waves
   (b) U waves
   (c) Peaked T waves
   (d) Short PR interval
3. *Which of the following medications are associated with an increased risk of hyperkalaemia?*
   (a) Lisinopril
   (b) Frusemide
   (c) Atenolol
   (d) Metformin

Case 7: A patient with hyponatraemia

A 71-year-old woman is recovering from an operation and is noted to have a serum sodium of 116 mmol/L, a potassium of 4.0 mmol/l, a urea of 8.0 mmol/L and a glucose of 5 mmol/L. She has marked peripheral oedema, an underactive thyroid (thyroid-stimulating hormone (TSH) is 23 mU/L), her jugular venous pressure is elevated and she is on frusemide (furosemide) 80 mg/day.

1. *What is her serum osmolality ?*
   (a) 153 milli-osmoles/kg
   (b) 253 milli-osmoles/kg
   (c) 249 milli-osmoles/kg
   (d) 116 milli-osmoles/kg

2. *What is this patient suffering from?*
   (a) Syndrome of inappropriate antidiuretic hormone secretion (SIADH) due to frusemide
   (b) SIADH
   (c) SIADH due to a postoperative pneumonia
   (d) None of the above

3. *She is mildly confused. What rate of correction of sodium should be aimed for?*
   (a) 1 mmol/hour
   (b) 2 mmol/hour
   (c) 0.5 mmol/hour
   (d) 5 mmol/hour

Case 8: A patient with a disorder of acid–base balance

A 58-year-old man is admitted to the ITU with coma and arterial blood gases showing a pH of 7.05, PCO_2 of 2.9 kPa and PO_2 of 11 kPa.

1. *Which of the following diagnoses are possible?*
   (a) Respiratory alkalosis with compensatory metabolic acidosis
   (b) Metabolic acidosis with compensatory respiratory alkalosis
   (c) Metabolic alkalosis
   (d) Respiratory failure

2. *Which of the following causes of this presentation are possible?*
   (a) Diabetic ketoacidosis
   (b) Milk alkali syndrome
   (c) Guillain–Barré syndrome
   (d) Vomiting due to pyloric stenosis

3. *His sodium is 140 mmol/L, chloride 98 mmol/L and bicarbonate 12 mmol/L. What is the anion gap?*
   (a) 10
   (b) 12
   (c) 22
   (d) 30

4. *Which of the following anions in the blood might explain this raised anion gap?*
   (a) Ketones
   (b) Bicarbonate
   (c) Chloride
   (d) Sodium valproate

Case 9: A patient with a urinary calculus

A 34-year-old man presents with an episode of renal colic.

1. *Which of the following tests could be undertaken to look for the aetiology of the calculus?*
   (a) Urinary Bence Jones protein
   (b) 24-hour urinary urinary calcium
   (c) Urinary vitamin B_6
   (d) Urinary copper

2. *He is found to have an elevated serum calcium. Which of the following diagnoses are possible?*
   (a) Hypoparathyroidism
   (b) Sarcoidosis
   (c) Hypothyroidism
   (d) Cystinuria

3. *Which of the following measures are recommended to reduce the occurrence of further calculi?*
   (a) Increase fluid intake to >3 L/day
   (b) Increase dietary intake of protein
   (c) Increase dietary sodium intake
   (d) Increase dietary oxalate

4. *Which of the following is a cause, with appropriate specific treatment, for renal calculi?*
   (a) Cystinuria: penicillamine
   (b) Hypercalciuria: thiazide diuretics
   (c) Urate calculi: allopurinol
   (d) All of the above

Case 10: A patient with nephrotic syndrome

A 33-year-old woman has developed marked swelling of her legs and a dipstick of urine shows a protein of +++, quantified at 10 g in 24 hours. Her creatinine is normal (72 μmol/L).

1. *What additional test is required to make a diagnosis of the nephrotic syndrome?*
   (a) Elevated serum cholesterol
   (b) Low serum albumin
   (c) Haematuria
   (d) Positive cytoplasmic antineutrophil cytoplasmic antibody (cANCA)

2. *Additional blood tests reveal elevated antinuclear antibodies and low complement components C3 and C4. What is the patient likely to be suffering from?*
   (a) Mesangiocapillary glomerulonephritis
   (b) Systemic lupus erythematosus (SLE)
   (c) Minimal change glomerulonephritis
   (d) IgA nephropathy

3. *Patients with the nephrotic syndrome are at risk of which of the following complications?*
   (a) Pulmonary embolism
   (b) Myeloma
   (c) Rheumatoid arthritis
   (d) Thyrotoxicosis

Case 11: A patient with glomerulonephritis

An 82-year-old woman becomes unwell and blood tests reveal renal failure with a creatinine of 667 μmol/L, although the latter was normal 5 days previously. A renal biopsy is performed.

1. *Which of the following histology findings are most consistent with this history?*
   (a) Amyloid
   (b) Diabetic nephropathy
   (c) Crescentic glomerulonephritis
   (d) Minimal change glomerulonephritis

Case 12: A man with heavy proteinuria and low serum protein

A 42-year-old man develops ankle swelling and tests reveal a creatinine of 72 μmol/L, serum albumin of 22 g/L and urinary protein loss of 8 g in 24 hours. He undergoes a renal biopsy.

1. *What are the possible histological diagnoses?*
   (a) Minimal change glomerulonephritis
   (b) Tubulointerstitial nephritis
   (c) Crescentic nephritis
   (d) Granuloma

Case 13: A patient with red cells in his urine

A 23-year-old man is found to have red cells in his urine on dipstick examination as part of a medical for entrance to the RAF. There is also one + of protein and his creatinine is 68 μmol/L.

1. *A renal biopsy is most likely to show which of the following?*
   (a) Amyloid
   (b) IgA nephropathy
   (c) Alport's syndrome
   (d) Wegener's granulomatosis

Case 14: A patient with general aches and nose bleeds

A 60-year-old man has been feeling unwell for the last month with general aches and pains and nose bleeds. Blood tests have revealed renal impairment with a creatinine of 330 μmol/L; his urine dipstick shows a blood of +++ and protein of +++.

1. *What blood test would point towards a diagnosis of Wegener's granulomatosis?*
   (a) Antineutrophil cytoplasmic antibodies (ANCA)
   (b) Anti scl-70 antibodies
   (c) Anti-Ro antibodies
   (d) Elevated complement levels (C3 and C4)
2. *A renal biopsy shows a crescentic nephritis. Which of the following treatments should be used?*
   (a) Cyclophosphamide and plasma exchange
   (b) Cyclophosphamide, plasma exchange, corticosteroids and chloroquine
   (c) Anticoagulation, cyclophosphamide, plasma exchange and corticosteroids
   (d) Cyclophosphamide, plasma exchange and corticosteroids

Case 15: A patient with a possible hereditary renal disorder

A 38-year-old man is seen in the outpatient clinic. He is concerned that he might have polycystic kidneys because his father had the condition and died suddenly of a stroke at the age of 56 years.

1. *What are the chances of him having the condition?*
   (a) 25%
   (b) 50%
   (c) 66%
   (d) 20%
2. *What causes of sudden death are more likely in patients with polycystic kidney disease?*
   (a) Subarachnoid haemorrhage
   (b) Ventricular tachycardia
   (c) Myocardial infarction
   (d) Cyst haemorrhage
3. *What diagnostic test should be undertaken to establish whether he has inherited polycystic kidney disease?*
   (a) Gene testing for mutations of polycystin-1
   (b) Renal ultrasound
   (c) Renal biopsy
   (d) Skin biopsy

Case 16: A patient with tubulointerstitial disease

A 48-year-old woman is found to have mild renal impairment during investigations for headache and malaise. She is taking ibuprofen, ranitidine, simvastatin, vitamin D and vitamin C.

1. *Which of the following features point towards a diagnosis of interstitial nephritis rather than a glomerulonephritis?*
   (a) Eosinophilia
   (b) Red cell casts in urine
   (c) 4 g/day proteinuria
   (d) A blood pressure of 190/105 mm/Hg
2. *During investigations she is found to have a single kidney. How common is this congenital variant?*
   (a) 1 in 10
   (b) 1 in 10 000
   (c) 1 in 1000
   (d) 1 in 5000
3. *Which of the following medications is the most likely culprit for interstitial nephritis?*
   (a) Vitamin C
   (b) Ibuprofen
   (c) Ranitidine
   (d) Simvastatin

Case 17: A patient with acute renal failure

A 25-year-old man has become rapidly unwell with diarrhoea, nausea, vomiting and breathlessness. Blood tests show a creatinine of 870 μmol/L.

1. *What other blood results should be sought urgently?*
   (a) Potassium, arterial blood gases and haemoglobin
   (b) Magnesium, phosphate and haemoglobin
   (c) Prostate-specific antigen and protein electrophoresis
   (d) Creatine kinase and troponin
2. *Additional blood tests show a platelet count of $33 \times 10^9/L$ and a Hb of 7.3 g/dL. Suggest a possible unifying diagnosis.*
   (a) Polycystic kidney disease
   (b) Acute lymphoblastic leukaemia
   (c) Haemolytic uraemic syndrome (HUS)
   (d) Myeloma
3. *Which of the following are indications for immediate dialysis treatment?*
   (a) Potassium of 5.5 mmol/L
   (b) Potassium of 7.2 mmol/L
   (c) pH of 7.35
   (d) Anaemia
4. *State which of the following are ECG changes of hyperkalaemia.*
   (a) J waves
   (b) U waves
   (c) Peaked T waves
   (d) All of the above

Case 18: A patient with chronic renal failure and dialysis

A 60-year-old man has been suffering from renal failure for many years and his creatinine has risen to 770 μmol/L. He weighs 68 kg.

1. *Which of the following symptoms might be due to his renal failure?*

(a) Vomiting, itch, nausea and impotence

(b) Jaundice, vomiting, itch, nausea and impotence

(c) Hiccoughs, vomiting, itch, nausea, impotence and breathlessness

(d) Iritis, vomiting, itch, nausea and impotence

2. *Investigations show anaemia with an Hb of 8.8 g/dL, a calcium of 1.9 mmol/L and a phosphate of 2.8 mmol/L. What treatment should he should receive?*

(a) Erythropoietin, α_1-hydroxylated vitamin D and calcium carbonate

(b) Erythropoietin, vitamin D and magnesium chloride

(c) Vitamin D and magnesium chloride

(d) Erythropoietin, vitamin D and calcium carbonate

3. *He is a candidate for renal replacement therapy with which of the following?*

(a) Cadaveric renal transplant, living related renal transplant, automated peritoneal dialysis, haemodialysis or continuous ambulatory peritoneal dialysis (CAPD)

(b) Automated pertoneal dialysis or haemodialysis

(c) Haemodialysis or CAPD

(d) Cadaveric renal transplant, living related renal transplant, automated peritoneal dialysis or haemodialysis

4. *What is his glomerular filtration rate (GFR) likely to be?*

(a) 20–30 mL/min

(b) 30–40 mL/min

(c) <15 mL/min

(d) 15–20 mL/min

Case 19: A patient with a renal transplant

A 41-year-old man received a kidney transplant from his brother 3 weeks ago for renal failure due to focal segmental glomerulosclerosis. His creatinine has been running in the range 120–125 μmol/L but has now risen to 190 μmol/L. He is taking prednisolone, tacrolimus, mycophenolate, aspirin and co-trimoxazole.

1. *State which of the following causes of impaired transplant function are possible.*

(a) Rejection, tacrolimus toxicity or mycophenolate toxicity

(b) Rejection, tacrolimus toxicity, mycophenolate toxicity or recurrent renal disease

(c) Rejection, tacrolimus toxicity or recurrent renal disease

(d) Tacrolimus toxicity, mycophenolate toxicity or recurrent renal disease

2. *He has a serum glucose of 12 mmol/L. Which of the following medications are associated with an enhanced incidence of diabetes mellitus post transplant?*

(a) Prednisolone, tacrolimus

(b) Mycophenolate, co-trimoxazole, aspirin

(c) Mycophenolate, co-trimoxazole

(d) Tacrolimus, aspirin

3. *Over the next 15 years, he is at substantially greater risk of which of the following?*

(a) Lymphoma and myocardial infarction

(b) Prostate cancer

(c) Prostate cancer and ulcerative colitis

(d) Thyrotoxicosis and systemic lupus erythematosus

4. *Following treatment, his renal function improves to a creatinine of 110 μmol/L. What is the chance of his transplant kidney working in 10 years' time?*

(a) 10–30%

(b) 20–30%

(c) 30–50%

(d) Over 60%

Case 20: Drugs and renal failure

You are contacted by the pharmacist in another hospital; she has a 68-year-old patient who has had abdominal surgery for colonic malignancy, and she is concerned about whether the drugs he is on are appropriate given his increasing creatinine.

1. *Which of the following drugs are excreted by the kidney and may accumulate dangerously in renal failure?*

(a) Gentamicin, digoxin, paracetamol

(b) Gentamicin, paracetamol, lithium, ferrous sulphate

(c) Lithium, digoxin, gentamicin, aciclovir

(d) Lithium, digoxin, ferrous sulphate

2. *Which of the following drugs can cause renal impairment and should be used in caution in patients with renal failure?*

(a) Erythropoietin, ferrous sulphate, angiotensin-converting enzyme (ACE) inhibitors

(b) α_1-Vitamin D, calcium carbonate

(c) Non-steroidal anti-inflammatory drugs (NSAIDs), cyclosporine, ACE inhibitors

(d) β-Blockers, erythropoietin, ferrous sulphate

Case 21: A patient with renal failure

A 64-year-old man with a creatinine of 330 μmol/L presents with a urinary tract infection and is given IV gentamicin. He is taking lisinopril and candesartan for blood pressure control, frusemide (furosemide) and spironolactone for heart failure, insulin for control of diabetes and simvastatin. He is given paracetamol and ibuprofen for pain relief and undergoes a CT scan of his abdomen with contrast. The next day his creatinine is 580 μmol/L.

1. *What agents may have contributed to the worsening of his renal failure?*

(a) Lisinopril, contrast, ibuprofen

(b) Lisinopril, contrast, ibuprofen, candesartan, gentamicin, insulin, paracetamol

(c) Lisinopril, contrast, ibuprofen, candesartan, gentamicin, simvastatin

(d) Lisinopril, contrast, ibuprofen, candesartan, gentamicin

2. *His potassium is 7.2 mmol/L. Which of the following agents are likely to have contributed to the hyperkalaemia?*

(a) Lisinopril, candesartan, spironolactone, frusemide

(b) Lisinopril, candesartan, spironolactone

(c) Lisinopril, candesartan, spironolactone, insulin

(d) Lisinopril, candesartan

Case 22: A patient with benign prostatic hypertrophy

A 74-year-old man has noted increasing difficulty passing urine, nocturia and general malaise. Blood tests show a prostrate-specific antigen (PSA) of 12 and a serum creatinine of 670 μmol/L.

1. *What other tests should be undertaken?*

(a) Renal tract ultrasound

(b) Plain abdominal X-ray

(c) Urine microscopy and culture

(d) Serum calcium

2. *He is offered but declines a transurethral resection of the prostate (TURP) operation. What drug treatments could be considered for benign prostatic hypertrophy?*
   (a) Finasteride
   (b) Frusemide (furosemide)
   (c) Gonadotrophin-releasing hormone (GnRH) analogues
   (d) Testosterone
3. *What test should be undertaken to examine for prostate cancer metastases?*
   (a) Chest X ray
   (b) CT of the head
   (c) Bone scan
   (d) Bone marrow

Case 23: A patient with a urinary tract infection

A 24-year-old woman has had thirst, polyuria, fevers and malaise for 5 days. A urine sample contains blood, protein, nitrite and leucocyte on dipstick testing. A specimen is sent for microscopy and culture. She had one previous urinary tract infection (UTI) 5 years ago.

1. *What other test should be undertaken?*
   (a) CT urogram
   (b) Blood glucose
   (c) Cystoscopy
   (d) Chest X-ray for tuberculosis
2. *Bacteria are seen on microscopy. Which of the following antibiotic treatments is appropriate?*
   (a) Intravenous gentamicin
   (b) Ciprofloxacin for 21 days
   (c) Oral amoxicillin for 5 days
   (d) Isoniazid
3. *She subsequently develops eight UTIs with Escherichia coli over the next 18 months. What tests should be undertaken?*
   (a) Tests for immunodeficiency and serum urea
   (b) Renal tract ultrasound and serum creatinine
   (c) Mantoux test and early morning urine
   (d) Urinary cystine and serum creatinine

Renal: Answers

Case 1: A patient with polyuria

1. (c) Urea/creatinine for chronic renal failure

Chronic renal failure can present with polyuria and nocturia and be detected by measurements of urea and creatinine. Polyuria can also be produced by elevated glucose in diabetes mellitus and in hypercalcaemia.

Further reading: Chapter 34 in Medicine at a Glance.

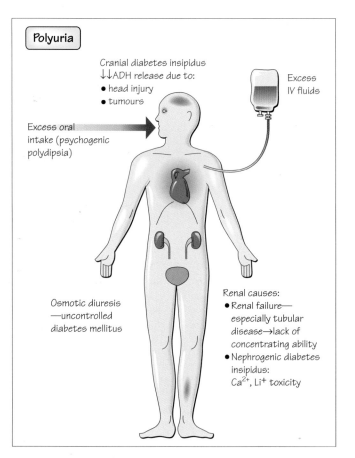

Figure 4.1.1 Features and causes of polyuria.

Case 2: A patient with oliguria

1. (e) All of the above

Gentamicin is a direct nephrotoxin. Ibuprofen a non-steroidal anti-inflammatory drug (NSAID) and lisinopril is an angiotensin-converting enzyme (ACE) inhibitor, both of which can jeopardize renal perfusion. The administration of radiographic contrast can produce deterioration in renal function known as contrast nephropathy.

2. (a) A rise in pulse rate from 80 beats/min lying to 120 beats/min standing

Tachycardia on standing is a sign of at least moderate hypovolaemia; the other clinical sign suggesting hypovolaemia is a postural fall in blood pressure, and this should always be measured in patients suspected of being fluid depleted. The other findings suggest fluid overload.

Further reading: Chapter 34.

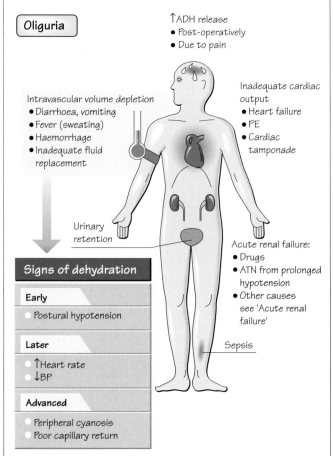

Figure 4.2.1 Clinical features of oliguria.

Case 3: A patient with dysuria

1. (d) Blood and urine cultures

The history suggests the likelihood of a pyelonephritis affecting her solitary kidney which might be obstructed. It will be vital to obtain a microbiological diagnosis with cultures to guide antibiotics. Imaging of the renal tract is required, most likely with ultrasound in the first instance. The concern is that she may have an obstructed and infected kidney with irreversible loss of renal substance.

Further reading: Chapter 35.

Case 4: A patient with haematuria

1. (d) Coughing up blood (haemoptysis)

The urinary features of glomerulonephritis are red cells, red cell casts, dysmorphic red cells and heavy proteinuria. There are several conditions in which renal failure and pulmonary haemorrhage occur, including Goodpasture's syndrome (antibasement membrane antibodies).

Further reading: Chapter 142.

Case 5: A patient with diabetes and anaemia

1. (c) 10–30 mL/min

The relationship between serum creatinine and glomerular filtration rate is shown in the graph below, for an 'average' patient:

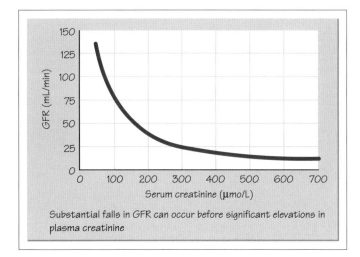

Substantial falls in GFR can occur before significant elevations in plasma creatinine

Figure 4.5.1 Relationship between GFR and creatinine.

There are however a number of problems with this, firstly, the normal GFR varies with age (falling by 7–10 mL/min for every decade increase in age from 20 years onward), secondly the relationship between GFR and creatinine is altered by body mass (particularly muscle): this can be accounted for by Cockcroft formula:

$$\text{Creatinine clearance, mL/min} = \{((140\text{-age}) \times \text{weight})/(72\ \text{Serum}_{\text{Creatinine}})\} \times 0.85 \text{ if female}$$

Related equations, derived from the Modification of Diet in Renal Disease (MDRD) study, do not use patients height or weight, and are now widely used to derive an estimated GFR. From the estimated GFR the "stage" of kidney disease can be determined according to Fig. 4.5.2 (from http://www.kidney.org/professionals/KLS/GFR.cfm#2). There are significant problems in such derived measures of GFR, the most important ones being that they all depend on patients being in a stable condition, without rapidly changing renal function (i.e. do not have acute renal failure) – this point is *crucial,* and is often forgotten – and secondly they assume that patients muscle mass is within the normal range, as gross deviations make the formulae ineffective.

2. (b) Serum creatinine, urine creatinine and 24-hour urine volume

Calculation of creatinine clearance is (urine volume ÷ urine creatinine) × plasma creatinine.

3. (a) Nephrotic syndrome

She has hypoalbuminaemia, nephrotic range proteinuria (4.5 g/24 hour) and oedema. Nephritic syndrome is acute renal impairment, usually considered to relate to a recent streptococcal sore throat, where the principle glomerular abnormalities are failure of filtration function and decreased ability to excrete salt and water (leading to fluid retention and hypertension). Protein loss is not a marked feature. Heart failure certainly can cause renal failure, though usually this is asymptomatic. However, heart failure sufficient to cause renal failure would have led to the heart failure symptoms, breathlessness, effort intolerance, not present here. Hypertensive nephropathy is not associated with this degree of proteinurea.

4. (c) Deficient erythropoietin production

At this low level of excretory renal function her kidneys are likely to be producing insufficient erythropoietin, and thus decreased production is likely to be the main mechanism explaining anaemia. However, the toxins that accumulate in renal failure are also known to shorten red cell lifespan, so

Stage	Glomerular filtration rate Values are normalized to an average surface area (size) of 1.73m²	Description	Management
I	90+	Normal renal function (but urinalysis, structural abnormalities or genetic factors indicate renal disease)	Observation and control of blood pressure
II	60–89	Mildly reduced renal function (Stage 2 CKD should not be diagnosed on GFR alone – but urinalysis, structural abnormalities or genetic factors indicate renal disease)	Observation, control of blood pressure and cardiovascular risk factors
IIIa	45–59	Moderate decrease in renal function, with or without other evidence of kidney damage	Observation, control of blood pressure and cardiovascular risk factors
IIIb	30–44	Moderate decrease in renal function, with or without other evidence of kidney damage	Observation, control of blood pressure and cardiovascular risk factors
IV	15–29	Severely reduced renal function	Planning for endstage renal failure
V	<15	Very severe (endstage) renal failure	Transplant or dialysis

Figure 4.5.2 Stages of chronic kidney disease. Use the suffix (p) to denote the presence of proteinuria when staging CKD.

decreased red cell survival may also be a contributory factor. Regardless, in most patients with this severity of renal failure, erythropoietin dramatically lessens anaemia and improves symptoms. Possible complications with erythropoietin therapy include: myalgia, 'flu like symptoms, hypertension, which may be severe.

Further reading: Chapter 140.

Case 6: A patient with hyperkalaemia

1. (b) Intravenous calcium gluconate, intravenous glucose and insulin

Hyperkalaemia requires immediate measures to stabilize the myocardium (intravenous calcium) and to lower the potassium (glucose/insulin enhance potassium uptake by cells). Failure to control hyperkalaemia promptly exposes patients to the risk of ventricular arrhythmias, especially if there is any 'structural' heart disease (such as left ventricular hypertrophy or coronary disease, clearly the former is quite likely in this woman with long standing hypertension). Should ventricular arrhythmias occur in this setting, leading to cardiac arrest, the patient is most unlikely to be successfully resuscitated until a normal or near normal potassium can be established.

2. (c) Peaked T waves

The ECG signs of hyperkalaemia are peaking of T waves, QRS widening, prolonged PR interval, loss of P waves and a sine wave appearance.

3. (a) Lisinopril

Angiotensin-converting enzyme (ACE) inhibitors, angiotensin II receptor blockers and spironolactone are the commonest drug causes of raised potassium. Loop diuretics such as frusemide tend to produce hypokalaemia.

Further reading: Chapter 136.

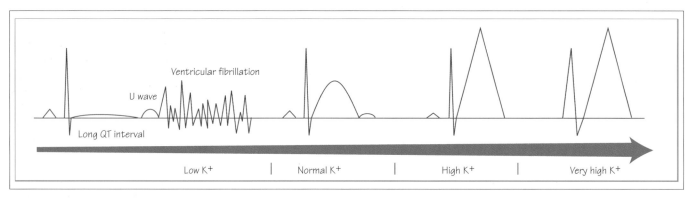

Figure 4.6.1 ECG features of hypo- and hyperkalaemia.

Case 7: A patient with hyponatraemia

1. (b) 253

Serum osmolality is calculated from: $(2 \times [Na]) + (2 \times [K]) +$ urea + glucose. A normal serum osmolality is 285–295 milli-osmoles/kg; in other words this patients serum is less osmotically active than normal.

2. (d) None of the above

The diagnostic criteria for SIADH are: (i) decreased osmolality; (ii) inappropriately concentrated urine; (iii) euvolaemia; (iv) elevated urinary sodium; and (v) no adrenal, thyroid or pituitary disease, and no renal dysfunction or diuretic use. This patient has oedema, abnormal thyroid function and is on diuretics and so does not have SIADH.

3. (c) 0.5 mmol/hour

Sodium should be corrected at less than 0.5 mmol/hour to prevent the development of central pontine myelinolysis. This is a rare potentially fatal complication of increasing serum sodium concentrations too rapidly in patients with chronic hyponatrae-mia. Those with high alcohol intakes are at greatest risk of the syndrome, as are those vitamin deficient for other reasons (e.g. hyperemisis gravidarum). Women are also at higher risk. CPM results in confusion (which can proceed to coma), spastic quadra-paresis, with eye signs, due to non-inflammatory damage to the pons. A locked-in syndrome can develop, which may not improve.

Further reading: Chapter 137.

Case 8: A patient with a disorder of acid–base balance

1. (b) Metabolic acidosis with compensatory respiratory alkalosis

The patient has an acidosis and a depressed CO_2 probably arising from compensatory hyperventilation.

2. (a) Diabetic ketoacidosis

Diabetic ketoacidosis is the only one of these conditions likely to produce a metabolic acidosis. Milk alkali syndrome, as the name suggests, leads to metabolic alkalosis due to the ingestion of excess amounts of alkali; likewise vomiting due to pyloric stenosis leads to loss of acid, and so a metabolic alkalosis. Guillain-Barré syn-drome can lead to type II respiratory failure (ventillatory failure), with hypercapnia, and so a respiratory acidosis, however, our patients pCO_2 is low, inconsistent with this being the diagnosis.

3. (d) 30

The anion gap is calculated as: [Na] – [Cl] – [bicarbonate]. The normal anion gap is 8-12 mEq/L; if it is increased, it implies that there is is loss of HCO_3^- without a concurrent increase in Cl^-. This is compensated for by an increase in non-measured cations; the com-monest are lactate, ketones (e.g. diabetic ketoacidosis), alcohol and its breakdown products, and a whole variety of toxins and drugs, including ethylene glycol (antifreeze), methanol, drug-induced lactic acidosis (e.g. metformin), aspirin in overdose amongst other conditions.

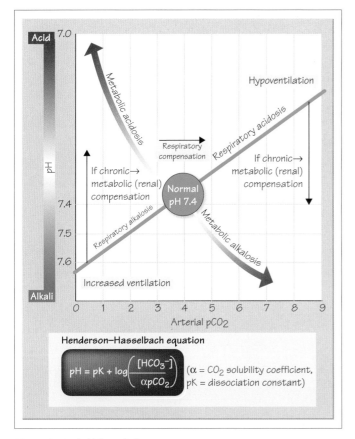

Henderson–Hasselbach equation

$$pH = pK + \log\left(\frac{[HCO_3^-]}{\alpha pCO_2}\right)$$

(α = CO_2 solubility coefficient, pK = dissociation constant)

Figure 4.8.1 Acid-base balance.

4. (a) Ketones

Ketones are the most likely cause of the raised anion gap acidosis.

Further reading: Chapter 138.

Case 9: A patient with a urinary calculus

1. (b) 24-hour urinary urinary calcium

It is important to determine the amount of calcium in the urine, as some 70% of patients with urinary calculi have hypercalciuria; this can be modified by treatments including, thiazide diuretics, reducing dietary sodium, and reducing dietary protein. Bence-Jones protein (immunoglobulin light chains in the urine) do not cause renal tract stones, though they certainly can be deposited within the renal parenchyma, leading to renal failure. Renal calculi are not a feature of Wilson's disease.

2. (b) Sarcoidosis

Sarcoidosis is the only one of these causes well known to produce hypercalcaemia. Though up to 50% of patients with sarcoidosis may have hypercalcaemia, in only 5% or so is it clinically relevant. Patients with sarcoidosis may have hypercalcaemia, largely due to disturbed vitamin D metabolism, so explaining why hypercalcaemia in sarcoidosis may be more common in the spring). It is felt that the sarcoid granulomas may have a crucial role in producing excess $1,25(OH)_2D_3$.

3. (a) Increase fluid intake to >3 L/day

The other measures would increase stone risk. Clearly the aim of increasing fluid intake is to increase urine volume, so diluting the concentration of calcium and any other calculogenic substances in the urine, so decreasing their tendency to precipiate out and produce stones. In tropical climates, though fluid intake is often much increased compared to temporate climates, the urine output may actually be decreased due to high levels of sweating, thus explaining the increased incidence of renal stones in the tropics.

4. (d) All of the above

Cystinuria is an inherited autosomal recessive condition, wherein the proximal portion of the tubule fails to resorb positively charged amino acids, particularly cysteine (also including histidine, lysine, ornithine, arginine), which if the urine is neutral or acid, allows amino-acid crystals to form, so producing renal tract stones. Alkalanising the urine helps, as does penicillamine. Hypercalciuria often responds to thiazide diuretics. Gout is a not uncommon cause of kidney stones, and responds moderately well to prophylaxis with allopurinol.

Further reading: Chapter 139.

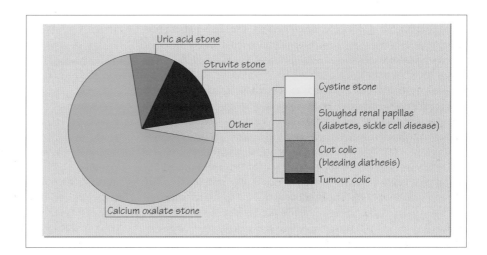

Figure 4.9.1 Causes of renal colic.

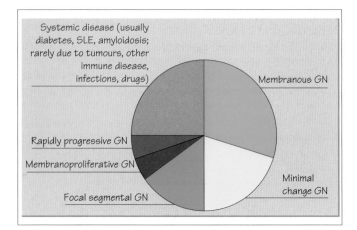

Figure 4.10.1 Causes of nephrotic syndrome in adults.

Case 10: A patient with nephrotic syndrome

1. (b) Low serum albumin

The nephrotic syndrome is the triad of oedema, proteinuria (>4.5 g in 24 hours) and hypoalbuminaemia. Hypercholesterolaemia is commonly present.

2. (b) Systemic lupus erythematosus (SLE)

SLE can cause the nephrotic syndrome; the complement consumption and antinuclear antibodies suggest this diagnosis. Renal biopsy is often undertaken in patients with SLE and renal involvement, as their can be so much variation in the histology (and so the mechanism of damage) which will require a tailored approach for therapy.

3. (a) Pulmonary embolism

Patients with the nephrotic syndrome are hypercoaguable and at greater risk of deep venous thrombosis, pulmonary embolism and renal vein thromboses.

Further reading: Chapter 140.

Case 11: A patient with glomerulonephritis

1. (c) Crescentic glomerulonephritis

Crescentic glomerulonephritis is the only disorder likely to produce such a rapid deterioration in renal function, and as such is often termed rapidly progressive glomerulonephritis (RPGN). Furthermore, the other diagnoses are most likely to produce a nephrotic syndrome picture, rather than the acute renal failure picture here though we do not have knowledge of the amount of proteinurea, and the serum protein levels to be conclusive. The importance in making a rapid diagnosis in crescentic glomerulonephritis is that the earlier treatment is started, the more likely is renal function to recover, and the less likely is there to be irreversible damage, and a requirement for long-term dialysis. In the setting of rapidly progressive renal failure due to crescentic glomerulonephritis, even a few days delay in treatment can mean the difference between renally independent living, and dialysis. The causes of RPGN include:

- Primary autoimmune renal illnesses
- Secondary to other autoimmune illnesses (up to 40% of cases), including Goodpasture's syndrome, Wegener's granulomatosis, systemic lupus erythematosis SLE

- Secondary to infections elsewhere, including infective endocarditis, hepatitis B infection
- Due to drugs

Treatment depends on removing the cause if possible, and often intense immunosuppressive therapy.

Further reading: Chapter 141.

Case 12: A man with heavy proteinuria and low serum protein

1. (a) Minimal change glomerulonephritis

He has the nephrotic syndrome, which is not seen with the other diagnoses.

Further reading: Chapter 140.

Cause of proteinuria as related to quantity	
Daily protein excretion	Cause
0.15 to 2.0 g	Mild glomerulopathies
	Tubular proteinuria
	Overflow proteinuria
2.0 to 4.0 g	Usually glomerular
>4.0 g	Always glomerular

Figure 4.12.1 Causes of proteinuria.

Case 13: A patient with red cells in his urine

1. (b) IgA nephropathy

IgA nephropathy is the commonest finding in well patients with incidentally noted microscopic haematuria, minimal proteinurua and normal renal function. As he is well, and there are no symptoms, signs or investigative findings of other disease, it might be argued that a renal biopsy is so likely to show IgA nephropathy, that it should not be performed, given the small but definite risks to biopsy. This is the sort of decision on which individual clinicians may have widely differing opinions! Idiopathic IgA nephropathy is by far the commonest form, though it can be secondary to cirrhosis, celiac disease and HIV infection. IgA is deposited in the mesangium of the glomerulus, leading to microscopic haematuria, sometimes macroscopic, particularly after respiratory tract infections. It is the commonest cause of glomerulonephritis world-wide. The course is often either of no progression, or very slowly progressive renal failure; after 10 years some 15% of affected patients are on dialysis, and after 20 years some 20% need renal replacement therapy.

Further reading: Chapter 141.

Case 14: A patient with general aches and nose bleeds

1. (a) Antineutrophil cytoplasmic antibodies (ANCA)

Two patterns of staining are found in vasculitis: one where staining is principally cytoplasmic (cANCA – the antigen is principally a proteinase) and the other where staining is principally perinuclear (pANCA – where the antigen is predominantly myeloperoxidase). scl-70 antibodies are seen in scleroderma, and anti-Ro antibodies and depressed C3 and C4 are seen in systemic lupus erythematosus (SLE).

2. (d) Cyclophosphamide, plasma exchange and corticosteroids

Treatment regimens usually include cyclophosphamide and corticosteroids and may include plasma exchange. Chloroquine is usually used in SLE, whilst anticoagulation is usually avoided given potential problems with pulmonary haemorrhage.
Further reading: Chapter 142.

Case 15: A patient with a possible hereditary renal disorder

1. (b) 50%

Autosomal dominant polycystic kidney disease (ADPKD) is inherited in an autosomal dominant fashion, so he has a 50% chance of inheriting the condition.

2. (a) Subarachnoid haemorrhage

Patients with polycystic kidneys have an enhanced incidence of Berry aneurysms which can rupture leading to subarachnoid haemorrhage.

3. (b) Renal ultrasound

Ultrasound will display multiple cysts in affected individuals. Gene testing is difficult because of the very large gene, multiple pseudogenes and different mutations in different pedigrees.
Further reading: Chapter 143.

Case 16: A patient with tubulointerstitial disease

1. (a) Eosinophilia

Eosinophilia may be a feature of interstitial nephritis; red cell casts, marked proteinuria and significant hypertension favour a diagnosis of glomerulonephritis.

2. (c) 1 in 1000

The frequency of a single kidney is about 1 in 1000; more commonly the left kidney is the absent one, and the incidence is increased in men. The single kidney is heavier than normal, and more vunerable to traumatic damage in contact sports, so the decision to participate in such sports should always be carefully evaluated. The long term outlook for most patients with single kidneys is very good, though there is a slightly higher frequency of proteinuria. Clearly, any disease process that may damage the kidneys, particularly if it involves ureteric obstruction must be even more rigorously treated than normal.

3. (b) Ibuprofen

Non-steroidal anti-inflammatory drugs are the commonest drugs producing interstitial nephritis.
Further reading: Chapter 144.

Case 17: A patient with acute renal failure

1. (a) Potassium, arterial blood gases and haemoglobin

The life-threatening derangements that could occur are hyperkalaemia, acidosis and hypoxia.

2. (c) Haemolytic uraemic syndrome (HUS)

Given the patient's young age, anaemia, thrombocytopenia, renal failure and diarrhoea, HUS is the most likely diagnosis.

3. (b) Potassium of 7.2 mmol/L

The indications for immediate dialysis in this context are hyperkalaemia ($K^+ > 6.5$ mmol/L), pulmonary oedema, acidosis (pH < 7.2), the presence of pericaridits or encephalopathy.

4. (c) Peaked T waves

The ECG changes of hyperkalaemia are peaked T waves, widened QRS, absent P waves and a sine wave appearance.
Further reading: Chapter 145.

Case 18: A patient with chronic renal failure and dialysis

1. (c) Hiccoughs, vomiting, itch, nausea, impotence and breathlessness

Hiccoughs, vomiting, itch, nausea, impotence and breathlessness are all symptoms of advanced renal failure. Jaundice and iritis are not.

2. (a) Erythropoietin, α_1-hydroxylated vitamin D and calcium carbonate

He requires correction of his anaemia with erythropoietin, and treatment with a phosphate binder (e.g. calcium carbonate) and with α_1-hydroxylated vitamin D.

3. (a) Cadaveric renal transplant, living related renal transplant, automated peritoneal dialysis, haemodialysis or continuous ambulatory peritoneal dialysis (CAPD)

There are no age or co-morbidity constraints to treatment. Age in itself is not a contra-indication to most forms of renal replacement therapy, but the very elderly patient tends to tolerate dialysis less well, and often has multiple co-morbidities decreasing the quality of their life, meaning that the decision to prolong life must be very carefully balanced against the quality of the life prolonged. This will need careful and sensitive communication with the patients and their family

4. (c) <15 mL/min

With a serum creatinine of 770 µmol/L, his GFR estimated by the Cockcroft–Gault equation is 8 mL/min.
Further reading: Chapter 146.

Case 19: A patient with a renal transplant

1. (c) Rejection, tacrolimus toxicity or recurrent renal disease

Mycophenolate does not commonly cause renal toxicity; rejection, tacrolimus toxicity and recurrent renal disease could all cause this presentation.

2. (a) Prednisolone, tacrolimus

Corticosteroids and the calcineurin inhibitors (cyclosporine and tacrolimus) are associated with an increased incidence of diabetes mellitus post transplant.

3. (a) Lymphoma and myocardial infarction

After a renal transplant, patients have a 20-fold increase risk in death from a myocardial infarction compared with age-matched controls and a greater than 20-fold risk of lymphoma.

4. (d) Over 60%

On average 75% of living related donor transplants will be functioning at 10 years.
Further reading: Chapter 147.

Case 20: Drugs and renal failure

1. (c) Lithium, digoxin, gentamicin, aciclovir

In all patients with renal failure, you should always be concerned, firstly, as to whether the drug may have caused the renal failure, and secondly whether the drug, or one of its active metabolites, are renally excreted, and so may accumulate and produce toxic side effects. The translation of this is; stop all unnecessary drugs in renal failure, always look up those that must be continued in the *British National Formulary* (*BNF*) to determine if the dose should be adjusted.

2. (c) Non-steroidal anti-inflammatory drugs (NSAIDs), cyclosporine, ACE inhibitors

Ferrous sulphate is not renally excreted. ACE inhibitors can provoke acute renal failure in patients with bilateral renal artery

stenosis; however in patients with renal failure without renal artery stenosis, they can be safely used to treat either hypertension or heart failure. Some β-blockers are renally excreted, including atenolol, whereas others need no dose adjustment in renal failure; follow the maxim, if a patient with renal failure is going to have a drug, always look that drug up in the *BNF* to ensure it is safe.
Further reading: Chapter 148.

Case 21: A patient with renal failure

1. (d) Lisinopril, contrast, ibuprofen, candesartan, gentamicin

Simvastatin, insulin and paracetamol are unlikely to have contributed to the worsening of his renal failure. The other agents (lisinopril, contrast, ibuprofen, candesartan, gentamicin) are all well recognized to cause deterioration in renal function.

2. (b) Lisinopril, candesartan, spironolactone

Angiotensin-converting enzyme (ACE) inhibitors, angiotensin II receptor blockers and potassium-sparing diuretics such as spironolactone and amiloride are all prone to produce elevated potassium.
Further reading: Chapter 148.

Case 22: A patient with benign prostatic hypertrophy

1. (a) Renal tract ultrasound

It is critical to establish whether urinary tract obstruction is the cause of his advanced renal failure.

2. (a) Finasteride

Finasteride is a 5α-reducatse inhibitor that inhibits the conversion of testosterone to its active metabolite and thereby reduces prostatic hypertrophy. However, it is very clear that this man desperately needs some form of mechanical relief to his obstructed urinary tract, and that all other interventions are much less effective. He needs a long careful conversation, outlining the high risks of non-surgical intervention, the likelihood of a reduced quality and quantity of life.

3. (c) Bone scan

Prostate cancer commonly metastasizes to bone and a bone scan is the most helpful investigation to detect this.
Further reading: Chapters 149 and 190.

Case 23: A patient with a urinary tract infection

1. (b) Blood glucose

The history of thirst and polyuria raises the possibility of diabetes. The other tests are not indicated in an uncomplicated UTI.

2. (a) Intravenous gentamicin

For uncomplicated UTIs, short duration (5 day or even single dose) antibiotic therapy is usually adequate.

3. (b) Renal tract ultrasound and serum creatinine

With a history of multiple UTIs, renal tract imaging should be performed to look for a predisposing structural abnormality and to assess level of renal function.
Further reading: Chapter 150.

5 Endocrinology: Cases and Questions

Case 1: A patient with a thyroid mass

A 60-year-old man has recently noticed a lump in the left side of his neck. On specific questioning he has not noticed any change in weight, shortness of breath or pain in the neck. His wife, however, feels his breathing is noisier than usual, and that his voice may have become a little rough. On examination there is a visible left-sided thyroid mass with no associated palpable lymph node enlargement. Initial investigations from general practice show normal thyroid biochemistry.

1. *Which is the most likely initial diagnosis?*
   (a) Graves' disease
   (b) Multinodular goitre
   (c) Thyroid cancer
   (d) Benign thyroid adenoma

2. *Fine needle aspiration cytology (FNAC) demonstrates abnormal cells. Which of the following is the commonest thyroid malignancy?*
   (a) Papillary
   (b) Anaplastic
   (c) Mcdullary
   (d) Follicular

3. *Which of the following abnormal investigations may be directly related to the thyroid lump?*
   (a) Serum catecholamines
   (b) Serum calcitonin
   (c) Urinary 5-hydroxyindoleacetic acid (5-HIAA)
   (d) Prolactin

4. *Primary definitive treatment in this case is likely to be which of the following?*
   (a) Recombinant thyroid-stimulating hormone (TSH)
   (b) Radioiodine
   (c) Chemotherapy
   (d) Surgical excision

Case 2: A tired patient with an enlarged thryoid gland

A 50-year-old woman is referred to outpatients because she feels tired all the time. On further questioning she has noticed constipation and thinning of her hair. On examination she appears pale, overweight and has a smoothly enlarged thyroid gland. Full blood count shows Hb of 10.5 g/dL and mean cell volume of 100 fL.

1. *On further examination she is most likely to demonstrate which of the following?*
   (a) Sinus tachycardia
   (b) Sinus bradycardia
   (c) Pigmentation of the skin creases
   (d) Exophthalmos

2. *What is the diagnostic significance of positive peroxidase antibodies?*
   (a) Addison's disease
   (b) Pernicious anaemia
   (c) Autoimmune thyroid disease
   (d) Thyroid cancer

3. *What are biochemistry tests likely to show?*

   (a) ↓ thyroxine (T4) and ↑ thyroid-stimulating hormone (TSH)
   (b) ↑ T4 and ↓ TSH
   (c) ↓ T4 and ↓ TSH
   (d) None of the above

4. *Which of the following drug treatments may also cause hypothyroidism?*
   (a) Digoxin
   (b) Aspirin
   (c) Insulin
   (d) Amiodarone

Case 3: A patient with an irregular heart beat

A.35-year-old woman is transferred to casualty with an irregular heart beat. On examination she is sweaty and warm, but finds it difficult to sit still! She is noted to have 'staring eyes', and cannot write her name and address legibly. On examination, the patient is in atrial fibrillation at a rate of 110 beats/min. She has difficulty raising her arms above her head. The thyroid gland is slightly enlarged and has an audible bruit.

1. *On examination, which of the following is she unlikely to show?*
   (a) Jaundice
   (b) Proptosis
   (c) Diplopia
   (d) Lidlag

2. *Biochemistry is most likely to show which of the following?*
   (a) Positive islet cell antibodies
   (b) ↑ thyroxine (T4) and ↑ thyroid-stimulating hormone (TSH)
   (c) ↑ T4 and ↓ TSH
   (d) ↓ T4 and ↑ TSH

3. *Following a likely diagnosis of Graves' disease, a thyroid uptake scan is performed. What does this show?*
   (a) A diffusely 'cold' gland due to reduced uptake
   (b) A diffusely 'hot' gland due to increased uptake
   (c) A single 'cold' nodule
   (d) Multiple 'hot' spots

4. *What is the appropriate first-line treatment of the underlying condition?*
   (a) Emergency thyroidectomy
   (b) Radio-iodine
   (c) Antithyroid drugs
   (d) Thyroxine

Case 4: A patient with confusion, weight loss and agitation

A 60-year-old woman is transferred as an emergency to casualty with confusion, weight loss and agitation. On examination she is cachetic and is sweating profusely. Her heart rate is 140 beats/min and she has difficulty breathing. An ECG shows atrial fibrillation, and chest X-ray demonstrates an enlarged heart with bibasal pleural effusions. A diffuse shadow is also noticed in the upper mediastinum. Further careful examination of the patient reveals a large scar previously 'hidden' underneath her necklace.

1. *Which is the likely diagnosis?*
   (a) Myxoedema coma
   (b) Diabetic ketoacidosis
   (c) Addison's disease
   (d) Thyroid storm

2. *The mediastinal shadow and scar are likely to be related to previous surgery for what?*
   (a) Thymoma
   (b) Phaeochromocytoma
   (c) Multinodular goitre
   (d) Parathyroid adenoma

3. *Initial treatment should include which of the following?*
   (a) Thyroxine
   (b) Radio-iodine
   (c) β-Blockers
   (d) Phenoxybenzamine

Case 5: A young man with anxiety attacks

A 30-year-old man has been attending the GP with anxiety attacks. On closer questioning these are typically associated with palpitations and sweating. During previous attendances no abnormality had been noticed on general examination. In particular, his BP was 110/70 mmHg and pulse 55 beats/min. On a third visit, however, he was noticed to be pale and sweaty with a BP of 180/120 mmHg and pulse 120 beats/min. He was referred with a possible diagnosis of phaeochromocytoma.

1. *The most appropriate initial urinary investigation should be which of the following?*
   (a) 5-Hydroxyindoleacetic acid (5-HIAA)
   (b) 5-Hydroxytryptamine (5-HT)
   (c) Catecholamines
   (d) Cortisol

2. *Which following statement is correct?*
   (a) A CT of the adrenal will show an adrenal cortical adenoma
   (b) Phaeochromocytomas are usually malignant
   (c) MRI of the adrenal is likely to show an adrenal medullary tumour
   (d) The diagnosis is commonest in the elderly

3. *Phaeos are known to be bilateral in a proportion of cases (approximately 10%). Which syndrome is unlikely to be associated?*
   (a) Multiple endocrine neoplasia (MEN) 2
   (b) Von Hippel–Lindau (VHL) syndrome
   (c) MEN 1
   (d) Neurofibromatosis

4. *Initial emergency management should be which of the following?*
   (a) Emergency surgery
   (b) Drug treatment with β-blockade followed by α-blockade
   (c) Glucocorticoid replacement
   (d) α-Blockade followed by β-blockade

Case 6: A tired patient with weakness and dizziness

A 25-year-old woman is referred to outpatients feeling 'tired all the time'. She has lost weight and feels dizzy on standing. She also describes muscle aches and weakness. On examination she appears suntanned although it is 8 months since her last holiday. She has postural hypotension of 90/50 mmHg when lying, but 75/40 mmHg on standing.

1. *You make a clinical diagnosis of Addison's disease. What is the most likely underlying cause?*
   (a) Past history of meningococcal septicaemia causing haemorrhagic infarction
   (b) Tuberculosis
   (c) Amyloid infiltration
   (d) Autoimmune adrenalitis

2. *Laboratory investigations are likely to show which of the following?*
   (a) Hypokalaemia
   (b) Hyperkalaemia
   (c) Hypernatraemia
   (d) Polycythaemia

3. *The appropriate diagnostic investigation is?*
   (a) Dexamethasone suppression test
   (b) 24-hour urinary cortisol
   (c) Mantoux test
   (d) Short synacthen test

4. *What is the appropriate long-term treatment?*
   (a) Glucocorticoid and mineralocorticoid replacement
   (b) Glucocorticoid replacement
   (c) Mineralocorticoid replacement
   (d) None of the above

Case 7: A patient with possible Cushing's syndrome

A 35-year-old woman is referred to outpatients with a 6–12-month history of weight gain (approximately 7 kg), amenorrhoea, hirsutism and a suggested diagnosis of Cushing's syndrome. Closer questioning reveals labile moods and difficulty sleeping. On examination you note a rounded face and acne. There are pink striae on the abdomen and axillae. Despite the weight gain, her legs and arms are relatively slim, and she has great difficulty climbing onto the couch. Her BP is 160/105 mmHg.

1. *GP screening investigations show increased 24-hour urinary free cortisol (UFC). Which of the following is unlikely to be a possible cause of this abnormal result?*
   (a) A diet rich in bananas and chocolate
   (b) Inhaled hydrocortisone treatment of asthma
   (c) Excess alcohol intake
   (d) Depression

2. *Which of the following statements is true for Cushing's syndrome (CS)?*
   (a) CS is commonest in the elderly
   (b) CS is usually associated with skin pigmentation
   (c) CS may cause short stature
   (d) CS is most commonly due to an adrenal tumour

3. *Which of the following investigations is not helpful in determining whether a patient has CS?*

(a) 24-hour UFC
(b) Overnight dexamethasone suppression test
(c) Pituitary MRI scan
(d) Midnight cortisol

4. *Which of the following tests is not useful in determining the cause of CS?*
(a) ACTH
(b) Oral glucose tolerance test (OGTT)
(c) Serum potassium
(d) Corticotrophin-releasing hormone (CRH) test

Case 8: A woman with possible acromegaly

A 52-year-old woman is referred to the hospital with a history of sweating and joint pains. She has a 10-year history of hypertension and more recently has been discovered to have impaired glucose tolerance. The striking feature on examination is her deep voice and oily skin. A shrewd medical student notices increased inter-dentate spacing and macroglossia, and suggests a possible diagnosis of acromegaly. Further questioning elicits increased shoe size, and the need to enlarge her wedding ring three times over the last 15 years.

1. *What test would be helpful in outpatients?*
(a) Growth hormone (GH)
(b) Oral glucose tolerance test (OGTT)
(c) Insulin growth factor 1 (IGF-1)
(d) Calcium
(e) Prolactin (PRL)

2. *Following confirmation of the diagnosis, what further investigation should be performed?*
(a) None
(b) Inferior petrosal sinus sampling (IPSS)
(c) MRI of the pituitary
(d) Dexamethasone suppression test
(e) Clomiphene test

3. *Initial treatment options are unlikely to include which of the following?*
(a) Dopamine agonists
(b) Radiotherapy alone
(c) Somatostatin agonists
(d) Pituitary surgery
(e) GH receptor analogues

Case 9: A patient with amenorrhoea

A 25-year-old woman is referred to the hospital with a 1-year history of amenorrhoea. Prior to this her periods were regular, although aged 17 she noticed amenorrhoea for 6 months while training for a marathon. Following the run she regained the weight she had lost, and reduced her running to three times a week with resumption of her normal menstrual pattern.

1. *The differential diagnosis is unlikely to include which of the following?*
(a) Pregnancy
(b) Turner's syndrome
(c) Polycystic ovary syndrome (PCOS)
(d) Hyperprolactinaemia
(e) Acromegaly

2. *If testing revealed elevated human chorionic gonadotrophin (hCG), which diagnosis is likely?*

(a) Anorexia nervosa
(b) Pregnancy
(c) PCOS
(d) Primary hypogonadism
(e) Pituitary microadenoma

3. *If testing revealed increased follicle-stimulating hormone (FSH), which diagnosis is likely?*
(a) Anorexia nervosa
(b) Pregnancy
(c) PCOS
(d) Primary hypogonadism
(e) Pituitary microadenoma

4. *If testing showed a body mass index (BMI) of 13 kg/m², which diagnosis is most likely?*
(a) Anorexia nervosa
(b) Pregnancy
(c) PCOS
(d) Primary hypogonadism
(e) Pituitary microadenoma

5. *If tests revealed increased testosterone, which is the most likely diagnosis?*
(a) Anorexia nervosa
(b) Pregnancy
(c) PCOS
(d) Primary hypogonadism
(e) Pituitary microadenoma

6. *If tests showed increased prolactin, which diagnosis is most likely?*
(a) Anorexia nervosa
(b) Pregnancy
(c) PCOS
(d) Primary hypogonadism
(e) Pituitary microadenoma

Case 10: A patient with hypercalcaemia

A 60-year-old woman is referred to outpatients for investigation. During a well-woman check, a routine biochemical profile has shown hypercalcaemia.

1. *It would be important to take a drug history because which of the following drugs may commonly cause hypercalcaemia?*
(a) Lithium
(b) Loop diuretics
(c) Steroid inhaler
(d) Vitamin E intoxication
(e) Bisphosphonates

2. *Although hypercalcaemia may be detected in asymptomatic individuals, all the following clinical features may be associated except which one?*
(a) Constipation
(b) Polyuria
(c) Carpopedal spasm
(d) Confusion
(e) Vomiting

3. *Which is the most likely diagnosis in the clinical case described above?*
(a) Malignancy
(b) Laboratory error
(c) Failure to correct for serum albumin
(d) Hyperparathyroidism
(e) Hyperthyroidism

4. *If there was a family history of hypercalcaemia, which of the following diagnoses would be likely?*
   (a) Albright's hereditary osteodystrophy
   (b) Autoimmune hyperparathyroidism
   (c) Pseudohyperparathyroidism
   (d) Familial hypercalciuric hypercalcaemia
   (e) DiGeorge syndrome
5. *Which following surprise result may indicate an alternative cause for the hypercalcaemia?*
   (a) Elevated cortisol
   (b) Increased thyroid-stimulating hormone (TSH)
   (c) Elevated amylase
   (d) Undetectable cortisol
   (e) Reduced magnesium

Case 11: A patient with excess hair growth

A 26-year-old woman has been referred to outpatients as she has seen her GP on several occasions with hair growth on the upper lip and lower abdomen. She has noticed an increased frequency of shaving her legs and under her arms. On examination she is moderately hirsute with facial acne.

1. *Which of the following is the most likely underlying diagnosis?*
   (a) Congenital adrenal hyperplasia
   (b) Polycystic ovary syndrome (PCOS)
   (c) Anorexia nervosa
   (d) Hypothyroidism
   (e) Androgen-secreting tumour
2. *Which hormone is unlikely to play a significant role in the diagnosis?*
   (a) Insulin
   (b) Prolactin
   (c) Dihydoepiandrosterone (DHEA)
   (d) Luteinizing hormone (LH)
   (e) Testosterone
3. *Which important feature in the presentation would support a tumour as the underlying cause?*
   (a) Deepening of the voice
   (b) Oligomenorrhoea
   (c) Amenorrhoea
   (d) A 6-month history of inability to conceive
   (e) Obesity
4. *Which associated condition/complication is not typically associated with PCOS?*
   (a) Hypertension
   (b) Adrenal crisis
   (c) Diabetes mellitus
   (d) Hyperlipidaemia
   (e) Endometrial hyperplasia

Case 12: A patient with type 2 diabetes mellitus

A 52-year-old man has recently been diagnosed with type 2 diabetes mellitus, and attends his local GP clinic. He takes no medication. His BP is 150/90 mmHg, HbA$_{1c}$ 8.5%, serum cholesterol 6 mmol/L and triglycerides 6 mmol/L.

1. *Which statement is not correct regarding the management of blood pressure in diabetes?*
   (a) BP-lowering treatment is initiated at all levels of BP in this age group
   (b) BP-lowering treatment is initiated if BP is >140/80 mmHg
   (c) Appropriate first-line treatment is angiotensin-converting enzyme (ACE) inhibitors
   (d) Evidence of renal or ocular abnormalities alter the targets
   (e) Ethnic origin is important
2. *Which is the appropriate initial drug treatment for elevated glucose?*
   (a) Sulphonylureas
   (b) Insulin secretagogues
   (c) Thiazolidinediones
   (d) Metformin
   (e) Acarbose
3. *Which statement is not true regarding cardiovascular risk management?*
   (a) Target cholesterol is <4 mmol/L
   (b) Triglycerides >4.5 mmol/L should be treated with fenofibrate
   (c) Fish oil should be administered to all aged >50 years
   (d) Aspirin should be administered to all aged >50 years
   (e) Simvastatin is usually first-line treatment

Case 13: A patient with possible diabetes mellitus

A 20-year-old man presents to his GP with a 2-week history of tiredness, thirst and polyuria. There is no history of weight loss but the patient is suspicious of a diagnosis of diabetes mellitus as several family members take tablets for glucose control. He appears well and physical examination is unremarkable. He is found to have glycosuria on dipstick. Random finger prick glucose is 10.7 mmol/L. A diagnosis of diabetes mellitus (DM) is suggested and he is referred to the local diabetes department.

1. *Which of the following statements is correct?*
   (a) A diagnosis of DM can be made on the information given in the above case scenario
   (b) A diagnosis of DM requires a formal oral glucose tolerance test (OGTT)
   (c) A diagnosis of DM is usually based on a fasting plasma glucose (FPG) of >7 mmol/L
   (d) A diagnosis of impaired fasting hyperglycaemia is based on a FPG of >7 mmol/l.
   (e) A diagnosis of impaired glucose tolerance is based on a FPG of >7 mmol/L.
2. *A formal diagnosis of diabetes mellitus is made in the patient. What is the likely underlying cause?*
   (a) Autoimmune pancreatic islet cell deficiency
   (b) Pancreatitis
   (c) Haemochromatosis
   (d) Cystic fibrosis
   (e) Maturity-onset diabetes in the young (MODY)
3. *Initial management should be which of the following?*
   (a) Weight loss
   (b) Insulin treatment
   (c) Sulphonylureas
   (d) Dietary advice
   (e) Metformin

4. *Which of the following statements is not true regarding treatment?*

(a) Sulphonylureas may be associated with weight loss

(b) Sulphonylureas may be associated with hypoglycaemia

(c) Metformin is contraindicated in patients with renal impairment

(d) Hepatotoxicity is a side effect of the thiazolidinediones

(e) Insulin may be associated with weight gain

Case 14: A patient with confusion and vomiting

A 50-year-old woman is transferred with a 7-day history of increasing confusion and vomiting. She is markedly dehydrated and is noted to be favouring her left side. Urgent investigations show a blood glucose of 50 mmol/L, urine dipstick 1+ ketones, arterial blood gas (ABG) bicarbonate 20 mmol/L and pH 7.35.

1. *What is the likely diagnosis?*

(a) Diabetic ketoacidosis (DKA) in a previously undiagnosed patient with type 2 diabetes

(b) Hyperosmolar non-ketotic confusion (HONK) in a patient with type 2 diabetes

(c) Lactic acidosis

(d) DKA in a patient with previously undiagnosed type 1 diabetes

(e) Urinary tract infection (UTI)

2. *Serum osmolality should be calculated according to which equation?*

(a) 2(cCreatinine + urea) + glucose + sodium

(b) 2(glucose + sodium) + urea

(c) 2(sodium + potassium) + glucose + urea

(d) 2(urea + glucose)

(e) 2(bicarbonate + glucose) + sodium

3. *Which following statement is true?*

(a) She will need life-long insulin treatment in view of the very high glucose levels

(b) DKA is uncommon in type 1 diabetes

(c) Following appropriate management mortality is low

(d) Undiagnosed diabetes mellitus is the commonest cause of DKA

(e) Most cases of HONK are associated with undiagnosed type 2 diabetes

4. *Which of the following statements is not true?*

(a) This patient may have had a cerebrovascular accident associated with a hypercoagulable state

(b) Myocardial infarction (MI) may be a precipitant/complication

(c) Some drugs may precipitate the condition

(d) Hypoglycaemic coma may also be a presenting feature of diabetes

(e) All patients with DKA require long-term insulin

Endocrinology: Answers

Case 1: A patient with a thyroid mass

1. (c) Thyroid cancer

Although it is not the commonest differential diagnosis of a thyroid lump, the likely diagnosis here is a malignancy because of the short history, age of the patient, and the association with possible recurrent laryngeal nerve palsy as suggested by the hoarse voice.

2. (a) Papillary

Papillary thyroid cancer constitutes >80% of thyroid cancer. It is more common in women, usually slow growing, and often spreads to the lower lymph nodes and structures. Follicular thyroid cancer constitutes 15% of thyroid cancer and is associated with vascular invasion and distant metastases. Anaplastic cancer is rare and is commonest in the elderly. It is associated with a very poor prognosis.

3. (b) Serum calcitonin

Elevated serum calcitonin is associated with the rare medullary thyroid cancer (MTC). Typically it accounts for only 5–10% of all thyroid cancer, and may also cause diarrhoea and flushing. It may be associated with a family history (either familial MTC or multiple endocrine neoplasia (MEN) type 2) with parathyroid adenoma and phaeochromocytoma.

4. (d) Surgical excision

Surgical excision should be performed by an experienced thyroid surgeon as part of a multidisciplinary group. Adjuvant treatment may be radioiodine or thyroxine suppression of TSH, depending on the extent of disease.

Further reading: Chapter 37 in Medicine at a Glance.

Case 2: A tired patient with an enlarged thryoid gland

1. (b) Sinus bradycardia

A sinus bradycardia, which is sometimes associated with small complexes on an ECG. The QT interval (corrected for heart rate) is often prolonged, though complicating ventricular arrhythmias are rare.

2. (c) Autoimmune thyroid disease

Autoimmune hypothyroidism is the commonest cause of primary hypothyroidism.

3. (a) ↓ thyroxine (T4) and ↑ thyroid-stimulating hormone (TSH)

Circulating T4 levels are reduced due to reduced thyroid production. Lack of negative feedback at the pituitary gland leads to an increase in TSH.

4. (d) Amiodarone

Due to its high iodine content and structural similarity to thyroxine, amiodarone treatment may cause either hypo- or hyperthyroidism. It is important to monitor thyroid function tests when patients receive amiodarone treatment. Hypothyroidism is more common (13% compared with 2%), and commoner in patients with thyroid autoantibodies. It is treated with T4 replacement.

Further reading: Chapter 155.

Case 3: A patient with an irregular heart beat

1. (a) Jaundice

The other eye signs are all associated with Graves' eye disease which is commonly found with Graves' disease of the thyroid – the commonest cause of hyperthyroidism.

2. (c) ↑ T4 and ↓ TSH

Circulating thyroid hormone levels (both triiodothyronine and T4) are elevated due to autoimmune stimulation of the thyroid gland. Increased thyroid hormone concentrations negatively feed

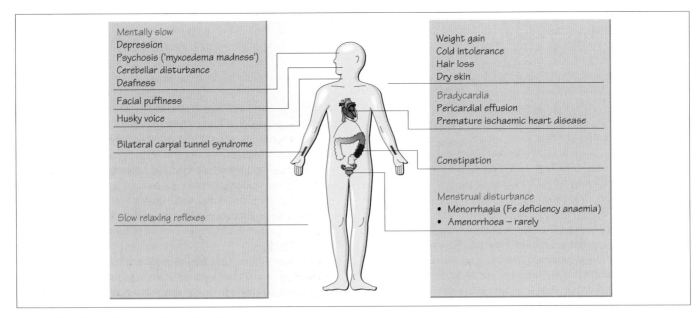

Figure 5.2.1 Clinical features of hypothyroidism.

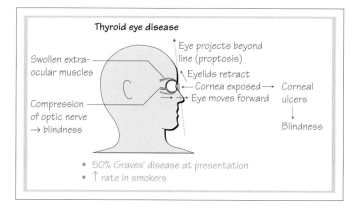

Figure 5.3.1 Features of thyroid eye disease.

back at the pituitary gland to suppress circulating TSH. A very rare exception is secondary hyperthyroidism due to a pituitary tumour secreting TSH – leading to ↑ T4 and ↑ TSH.

3. (b) A diffusely 'hot' gland due to increased uptake

This is due to diffuse stimulation of the whole gland by thyroid antibodies. The aim of the scan is to determine the anatomical basis of hyperthyroidism (which thereby helps determine aetiology and so treatment), that is to say, is it a single hot nodule (when there is a possibility of an adenoma or carcinoma), multiple diffuse nodules, diffusely hot, as in Graves' disease, or patchily hot, as is often the case with Hashimotos thyroiditis.

4. (c) Antithyroid drugs

Give either carbimazole or propylthiouracil. It is essential to warn the patient of the possible risk of agranulocytosis (0.1%). Thyroid function tests should be rechecked after approximately 6–8 weeks.

Further reading: Chapter 156.

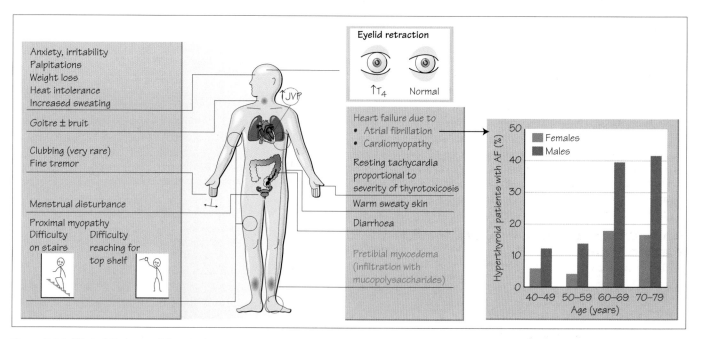

Figure 5.3.2 Clinical features of thyrotoxicosos.

Case 4: A patient with confusion, weight loss and agitation

1. (d) Thyroid storm

This is a rare emergency with a high mortality. The pointers to severe hyperthyroidism include; substantial weight loss (50% of patients with thyroid storm have lost > 15kg), atrial fibrillation (though this would go with any patient with hyperthyroidism), profuse sweating (the differential diagnosis therefore includes sepsis; however, sepsis is usually easily diagnosed from simple blood tests and investigations). The previous presumed thyroid surgery and upper mediastinal mass are highly suggestive of a thyroid problem. The enlarged heart and pleural effusions suggest that hyperthyroidism-induced heart failure is complicating the picture

2. (c) Multinodular goitre

Hyperthyroidism may arise in a long-standing goitre, which may regrow following previous surgery. Alternatively, patients may develop recurrent symptoms following discontinuation of long-term antithyroid medication causing a flare up of the disease. Amiodarone therapy may also cause hyperthyroidism in a pre-existing goitre, and rarely thyroid storm.

3. (c) β-Blockers

β-Blockers may be required in high dose. Other treatment will include fluid and electrolyte management, often in the intensive therapy unit, and antithyroid drugs and glucocorticoids to inhibit thyroid hormone synthesis.

Further reading: Chapter 156.

Case 5: A young man with anxiety attacks

1. (c) Catecholamines

Catecholamine metabolites will be detectable in the urine. Older investigations included vanillylmandelic acids; however this has been superseded as catecholamines are less likely to be interfered with by diet, etc. Typically, three sets of 24-hour urines for catecholamines are ordered, the first two to be done whenever convenient, the third starting immediately after an attack.

2. (c) MRI of the adrenal is likely to show an adrenal medullary tumour

Phaeochromocytomas ('phaeos') are most commonly found in the adrenal medulla. The adrenal cortex synthesizes steroid hormones, and tumours lead to steroid hypersecretion, e.g. Cushing's syndrome or Conn's syndrome. Phaeos are commonest in the age group 30–50 years, and have an equal sex incidence. An *aide mémoire* states that 10% are likely to be malignant, 10% multiple and 10% bilateral.

3. (a) Multiple endocrine neoplasia (MEN) 2

MEN 2 includes hyperparathyroidism, phaeos and medullary thyroid cancer and is associated with the RET proto-oncogene on chromosome 10. In contrast MEN 1 most commonly consists of primary hyperparathyroidism, a pituitary tumour and pancreatic tumours. It is an autosomal condition associated with a mutation on chromosome 11. VHL syndrome (renal cell cancer, cerebellar haemangiomas, retinal angiomas, pancreatic cysts) and neurofibromatosis may both be associated with phaeos and these patients should be screened appropriately.

4. (d) α-Blockade followed by β-blockade

The usual drugs are phenoxybenzamine (an α-blocker) and propanolol (a β-blocker). This is to protect the patient from the effects of massive catecholamine release during surgical manipulation of the tumour.

Further reading: Chapter 158.

Case 6: A tired patient with weakness and dizziness

1. (d) Autoimmune adrenalitis

Autoimmune adrenalitis accounts for approximately 70% cases in the developed world. While the other three conditions may all cause adrenal failure they are much less common. However, on a world-wide basis, tuberculosis is still probably the most common cause.

2. (b) Hyperkalaemia

Hyperkalaemia is due to mineralocorticoid deficiency. Other commonly detected initial abnormal tests may include eosinophilia and normochromic normocytic anaemia, hyponatraemia and elevated urea.

3. (d) Short synacthen test

A lack of a normal cortisol rise following adrenal stimulation with synthetic adrenocorticotrophic hormone (ACTH) is found in adrenal failure. Elevation of ACTH and positive adrenal cortical antibodies are commonly demonstrated.

4. (a) Glucocorticoid and mineralocorticoid replacement

A usual regimen would be thrice daily hydrocortisone (waking, midday and late afternoon) and daily fludrocortisone. Replacement should be titrated to avoid overtreatment, associated with weight gain, hypertension and oedema. During intercurrent illness, or stress of surgery or pregnancy, cortisol requirements increase and

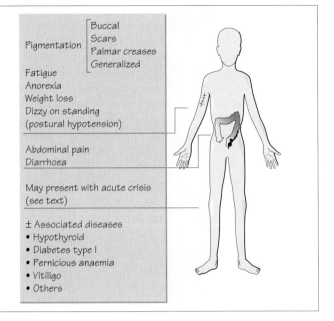

Figure 5.6.1 Features of Addison's disease.

patients may require parenteral replacement. Patient education is essential – including a Medic-Alert and a steroid card.

Further reading: Chapter 158.

Case 7: A patient with possible Cushing's syndrome

1. (a) A diet rich in bananas and chocolate

Bananas and chocolate interfere with urinary vanillylmandelic acid. Exogenous hydrocortisone (less so with prednisolone and none with dexamethasone) may increase UFC. Severe depression and alcohol excess are both causes of pseudo-Cushing's syndrome, which may produce false-positive screening investigations.

2. (c) CS may cause short stature

Rarely CS may present in childhood with short stature due to glucocorticoid-induced growth arrest. It is commonest in women, aged 20–40 years, and the commonest underlying cause is an adrenocorticotrophic hormone (ACTH)-secreting pituitary tumour. Pigmentation of the skin is due to very high ACTH and is usually associated with Nelson's syndrome or ectopic ACTH secretion by a tumour.

3. (c) Pituitary MRI scan

MRI of the pituitary may be abnormal and demonstrate a microadenoma in 10% of the population (usually an incidentaloma of no clinical relevance). MRI of the pituitary may also be normal in up to 20% cases of patients with pituitary-dependent CS. The other tests are all useful in screening for CS.

4. (b) Oral glucose tolerance test (OGTT)

Glucose intolerance is associated with all causes of CS. Pituitary-dependent disease is typically associated with suppression of basal cortisol on high-dose dexamethasone suppression testing, an exaggerated rise in ACTH with CRH, and lateralization on inferior petrosal sinus testing. In contrast, ectopic ACTH secretion is virtually always associated with hypokalaemia. In adrenal causes of CS, ACTH is suppressed in contrast to elevation in both ectopic and pituitary-dependent disease.

Further reading: Chapter 158.

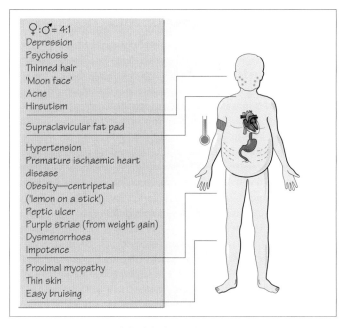

Figure 5.7.1 Features of Cushing's syndrome.

Case 8: A woman with possible acromegaly

1. (b) Oral glucose tolerance test (OGTT)

Random GH testing is not useful as a normal individual secretes pulses of GH throughout the day, which are difficult to differentiate from elevated GH in acromegaly. The OGTT shows a lack of the normal suppression of GH with a glucose load in acromegaly and is used to diagnose acromegaly. IGF-1 has a long half-life and is elevated in patients with acromegaly. Calcium concentrations may rise because GH increases renal α-hydroxylase activity, or because of associated primary hyperparathyroidism. PRL co-secretion by a GH-secreting tumour is found in a minority of cases of acromegaly.

2. (c) MRI of the pituitary

MRI of the pituitary usually demonstrates a tumour. A pituitary adenoma is the cause in >95% cases. Macroadenomas (>1 cm in diameter) are commoner than microadenoma in acromegaly, and may be associated with visual field defects. Very rare causes include pituitary cancer and GH-releasing hormone (GHRH)-secreting carcinoid tumours.

3. (b) Radiotherapy alone

Radiotherapy does usually lower GH, but only slowly. Due to the increased mortality, as demonstrated by the impaired glucose tolerance and hypertension in this patient, more immediately effective treatments are appropriate if the patient is fit.

Further reading: Chapter 154.

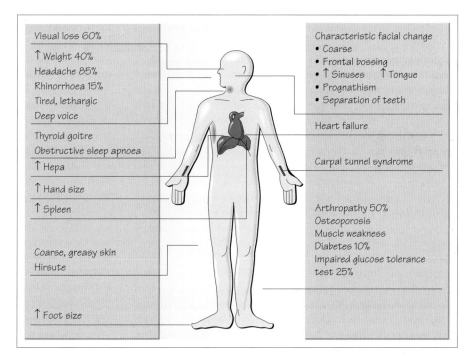

Figure 5.8.1 Features of acromegaly.

Case 9: A patient with amenorrhoea

1. (b) Turner's syndrome

Turner's syndrome is the commonest genetic cause of primary hypogonadism and is associated with primary amenorrhoea (lack of menstruation by age 16 years), in addition to the typical phenotype of short stature, webbed neck, cubitus valgus, autoimmune hypothyroidism, coarctation of the aorta, and renal and ENT abnormalities. Pregnancy, PCOS, increased prolactin and acrome-galy (due to hypopituitarism secondary to a pituitary macroadenoma) are all possible causes.

2. (b) Pregnancy

Human chorionic gonadotrophin (hCG) is made in the placenta, and acts to maintain the corpus luteum of the ovary, and so maintains the progesterone levels that are crucial to the maintance of pregnancy. Pathologically, it is however also made by some cancers and other tumours including; choriocarcinoma, germ cell tumours, hyatidiform mole, teratoma with elements of choriocarcinoma (very rare), and islet cell tumours, and in some men with testicular tumours. However, it does not occur in the other conditions listed.

3. (d) Primary hypogonadism

True elevated gonadotrophins are associated with primary ovarian failure which may be genetic or acquired. In this case, acquired premature ovarian failure is possible.

4. (a) Anorexia nervosa

Anorexia nervosa leads to secondary hypogonadism with a failure of gonadotrophin secretion.

5. (c) PCOS

PCOS is associated with increased testosterone but is more commonly associated with oligomenorrhoea (<9 periods/year).

6. (e) Pituitary microadenoma

Hyperprolactinaemia is usually associated with a microadenoma (rather than macroadenoma) of the pituitary. Examination may demonstrate galactorrhoea. A differential diagnosis of increased prolactin includes stress, PCOS and hypothyroidism. Dopamine agonist treatment is usually effective in restoring menses and fertility.

Further reading: Chapters 154 and 160.

Case 10: A patient with hypercalcaemia

1. (a) Lithium

Lithium, thiazide diuretics, vitamin D and rarely vitamin A may cause hypercalcaemia; loop diuretics are sometimes used in the emergency treatment of hypercalcaemia, and bisphosphonates likewise are routine treatment for many forms of hypercalcaemia.

2. (c) Carpopedal spasm

Carpopedal spasm is associated with hypocalcaemia, either genuine, or much more likely in clinical practise, functional hypocalcaemia induced by hyperventilation and low pCO_2 levels. All the other features are found in hypercalcaemia.

3. (d) Hyperparathyroidism

Primary hyperparathyroidism is the commonest cause of hypercalcaemia in the so-called asymptomatic patient. Malignancy is the other common cause but is usually, although not always, associated with specific symptoms as it is typically a late manifestation of malignancy. The common tumours associated with hypercalcaemia are multiple myeloma, squamous cell carcinoma and breast cancer.

4. (d) Familial hypercalciuric hypercalcaemia

Familial hypercalciuric hypercalcaemia accounts for approximately 2% of asymptomatic hypercalcaemia, and is an autosomal dominant condition due to a mutation in the calcium-sensing receptor. Patients have low 24-hour urine calcium excretion. Albright's hereditary osteodystrophy and DiGeorge syndrome are both associated with hypocalcaemia. Autoimmune hypoparathyroidism and pseudohypoparathyroidism are also causes of hypocalcaemia.

5. (d) Undetectable cortisol

Rarely, Addison's disease may cause hypercalcaemia. Other causes include hyperthyroidism (suppressed TSH). Serum amylase may be elevated in pancreatitis and hypocalcaemia. Hypomagnesaemia may lead to defective parathyroid hormone secretion and hypocalcaemia.

Further reading: Chapter 157.

Case 11: A patient with excess hair growth

1. (b) Polycystic ovary syndrome (PCOS)

PCOS causes approximately 95% of cases of hirsutism. Congenital adrenal hyperplasia and androgen-secreting tumours cause <1% of androgen-dependent hair growth, while hypothyroidism and anorexia nervosa are causes of androgen-independent hair growth.

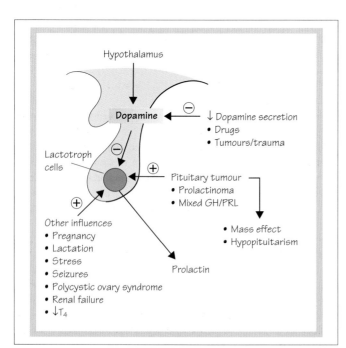

Figure 5.9.1 Features of hyperprolactinaemia.

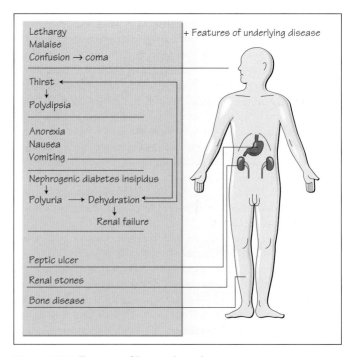

Figure 5.10.1 Features of hypercalcaemia.

2. (b) Prolactin

The ovary is the main source of the androgens testosterone and androstenedione, under LH control, whereas DHEA is the main adrenal androgen, which is adrenocorticotrophic hormone (ACTH) dependent. Hyperinsulinaemia is commonly found in PCOS.

3. (a) Deepening of the voice

Frontal balding, deepening of the voice and cliteromegaly are all signs of virilization. An associated short history would also point to a possible androgen-secreting tumour. Oligomenorrhoea, amenorrhoea, infertility due to anovulation and obesity are common in PCOS.

4. (b) Adrenal crisis

Adrenal crisis is associated with congenital adrenal hyperplasia (21-hydroxylase deficiency most commonly). Metabolic syndromes associated with hyperinsulinaemia and endometrial hyperplasia (visible on ultrasound) due to anovulation are all associated with PCOS.

Further reading: Chapter 160.

Case 12: A patient with type 2 diabetes mellitus

1. (a) BP-lowering treatment is initiated at all levels of BP in this age group

BP-lowering agents are initiated if BP is confirmed to be >140/80 mmHg or >130/80 mmHg if there is evidence of end-organ damage. ACE-I is appropriate first-line treatment unless the patient is Afro-Caribbean or pregnant. Second-line agents include calcium channel blockers and thiazide diuretics.

2. (d) Metformin

Metformin is first-line treatment except in patients with significant renal impairment and cardiac failure. Sulphonylureas are appropriate second-line treatment. Insulin is commenced if the HbA_{1c} remains above 7.5%. Acarbose, insulin secretagogues and thiazolidinediones may be used if other treatments are inappropriate due to intolerance or lifestyle.

3. (c) Fish oil should be administered to all aged >50 years

Option (c) is only indicated if the other measures fail. Aspirin 75 mg is indicated in all patients aged >50 years and younger if there is also cardiovascular/renal disease. Following the investigation of possible secondary causes of increased triglycerides (alcoholic liver disease, hypothyroidism, failure to control hyperglycaemia, renal failure), fenofibrate should be administered. Simvastatin is the first-line treatment in all patients aged >40 years and in younger patients if there is evidence of significant cardiovascular risk. The target cholesterol is <4 mmol/L.

Further reading: Chapter 152.

Case 13: A patient with possible diabetes mellitus

1. (c) A diagnosis of DM is usually based on a fasting plasma glucose (FPG) of >7 mmol/L

A diagnosis of DM is made on a FPG of >7 mmol/L or a random glucose of >11.1 mmol/L in a symptomatic individual in the absence of intercurrent illness. Impaired fasting hyperglycaemia is diagnosed if the FPG is 6–6.9 mmol/L, and impaired glucose tolerance if the FPG is <7 mmol/L but the 2-hour post-glucose load is 7.8–11.1 mmol/L.

2. (e) Maturity-onset diabetes in the young (MODY)

Several family members are affected and managed without insulin suggesting type 2 diabetes caused by the autosomal dominant MODY syndrome, which typically presents in young adults. Autoimmune pancreatic islet cell deficiency is unlikely as this leads to type 1 diabetes. The patient has no clinical features to suggest the other possible secondary causes of diabetes listed.

3. (d) Dietary advice

Weight loss is necessary in overweight individuals. Dietary advice and monitoring of glucose control for 3 months is the usual first step. Drug treatment may be required if there is failure of control. Metformin is first-line treatment and sulphonylureas would be second-line treatment. Insulin is required in all patients with type 1 diabetes, and some patients with MODY.

4. (a) Sulphonylureas may be associated with weight loss

Both sulphonylureas and insulin are associated with weight gain and hypoglycaemia. Metformin is contraindicated if the creatinine is >14 nmol/L. Lactic acidosis is rare with metformin, but there is an increased risk when radiological contrast media are used. Metformin should therefore be stopped prior to these investigations. Thiazolidinediones are associated with hepatotoxicity and checking liver biochemistry prior to treatment is advisable.

Further reading: Chapter 151.

Case 14: A patient with confusion and vomiting

1. (b) Hyperosmolar non-ketotic confusion (HONK) in a patient with type 2 diabetes

HONK is indicated with a glucose of 30–50 mmol/L and a lack of significant acidosis in this age group. DKA occurs in patients with type 1 diabetes due to absolute insulin deficiency. In this case ketonuria is mild (probably due to lack of food intake). In DKA one would expect a pH < 7.3 and bicarbonate <15 mmol/L. Lactic acidosis is a complication of metformin treatment.

2. (c) 2(sodium + potassium) + glucose + urea

The appropriate formula is serum osmolality = 2(sodium + potassium) + glucose + urea. The normal serum osmolality is 275-299 milli-osmoles per kilogram. If in this case her Na was 150 mmol/L, her K was 5 mmol/L, and urea 20 mmol/L, not unreasonable numbers, then the osmolality would be 380, clearly very substantially raised.

3. (e) Most cases of HONK are associated with undiagnosed type 2 diabetes

Two-thirds of cases of HONK occur in previously undiagnosed patients with type 2 diabetes, whereas the commonest precipitant of DKA is infection. Mortality is reported as being up to 50% (higher than in DKA, where it is 10%). Many patients with HONK are successfully managed in the long term with oral hypoglycaemic agents.

4. (d) Hypoglycaemic coma may also be a presenting feature of diabetes

Hypoglycaemia is a complication of the treatment of diabetes. Patients with HONK are hypercoagulable and at an increased risk of venous thrombosis. Precipitants include high sugar intake, intercurrent infection and MI, and drugs such as glucocorticoids, phenytoin and thiazide diuretics. DKA occurs due to an absolute absence of insulin due to pancreatic failure and is only seen in patients with type 1 diabetes who will therefore need life-long insulin treatment.

Further reading: Chapter 153.

6 Infectious Disease: Cases and Questions

Case 1: A red, sore venflon site

A 35-year-old woman has been an inpatient in hospital for 5 days. She is on treatment for severe community-acquired pneumonia and had 48 hours of intravenous antibiotics which has now been changed to oral. She is clinically improving. As an on-call doctor you have been asked to assess her because she is febrile. She complains of a red sore arm. You note that she still has a venflon *in situ*. On examination she has a temperature of 38.2°C, a heart rate of 105 beats/min and an arterial blood pressure of 105/70 mmHg. Her skin is red, tender, swollen and indurated around her venflon site.

1. *Which of the following non-specific barriers could have been breached in this scenario?*
   (a) Biological barrier
   (b) Physical barrier
   (c) Chemical barrier
2. *Which of these factors is most likely to have promoted her illness?*
   (a) Her immune status
   (b) Her age
   (c) The switch from intravenous to oral antibiotics
3. *What is the most likely pathogen causing the infection?*
   (a) *Staphylococcus aureus*
   (b) *Escherichia coli*
   (c) *Enterococcus*
4. *What initial steps should you take in her management?*
   (a) Isolate in a side room
   (b) Commence on empirical antibiotics
   (c) Remove the infected venflon

Case 2: A young man with a sore throat and dark urine

A 20-year-old man had a sore throat 1 week ago. He was treated with antibiotics in the community and his symptoms improved. He presented 10 days later to A&E with dark urine and abdominal pain. On examination he appeared relatively well at rest. He was afebrile and had a normal blood pressure. There were no murmurs heard on examination. The following results were available to you:

Hb	13 g/L
WCC	12×10^9/L
Platelets	240×10^9/L
CRP	40 mg/L
ESR	59 mm/h
Na	138 mmol/L
K	4.1 mmol/L
Urea	8 mmol/L
Creatinine	120 μmol/L
LFTs	Normal

Urinalysis: microscopic haematuria, protein ++
Blood culture: no growth
ASO titre: positive

1. *What is the significance of a positive antistreptolysin (ASO) titre?*
   (a) Current or past infection with group A *Streptococcus*
   (b) Current or past infection with Epstein–Barr virus
   (c) Current or past infection with *Enterococcus*

2. *What is the unifying diagnosis?*
   (a) Subacute bacterial endocarditis
   (b) Post-streptococcal glomerulonephritis
   (c) Glandular fever
3. *This patient initially had tonsillitis, due to bacterial infection of the tonsils; what is the mechanism of the renal damage from this infection?*
   (a) Sepsis
   (b) Autoimmune phenomena
   (c) Systemic thromboembolic phenomena
4. *If a renal biopsy was performed, what would you expect to see under light microscopy?*
   (a) Minimal change
   (b) Membranous nephropathy
   (c) Mesangial proliferation

Case 3: A patient with flu-like symptoms and a rash

A 25-year-old man who was previously fit and well presented with a 4-day history of headache, myalgia and arthralgia followed by a dry cough. He initially thought he had the flu but his symptoms progressed. He then developed a generalized rash on his trunk, which led to his admission. He denied having a fever and had not travelled recently. He did not take any medication or use illicit drugs.

On examination he was jaundiced, had a temperature of 37.8°C, a heart rate of 110 beats/min, an arterial blood pressure of 105/70 mmHg, and a respiratory rate of 25 breaths/min with an oxygen saturation of 93% on air. He had bronchial breathing in his right upper lobe, normal heart sounds and a soft abdomen with no evidence of organomegly. Central nervous system examination was normal and there was no meningism or papilloedema on fundoscopy. On close scrutiny of the rash on his trunk you see multiple target lesions.

His blood results are below.

Hb	9 g/dL
WCC	12×10^9/L
Neutrophils	10×10^9/L
Platelets	600×10^9/L
CRP	198 mg/L
ESR	60 mm/h
Clotting	Normal
Direct Coombs' test	Positive
Na	145 mmol/L
K	3.7 mmol/L
Urea	10 mmol/L
Creatinine	115 mmol/L
Albumin	27 g/L
Bilirubin	50 μmol/L
ALT	23 U/L
ALP	60 U/L
γ-GT	60 U/L

1. *Which of these blood markers most strongly suggest a bacterial infection?*
   (a) Raised C-reactive protein (CRP)
   (b) Neutrophilia
   (c) Raised erythrocyte sedimentation rate (ESR)

2. *What is the most likely explanation for the jaundice?*
   (a) Haemolytic anaemia
   (b) Gilbert's syndrome
   (c) Hepatitis
3. *What is the most appropriate investigation?*
   (a) Urine dipstick
   (b) Abdominal ultrasound
   (c) Chest radiograph
4. *This man was clinically diagnosed with Mycoplasma pneumonia; what is the definitive test to establish diagnosis?*
   (a) Acute and convalescent serology
   (b) Blood culture
   (c) Skin biopsy

Case 4: A young patient with fever and heart murmur

A 14-year-old African boy is referred with a 2-week history of fever and night sweats. He had a sore throat and scarlet fever 2 months ago and recovered from this. In the last 2 weeks he has developed a painful right knee and wrist and noticed a painless nodule on his elbow. His mother was particularly concerned by his clumsiness as he kept on dropping things and unpredictably flinging his arms. This boy had a previously unremarkable childhood and was up to date with all his vaccinations. He has no family history of neurological conditions.

On examination he had a low-grade fever but was haemodynamically stable. His chest was clear. However, he had a mid-diastolic murmur. He had a swollen and tender right knee but the signs on the right wrist had resolved. There was a painless mobile nodule on his right elbow. Examination of the central nervous system was unremarkable although occasional involuntary movement of the left hand was observed.

The following results are obtained:
Hb   12.5 g/dL
WCC   13 × 10⁹/L
                (80% neutrophils)
Platelets   400 × 10⁹/L
CRP   105 mg/L
ESR   90 mm/h
U&Es   Normal
LFTs   Normal
ANA + rheumatoid factor: negative
Monospot test: negative
X-ray of right knee: normal
ECG: sinus rhythm, prolonged PR interval

1. *What two further investigations would you request?*
   (a) Antistreptolysin O (ASO) titre and echocardiogram
   (b) Chest radiograph and blood culture
   (c) Joint aspiration and blood culture
2. *What is the significance of his history of scarlet fever?*
   (a) Previous streptococcal infection
   (b) Immunosuppression
   (c) Previous staphylococcal infection
3. *What is the diagnosis?*
   (a) *Streptococcus* septicaemia
   (b) Subacute bacterial endocarditis
   (c) Rheumatic fever
4. *What is the explanation for his involuntary arm movements?*

   (a) Brain abscess
   (b) Stroke
   (c) Sydenham's chorea

Case 5: A patient with presumed infection

A 56-year-old lady presented to A&E with malaise and a fever. She was discharged 1 month ago following emergency surgery for a fractured neck of the femur. The procedure had been event free and she was now mobilizing with crutches. She complained of pain and swelling of her right leg and found walking increasingly difficult. She had no chest symptoms. She had a past history of breast cancer but has been in remission for 10 years with regular follow-up. Other than analgesia she is not on regular medication. She is not aware of any conditions that run in the family.

On examination she was febrile at 38°C with a heart rate of 95 beats/min, an arterial blood pressure of 115/70 mmHg, respiratory rate of 18 breaths/min with an oxygen saturation of 99% on air. Cardiovascular, abdominal and respiratory examinations were unremarkable. She had an asymmetrical swelling of her right leg extending to her mid-thigh. This area was red and she was exquisitely tender around the calf and the pain was exacerbated by forced foot dorsiflexion.

The following results were obtained:
Hb   13 g/L
WCC   10 × 10⁹/L
Platelets   240 × 10⁹/L
CRP   20 mg/L
ESR   20 mm/h
D-dimer   Elevated
Na   138 mmol/L
K   4.1 mmol/L
Urea   4 mmol/L
Creatinine   120 μmol/L
LFTs   Normal
Blood culture: no growth

1. *What further investigation would you request*
   (a) CT pulmonary angiogram (CTPA)
   (b) Ultrasound Doppler scan of her left leg
   (c) Blood culture
2. *Which of these risk factors increases her probability of a thromboembolic event?*
   (a) Recent pelvic surgery
   (b) History of breast cancer
   (c) Age
3. *What is the most likely diagnosis?*
   (a) DVT
   (b) Cellulitis
   (c) Ruptured Baker's cyst
4. *If this lady had a family history of DVT/PE, what additional test would you recommend?*
   (a) Activated protein C resistance
   (b) Thrombin time
   (c) Bleeding time

Case 6: A patient with presumed infection and confusion

A 55-year-old woman had been previously fit and well. She was brought into hospital via ambulance with acute confusion and drowsiness. You were told by her son that she had a preceding history of headache, malaise and numerous cold sores on her lip. She had no past medical history, no recent foreign travel and did not take any regular medication.

On examination she had a temperature of 39°C, a heart rate of 100 beats/min and an arterial blood pressure of 110/80 mmHg. Her respiratory rate was 18 breaths/min with an oxygen saturation of 98% on air. She was restless and very confused. Her Glasgow Coma Score was 11 (eye 4; voice 2; motor 5). She was unable to cooperate with a neurological examination, however you observed that she was moving all four limbs equally, both plantar reflexes were down-going and there was no meningism or rash. You also observed numerous herpetic lesions on her lips. Examination of her respiratory, cardiovascular and abdominal system was unremarkable.

The following results are obtained:

Hb	13 g/L
WCC	20 × 10⁹/L
Platelets	240 × 10⁹/L
CRP	220 mg/L
ESR	60 mm/h
U&Es	Normal
LFTs	Normal
CSF	
Appearance	Cloudy
Microscopy	No organisms seen
WCC	2000 cells/mm³ (98% lymphocyte)
RCC	30 cells/mm³
Biochemistry	
Protein	0.7 g/L
Glucose	>50% plasma level

Blood culture: no growth

Chest X-ray: clear

1. *What is the significance of the herpetic lesions?*
   (a) Herpes simplex virus (HSV) infection
   (b) Cytomegalovirus (CMV) infection
   (c) Echovirus infection
2. *Her cerebrospinal fluid (CSF) profile is suggestive of what type of CNS infection?*
   (a) Bacterial
   (b) Viral
   (c) Tuberculosis (TB)
3. *What is the unifying diagnosis?*
   (a) Pneumococcal meningitis
   (b) *Listeria* meningitis
   (c) HSV encephalitis
4. *What investigation would be diagnostic in this patient?*
   (a) CSF HSV polymerase chain reaction (PCR)
   (b) Blood culture
   (c) Meningococcal PCR

Case 7: A patient in hospital with abdominal pain and diarrhoea

A 75-year-old man was admitted to hospital 1 week ago with cellulitis of his right leg. He was treated with a course of antibiotics and his leg was clinically improving. He is known to have hypertension and diabetes. Whilst on call you were asked to assess this gentleman. He complained of diarrhoea and abdominal pain and felt unwell. He passed five large bouts of brown/green watery stool over the last 12 hours. There was no evidence of blood in his stool.

On examination he had a temperature of 38°C, a heart rate of 100 beats/min and an arterial blood pressure of 105/80 mmHg. His respiratory rate was 18 breaths/min with an oxygen saturation of 98% on air. He had generalized abdominal tenderness but there was no evidence of peritonism.

His blood results were available to you:

Hb	13 g/L
WCC	30 × 10⁹/L
	(80% neutrophils)
Platelets	240 × 10⁹/L
CRP	20 mg/L
ESR	20 mm/h
D-dimer	Elevated
Na	138 mmol/L
K	4.1 mmol/L
Urea	12 mmol/L
Creatinine	120 μmol/L
LFTs	Normal

1. *How is the diagnosis most likely to be established?*
   (a) Blood culture
   (b) Abdominal X-ray
   (c) Stool sample
2. *What is the most likely pathogen involved in this process?*
   (a) *Clostridium difficile*
   (b) Norovirus
   (c) *Campylobacter*
3. *Which is the more likely complication to occur as a result of this infection?*
   (a) Endocarditis
   (b) Toxic megacolon
   (c) Arthritis
4. *What initial steps would you take in managing this patient?*
   (a) Isolate in a side room
   (b) Contact the Consultant in Communicable Disease Control (CCDC)
   (c) Commence on ciprofloxacin

Case 8: A man in hospital with a temperature

A 79-year-old man is known to have advanced Parkinson's disease. He was initially admitted with reduced mobility. His anti-Parkinson medication had been altered and his mobility was improving with physiotherapy input. He had no other past medical history and was a non-smoker. On the fourth day of admission he started to spike a temperature and became unwell. He was short of breath, sweaty and complained of right-sided pleuritic chest pain.

On examination he was febrile, tachypneoic and tachycardic and had an oxygen saturation of 93% on air. He had bronchial breathing on the right lower zone of his chest, and there was no wheeze. Heart sounds were normal and his abdominal system was unremarkable.

The following arterial blood gas (on air) results were obtained:

pH	7.36
PCO₂	6.55 kPa
PO₂	8.65 kPa
HCO₃	28 mmol/L
Base excess	4 mmol/L

Chest X-ray: right lower lobe consolidation, no evidence of hyperinflation

ECG: sinus tachycardia, no evidence of ischaemia

1. *What type of pneumonia is this patient likely to have developed?*
   (a) Atypical
   (b) Aspiration
   (c) Community acquired
2. *What initial steps would you take in his management?*
   (a) Isolate in a side room
   (b) Make him nil by mouth (NBM)
   (c) Test his urine for *Legionella* antigen
3. *What is the significance of the right lower lobe being affected?*
   (a) It is the best oxygenated lobe, therefore aerophilic organisms tend to cause infection here
   (b) The right main stem bronchus is of a larger calibre and more vertical, therefore the right middle and lower lobes are prone to aspiration pneumonitis
   (c) Parkinson's disease causes weakness to the lower intercostal muscles, therefore the lower lobes are poorly ventilated and prone to infection
4. *What is the best antibiotic regimen?*
   (a) Amoxicillin
   (b) Ciprofloxacin
   (c) Tazocin

Case 9: A young man with a fever of unknown origin

A 25-year-old labourer had an 8-week history of feeling unwell. His symptoms initially started with right-sided otitis media which did not resolve with antibiotics; he then developed right-sided Bell's palsy with minimal improvement with prednisolone and aciclovir. During this time he experienced intermittent fevers, night sweats and lost 6 kg in weight. He presented to A&E with a 2-day history of breathlessness, haemoptysis and a fever. There was no history of foreign travel.

On examination he was found to be febrile and hypoxic with a PaO_2 of 8 kPa on air. He had a complete right VII nerve palsy and reduced hearing on the right; the rest of the CNS examination was normal. There were no vesicles in his external auditory canal. Bronchial breathing was heard bi-basally and his heart sounds were normal.

The following results were obtained:

Hb	13 g/dL
WCC	17×10^9/L
	(80% neutrophils)
Platelets	240×10^9/L
CRP	240 mg/L
ESR	90 mm/h
Clotting	Normal
U&Es	Normal
LFTs	Normal

Chest radiograph: multiple coin-shaped cavitating lesions in both lung fields
Sputum analysis: negative for acid-fast bacilli
HIV test: negative
Blood culture: no growth
Urinalysis: blood ++
c-ANCA: positive (high titre)

1. *What is the likely cause of his fevers?*
   (a) Infection
   (b) Vasculitis
   (c) Neoplastic

2. *What is the likely cause of his multiple cavitating lung lesions?*
   (a) Abscess
   (b) Pulmonary metastasis
   (c) Pulmonary haemorrhage
3. *What is the likely explanation for the microscopic haematuria?*
   (a) Urinary tract infection (UTI)
   (b) Renal stones
   (c) Glomerulonephritis
4. *What is the underlying diagnosis?*
   (a) Wegener's granulomatosis
   (b) Glomerular basement membrane disease
   (c) Subacute bacterial endocarditis

Case 10: A patient with respiratory problems and fever

A 60-year-old environmental officer presented to his district general hospital with acute lower respiratory tract symptoms and fever. He admitted to non-specific symptoms such as weight loss, reduced appetite and lethargy 2 months prior to his acute illness. There was no history of foreign travel. He had raised inflammatory markers and a right pleural effusion on his chest radiograph. He had no cardiac murmurs on examination. His pleural effusion was tapped and found to be sterile. However he was commenced on antibiotics.

Routine bloods revealed abnormal liver function tests, this initiated a liver ultrasound. He had multiple cystic/solid lesions in his liver which were thought to be abscesses. These were drained and, again, the sample was sterile. Serology for amoeba/hydatid was negative. By this time multiple blood cultures had been sent and were all negative. In total he had 4 weeks of appropriate antibiotics and his symptoms had not resolved nor had his liver lesions regressed. He continued to have spike fevers.

1. *What further investigation would help?*
   (a) Biopsy of liver tissue
   (b) Echocardiogram
   (c) Blood culture
2. *He had a CT of the chest/abdomen and pelvis. This showed multiple lung nodules, right pleural effusion, multiple liver lesions and slight thickening of the distal oesophagus. What is the likely diagnosis?*
   (a) Disseminated bacterial infection
   (b) Metastatic disease
   (c) Systemic granulomatosis
3. *Given the CT findings, what further investigations would you arrange?*
   (a) Gastroscopy
   (b) Bronchoscopy
   (c) Barium swallow
4. *Given his history and CT findings, how would you manage this patient?*
   (a) Continue with antibiotics
   (b) Refer to the gastrointestinal surgeons
   (c) Refer to the oncologist

Case 11: A patient with a fever and rash

A 17-year-old student was brought to the A&E department pyrexial and obtunded. Prior to this acute presentation he had flu-like symptoms. On examination he was drowsy and had a Glasgow Coma Score (GCS) of 9 (eye 2; voice 2; motor 5) and febrile. He had a regular heart rate of 115 beats/min, arterial blood pressure of 105/77 mmHg and normal heart sounds. His abdomen was soft and non-tender. The patient showed mild photophobia and neck stiffness and was Kernig positive. There was no focal neurology and fundoscopy was normal. On his trunk and thigh he had a petechial rash that was non-blanching.

The following results were obtained

Hb	10 g/dL
WCC	18×10^9/L (80% neutrophils)
Platelets	90×10^9/L
CRP	380 mg/L
ESR	90 mm/h
Na	138 mmol/L
K	5 mmol/L
Urea	10 mmol/L
Creatinine	80 µmol/L
LFTs	Normal
PT	20 sec
APTT	50 sec
Fibrinogen	0.5
D-dimer	Elevated

1. *Which of these investigations would be most appropriate?*
    (a) Blood culture
    (b) CT of the head
    (c) Lumbar puncture
2. *Taking into account his blood result and the observed rash, what complication has occurred?*
    (a) Systemic embolic phenomena
    (b) Disseminated intravascular coagulation (DIC)
    (c) Severe sepsis
3. *What is the diagnosis?*
    (a) Pneumococcal meningitis
    (b) Meningococcal meningitis
    (c) Viral meningitis
4. *Which of these investigations is least likely to establish a diagnosis?*
    (a) Polymerase chain reaction (PCR)
    (b) Skin scraping of petechiae
    (c) Antistreptolysin O (ASO) titre

Case 12: A patient with a fever and rash

A 22-year-old woman presents to her GP with malaise, arthralgia and fever. She mentioned a raised painful rash on both her shins. She denies any respiratory or gastrointestinal symptoms. She is not on any medication and there is no history of foreign travel. On examination she has a low-grade fever and has tender erythematous nodules present on both anterior shins.

1. *What rash has she got?*
    (a) Erythema multiforme
    (b) Erythema nodosum
    (c) Erythema marginatum
2. *What is the most important investigation to perform?*
    (a) Chest radiograph
    (b) Erythrocyte sedimentation rate (ESR)
    (c) Urine dipstick
3. *Which of the following conditions is least likely to cause painful erythematous nodules?*
    (a) Streptococcal infection
    (b) Sarcoidosis
    (c) Aspirin

4. *A skin biopsy is taken; what would expect to see under light microscopy?*
    (a) Lymphoclastic vasculitis
    (b) Panniculitis
    (c) Neutrophilic infiltration of the epidermis

Case 13: An HIV-infected patient with fever

A 27-year-old man was recently found to be HIV positive. He presented with HIV encephalopathy and, following successful rehabilitation, he was discharged home and commenced on anti-retroviral treatment. His CD4 count at the time was 5 and he had a high viral load. He represented 2 weeks later with malaise, fever and vomiting. He had been adherent with his medication. He denied having diarrhoea.

On examination he had a temperature of 39°C, a heart rate of 100 beats/min and an arterial blood pressure of 110/80 mmHg. His respiratory rate was 18 breaths/min with an oxygen saturation of 98% on air. He had evidence of oral *Candida* and cervical and inguinal lymphadenopathy. He had a normal heart sound and a clear chest. His abdomen was soft but he had a moderately sized hepatosplenomegaly. Neurological examination was unremarkable and there was no evidence of retinal scarring or papilloedema on fundoscopy. There was no visible rash.

The following results are available to you:

Hb	8 g/dL
WCC	2×10^9/L
Platelets	90×10^9/L
CRP	250 mg/L
ESR	90 mm/h
Na	138 mmol/L
K	5 mmol/L
Urea	16 mmol/L
Creatinine	140 µmol/L
LFTs	Normal

Chest radiograph: normal
Blood culture: normal
Lactate dehydrogenase: normal
Cryptococcal antigen: negative
Cytomegalovirus PCR: undetected

1. *Which of the following investigations is least useful?*
    (a) Bone marrow biopsy
    (b) Liver biopsy
    (c) Renal biopsy
2. *This presentation could be an immune reconstitution illness, what does this mean?*
    (a) Febrile illness secondary to the anti-retroviral therapy
    (b) As the immune system improves on anti-retroviral therapy, previously ignored immune targets are recognized
    (c) Adverse drug reaction
3. *What is the most likely pathogen?*
    (a) Cytomegalovirus (CMV)
    (b) Cryptococcosis
    (c) *Mycobacterium avium* complex (MAC)
4. *What is the likely explanation for his pancytopenia?*
    (a) Lymphoma
    (b) Severe bacterial sepsis
    (c) Marrow infiltration by MAC

Case 14: A patient with a fever, sore throat and rash

A 35-year-old businessman presented to his GP with an acute onset of fever, sore throat and a rash across his trunk. He also complained of muscle ache and loose stool. He has frequented Thailand in the last 6 months to establish business links. He was last there 6 weeks ago. He admitted to having sex with a prostitute during this visit. He is married with a 1-month-old baby.

On examination he was febrile and there was evidence of oral *Candida*. He had cervical and inguinal lymphadenopathy and a maculopapular rash on his trunk. His tonsils were swollen and red. His chest was clear and abdominal examination was unremarkable. He had mild lymphopenia, but otherwise his full blood count/urea and electrolytes/liver function tests were normal. He also had a negative monospot test.

1. *What is the likely diagnosis?*
   - (a) Glandular fever
   - (b) HIV seroconversion
   - (c) Viral hepatitis
2. *What should you do next?*
   - (a) Offer an HIV test and counselling
   - (b) Reassure him and offer a review date in a month's time
   - (c) Send him home with antivirals
3. *He has two HIV-positive test results, what do you do next?*
   - (a) Refer to genitourinary medicine for a sexually transmitted infection (STI) screen and general management of his illness
   - (b) Commence on anti-retroviral
   - (c) Manage in the community because he has a high CD4 count
4. *What action would the specialist team need to take?*
   - (a) Inform the Consultant in Communicable Disease Control (CCDC)
   - (b) Offer an HIV test to his wife and baby
   - (c) Give smoking cessation advice

Case 15: A traveller with diarrhoea and fever

A 25-year-old backpacker had been travelling in Malawi for a month and arrived back in the UK 3 weeks ago. He had been fully vaccinated prior to his travels and was diligent in taking his malaria tablets. He stayed in semi-rural areas and ate local cuisine. He developed bloody diarrhoea 2 weeks after arriving back and became increasingly lethargic with occasional rigors. Despite eating lots he could not keep his weight on. There was no rash or abdominal pain. There was no history of sexual contact whilst in Malawi. He has never had diarrhoea before and there is no family history of inflammatory bowel disease.

Examination revealed a low-grade fever but was otherwise normal. There was no rash, lymphadenopathy or organomegaly on abdominal examination. He was not jaundiced. He was HIV negative, his blood culture was negative and three thick films for malaria parasites were negative.

1. *Which of the following pathogens does not typically cause bloody diarrhoea?*
   - (a) *Salmonella typhi*
   - (b) Amoeba
   - (c) Norovirus

2. *Which investigation would help to establish a diagnosis?*
   - (a) Stool microscopy
   - (b) Blood culture
   - (c) Abdominal X-ray
3. *What complication is most likely to occur post-infection?*
   - (a) Endocarditis
   - (b) Lactose intolerance
   - (c) Encephalitis
4. *How would you manage this patient?*
   - (a) Amoxicillin
   - (b) Flexi-sigmoidoscopy
   - (c) Metronidazole

Case 16: A traveller with jaundice

A 22-year-old male backpacker went travelling in Thailand for 6 weeks. He had now been back in the UK for 2 weeks. The decision to travel was spontaneous so he had no vaccinations nor did he take malaria chemoprophylaxis. He stayed in semi-rural areas and ate local cuisine and his alcohol intake was minimal. He is an ex-smoker. Since his return, he has had a fever and flu-like symptoms, which slowly improved but a week later he became jaundiced. Though he felt better he presented to his GP concerned by his skin discolouration. There was no rash, diarrhoea or chest symptoms. He had no sexual contacts during this time. He does not take regular medication and denies illicit drug use.

The following blood results were available to you:

Bilirubin	60 μmol/L
ALT	1230 U/L
ALP	200 U/L
γ-GT	150 U/L
Albumin	27 g/L

Malaria screen: negative
HIV: negative

1. *What blood test would you perform?*
   - (a) Blood culture
   - (b) Hepatitis serology
   - (c) Serum paracetamol levels
2. *What other investigation would you perform?*
   - (a) Abdominal X-ray
   - (b) Liver ultrasound scan
   - (c) Liver biopsy
3. *What is the likely diagnosis?*
   - (a) Hepatitis A
   - (b) Hepatitis C
   - (c) Leptospirosis
4. *What future advice would you give to this man?*
   - (a) Offer hepatitis A vaccination for his next trip abroad
   - (b) Emphasis the importance of malaria prophylaxis
   - (c) Smoking cessation advice

Case 17: A patient with fever and joint pain

A 34-year-old banker presented to his GP with a 5-day history of fever and joint pain. He is currently single but has had unprotected sexual intercourse with two female partners in the last 6 months. He recalls having a slight urethral discharge about 1 month ago but this was self-limiting so he did not pursue it. On examination he had a low-grade fever and a hot right knee effusion and a pustular rash surrounds the joint. He has previously been well.

The following results were available to you:

Haematology profile	Normal
Biochemical profile	Normal
Glucose	Normal
CRP	240 mg/L
Rheumatoid factor	Negative
Autoantibody screen	Negative
HIV	Negative
Hepatitis screen	Negative

Joint aspirate: turbid fluid, no organisms, no crystals

1. *What investigation would you next initiate?*
   (a) Urethral swab and divided urine sample
   (b) Chest X-ray
   (c) Joint aspirate and culture
2. *Which of the following complications is least likely to occur following a urethritis infection?*
   (a) Hepatitis
   (b) Uveitis
   (c) Gastritis
3. *What is the likely diagnosis?*
   (a) Reiter's syndrome
   (b) Secondary syphilis
   (c) Gonococcal arthritis
4. *How would you manage this patient?*
   (a) Reassurance
   (b) Commence on ciprofloxacin
   (c) Therapeutic joint aspiration

Case 18: A patient with vaginal discharge

A 35-year-old female has attended the genitourinary clinic. She complained of a 2-week history of foul-smelling vaginal discharge. She had tried over-the-counter Canesten pessaries several times without success. She finds the smell disturbing and sexual intercourse with her partner of 10 years has become increasingly difficult because of the pain. She is otherwise well.

On examination she had a soft and non-tender abdomen. You perform a speculum examination and find that she has a malodorous grey discharge, and a markedly inflamed vaginal wall. However, there was no adnexal tenderness or cervical excitation. The pH of the discharge was 5.

1. *What simple test could you do to the discharge sample to help differentiate the pathogen?*
   (a) Test for a fishy odour with potassium hydroxide (KOH)
   (b) Test for effervescence with calcium carbonate
   (c) Test for brown discolouration with NaCl
2. *What is the likely cause of her discharge?*
   (a) Physiological
   (b) *Chlamydia*
   (c) *Trichomonas*
3. *What other investigation would help to establish a diagnosis?*
   (a) Blood culture
   (b) Urine test
   (c) High vaginal swab for microscopy and culture
4. *How would you treat this condition?*
   (a) Topical or systemic azole
   (b) Metronidazole
   (c) Doxycycline

Case 19: A patient with malaise and fever following a tick bite

A 46-year-old woman attended her general practice with a 1-week history of malaise, general body ache and fever. Further questioning revealed that she had been in the New Forest 3 weeks ago and recalls been bitten on her leg. A week later she developed an expanding rash. She denied any respiratory, gastrointestinal or cardiovascular symptoms.

Examination revealed a low-grade pyrexia of 37.5°C. You note a non-tender, erythematous, annular rash on her right buttock. Examination of her cardiovascular, respiratory, musculoskeletal and central nervous system was normal.

1. *What is the likely diagnosis?*
   (a) Influenza B
   (b) Lyme disease
   (c) Cellulitis
2. *What is the name of the rash?*
   (a) Erythema marginatum
   (b) Erythema chronicum migrans
   (c) Erythema multiforme
3. *What pathogen is responsible for this disease process?*
   (a) *Borrelia burgdorferi*
   (b) *Brucella abortus*
   (c) Streptococcal pneumonia
4. *Which is the best antibiotic to use in this patient?*
   (a) Ciprofloxacin
   (b) Gentamycin
   (c) Doxycycline

Case 20: A farmer with night sweats and a large spleen

A 62-year-old cattle farmer was admitted to your hospital with a 3-week history of malaise, muscle ache and night sweats. He had unintentionally lost 3 kg in weight over this period. On examination he was febrile, with a heart rate of 105 beats/min and an arterial blood pressure of 120/80 mmHg. He had cervical lymphadenopathy and a palpable splenic tip. He had right sacroiliac tenderness but this did not hinder his range of movement. Examination of his chest and central nervous system was normal. He had a tender macular lesion about 4 × 3 cm on both shins. He had an ECG which showed a sinus tachycardia and his chest radiograph was clear.

The following results are available:

Hb	10.5 g/dL
WCC	2×10^9/L
	(75% neutrophils)
Platelets	220×10^9/L
CRP	190 mg/L
ESR	40 mm/h
U&Es	Normal
LFTs	Normal
Calcium	Normal

1. *What is the likely pathogen causing this disease process?*
   (a) *Leptospira interrogans*
   (b) *Mycobacterium tuberculosis*
   (c) *Brucella abortus*
2. *What investigation would help to make a diagnosis?*
   (a) X-ray of the pelvis, to examine the sacro-iliac joints further
   (b) Blood culture
   (c) Montoux test

3. *What would you expect to see on a Gram stain?*
   (a) Gram-positive cocci
   (b) Gram-negative coccobacillus
   (c) Gram-positive rods
4. *What rash has this patient got?*
   (a) Erythema nodosum
   (b) Erythema ab igne
   (c) Erythema multiforme

Case 21: A febrile traveller returning from the Gambia

A 40-year-old woman had come back from the Gambia 2 weeks ago. She presented to A&E with a 4-day history of general lethargy, fever and muscle ache. She stayed in a semi-rural area and ate local cuisine. She denied any sexual contact during her trip. She had taken doxycycline as chemoprophylaxis for malaria but missed a few doses. She had been bitten by mosquitoes on numerous occasions.

On examination she was febrile, tachycardic with a heart rate of 110 beats/min and had an arterial blood pressure of 115/80 mmHg. Her respiratory rate was 18 breaths/min with an oxygen saturation of 99% on air. She had a clear chest, normal heart sounds and a soft and non-tender abdomen.

The following results were available to you:

Hb	9.4 g/dL
WCC	14×10^9/L
Platelets	100×10^9/L
ESR	40 mm/h
U&Es	Normal
Albumin	29 g/L
Bilirubin	50 µmol/L
ALT	Normal
ALP	Normal

1. *How is the diagnosis most likely to be established?*
   (a) Blood culture
   (b) Thick and thin blood films
   (c) Urine for microscopy and culture
2. *What is the likely cause of her anaemia?*
   (a) Vitamin B_{12} deficiency
   (b) Haemolysis
   (c) Haemorrhage
3. *Which condition could confer some protection against severe malaria?*
   (a) Being pregnant
   (b) Glucose-6-phosphate dehydrogenase (G6PD) deficiency
   (c) Being splenectomized
4. *What is the usual incubation period for falciparum malaria?*
   (a) 24–48 hours
   (b) 10–14 days
   (c) 6–8 months

Case 22: A young man returning from sub-Saharan Africa unwell and drowsy

A 20-year-old Caucasian boy has just come back from a gap year in southern Africa. Prior to his trip he had been vaccinated for yellow fever/typhoid/tetanus and hepatitis A. He had good intentions of taking his malaria chemoprophylaxis but stopped it after 2 months.

He was brought into your hospital very unwell and drowsy. You were unable to take a history but on examination you found that he had a temperature of 39°C, heart rate of 120 beats/min and an arterial blood pressure of 95/70 mmHg. He had a respiratory rate of 25 breaths/min and his oxygen saturation was 98% on air. His chest was clear and there were no added heart sounds. He had a moderately enlarged spleen. There was no visible rash and he was Kernig negative. He had a normal central nervous system examination and there was no papilloedema on fundoscopy.

The following results were available to you:

Hb	8.4 g/dl
WCC	14×10^9/L
	(75% neutrophils)
Platelets	15×10^9/L
CRP	300 mg/L
ESR	40 mm/h
U&Es	Normal
Albumin	25 g/L
Bilirubin	50 µmol/L
ALT	Normal
ALP	Normal

Chest radiograph: normal
ECG: sinus tachycardia
Blood film: *Plasmodium* species identified with a parasite count of 15%

1. *What is Kernig's sign?*
   (a) Pain or resistance on passive extension of the knee with a flexed hip and with the patient lying in a supine position
   (b) Involuntary lifting of the leg when lifting the patient's head
   (c) Pressure on the cheeks leads to rising and flexion of the forearm
2. *What is the likely pathogen?*
   (a) *Plasmodium vivax*
   (b) *Plasmodium falciparum*
   (c) *Plasmodium malariae*
3. *This man was classified as having severe malaria. Which of the following is a marker of severity?*
   (a) Hypoglycaemia
   (b) Thrombocytopenia
   (c) Splenomegaly
4. *He was immediately commenced on IV quinine. What ECG abnormality should you be aware of whist he is on treatment?*
   (a) First degree heart block
   (b) Atrial bigeminy
   (c) Long QT syndrome

Case 23: A patient with asthma and a fever

A 35-year-old man has had poorly controlled asthma for the last year with repeated hospital admissions. He presented to hospital on this occasion with a fever and a cough with excessive mucous expectoration. He was unable to talk in complete sentences, was wheezy, had a heart rate (HR) of 115 beats/min, a respiratory rate (RR) of 30 breaths/min and an oxygen saturation of 92% on air; his arterial blood pressure was 90/60 mmHg. He had peripheral eosinophilia and his chest radiograph showed left upper zone consolidation and tramlines were noted on the left midzone.

1. *Which of these features describes acute severe asthma?*
   (a) HR 110 + RR > 25 + unable to speak in complete sentences
   (b) HR 100 + RR 20 + peak flow 70% of predicted
   (c) HR 50 + exhaustion + silent chest
2. *How is it best to manage this patient in the acute setting?*
   (a) Oxygen + bronchodilators + steroids + antibiotics + anaesthetic/ITU assessment
   (b) Oxygen + bronchodilators + steroids + antifungals
   (c) Oxygen + bronchodilators
3. *What diagnosis underlies his repeated admissions and poor control?*
   (a) Allergic bronchopulmonary aspergillosis (ABPA)
   (b) Pulmonary vasculitis
   (c) Poor compliance
4. *What is the disease mechanism of allergic bronchopulmonary aspergillosis (ABPA)?*
   (a) Type I and III hypersensitivity reaction
   (b) Direct invasion of *Aspergillus* on the lung parenchyma
   (c) Type IV hypersensitivity reaction
5. *What is the significance of tramlines on the chest radiograph?*
   (a) Collapse of lung tissue secondary to mucus plugging
   (b) Evidence of bronchiectasis
   (c) Pulmonary congestion

Case 24: An HIV-positive patient with vomiting and fever

A 30-year-old HIV-positive man has a poor adherence to his anti-retroviral treatment. He has a CD4 count of 45/mm³. He attended clinic with a 2-week history of persistent vomiting, fever and an intense headache. Examination revealed a pyrexia of 38°C, a heart rate of 115 beats/min and an arterial blood pressure of 110/70 mmHg. He had no focal neurology or meningism, nor did he have evidence of papilloedema on fundoscopy. He had hepatosplenomegaly, although his chest was clear.

He was admitted to hospital for investigation and the following results were available to you:

CSF

Appearance	Clear
Microscopy	No organisms seen
WCC	2 cells/mm³
RCC	10 cells/mm³
Biochemistry	
Protein	0.45 g/L
Glucose	>50%
Cryptococcal antigen	Positive >1 in 256
CMV/VZV/HSV/EBV PCR	Not detected
Syphilis serology	Negative
Toxoplasma serology	Negative

Blood culture: positive for *Cryptococcus* sp.
CT of the head: normal

1. *Which staining method would have been used in the cerebrospinal fluid (CSF) and blood sample to detect the cryptococcal pathogen?*
   (a) Gram stain
   (b) Giemsa stain
   (c) Indian ink stain
2. *Which cryptococcal species is most likely to be responsible for his illness?*
   (a) *Cryptococcus neoformans* var. *gatti*
   (b) *Cryptococcus neoformans* var. *neoformans*
   (c) *Cryptococcus albidus*
3. *What delayed complication should a clinician be alert to in a patient with cryptococcal meningitis?*
   (a) Hydrocephalus
   (b) Disseminated intravascular coagulation (DIC)
   (c) Pericarditis
4. *What is the most appropriate therapy?*
   (a) Amphotericin B + flucytocine as initial therapy followed by fluconazole
   (b) Amphotericin B alone
   (c) Amphotericin B + flucytocine

Case 25: A refugee with night sweats and haemoptysis

A 35-year-old refugee from Eritrea had a 4-month history of night sweats and weight loss. Recently he had become more short of breath and had haemoptysis. He shared a room with four other family members. He has lived in the UK for 6 months. Though he remained haemodynamically stable he had a temperature of 38°C. Bronchial breathing was heard in the right upper zone of his chest. He had a mantoux test which was read 48 hours later and found to be strongly positive. He had a chest X-ray (Fig. 6.25.1) and his sputum showed acid-fast bacilli.

1. *What does a positive mantoux test mean?*
   (a) Indurated area >5 mm after 48 hours
   (b) Indurated area >10 mm after 48 hours
   (c) Indurated area >15 mm after 48 hours
2. *What initial management steps should you take?*
   (a) Isolate the patient in a negative pressure room
   (b) Commence on antibiotics
   (c) Commence on anti-TB medication
3. *Given this man's diagnosis, what public health action should you take?*

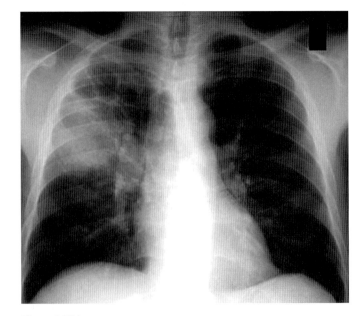

Figure 6.25.1

(a) Inform the Consultant in Communicable Disease Control CCDC
(b) Advice on smoking cessation
(c) Offer BCG (bacilli Calmette-Guérin) vaccination to everyone he has had contact with over the last month

4. *Which pathogen does not typically cause a cavitating lung lesion?*
   (a) *Mycobacteria* tuberculosis
   (b) *Staphylococcus aureus*
   (c) *Haemophilus* influenza

Case 26: A patient with abdominal pain and vomiting

A 33-year-old man from Somalia presented to A&E with recurrent right upper quadrant abdominal pain and vomiting. He has lived in the UK for 12 years and last visited Somalia 4 years ago. On further questioning he admitted to unintentional weight loss of over 6 kg and occasional night sweats. He denied having any chest symptoms. He was not jaundiced and was free from diarrhoea. On examination a 2×2 cm right axillary lymph node was palpable. He was also tender in his right upper quadrant but neither his liver nor spleen was enlarged. He was Murphy's negative.

His blood results showed an abnormal liver function test:

FBC	Normal
U&Es	Normal
Clotting	Normal
Bilirubin	35 μmol/L
ALT	400 U/L
ALP	190 U/L
γ-GT	100 U/L

Hepatitis A/B/C: negative
HIV: negative
Autoimmune screen: negative
Mantoux test: positive

He had a CT of the liver with contrast which showed intrahepatic duct dilatation and enlarged lymph nodes at the porta hepatis. His common bile duct was normal and he had a normal head of the pancreas and gall bladder. A fine needle aspiration of the lymph node showed features consistent with a caseating granuloma.

1. *This patient was Murphy's negative; what is he likely not to have?*
   (a) Cholecystitis
   (b) Hepatitis
   (c) Head of pancreas carcinoma

2. *Which of these conditions does not typically form a caseating granuloma?*
   (a) *Mycobacterium* tuberculosis
   (b) Cryptococcosis
   (c) Sarcoidosis

3. *What other investigations would give a definitive diagnosis of TB?*
   (a) Culture of a sample from the lymph node
   (b) Chest radiograph
   (c) Liver ultrasound

4. *The decision was made to commence him on anti-TB medication; which is the best treatment option?*
   (a) Isoniazid + rifampicin + pyrazinamide + ethambutol for 6 months

(b) Isoniazid + rifampicin for 6 months with pyrizinamide + ethambutol for the first 2 months
(c) Isoniazid + rifampicin + pyrizinamide + ethambutol for 12 months

Case 27: A young man with a sore throat

A 30-year-old man presented to hospital with a 7-day history of sore throat, fever and malaise. He had been previously fit and well. There was no history of recent travel. On examination he looked unwell. He was sweaty and had warm peripheries. He had a temperature of 39°C, arterial blood pressure of 90/60 mmHg and a heart rate 115 beats/min. His respiratory rate was 22 breaths/min with an oxygen saturation of 97% on air. Examination of his chest and abdomen was unremarkable and he had normal heart sounds. He also had swollen inflamed tonsils with purulent exudates.

You arrange for some investigation and the results are as follows:

Hb	15 g/dL
WCC	18×10^9/L (80% neutrophils)
Platelets	240×10^9/L
CRP	170 mg/L
ESR	60 mm/h
Na	142 mmol/L
K	3.5 mmol/L
Urea	6 mmol/L
Creatinine	110 μmol/L

Throat swab: Gram-positive cocci
Blood film: Gram-positive cocci
MSU: normal
Chest X-ray: normal

1. *Which diagnosis best fits this clinical scenario?*
   (a) Toxic shock syndrome
   (b) Glandular fever
   (c) Tonsillitis

2. *What is the likely pathogen?*
   (a) *Listeria*
   (b) Group A *Streptococcus*
   (c) *Staphylococcus aureus*

3. *What should be your initial approach to managing this patient?*
   (a) Fluid resuscitation
   (b) Isolate the patient
   (c) Commence on antibiotics

4. *What complication of tonsillitis should you be alert to?*
   (a) Quinsy
   (b) Thrombocytopenia
   (c) Hypoglycaemia

Case 28: An elderly woman with fever and right upper quadrant pain

An 80-year-old woman was admitted to your ward with a 1-week history of malaise, fever and right upper quadrant pain. Over the last year she has experienced upper abdominal discomfort and her appetite has been poor as a result. She is a non-smoker and drinks 10 units of alcohol per week. There is no recent travel history. On examination she looked unwell and was jaundiced. Her temperature was 38°C, heart rate 103 beats/min and arterial blood pressure 105/70 mmHg. She was tender in the right upper quadrant with a palpable liver edge. She also had a non-blanching rash on her trunk and upper legs.

The following results are available to you:

Hb	13 g/dL
WCC	18×10^9/L
Platelets	90×10^9/L
CRP	360 mg/L
ESR	60 mm/h
Na	135 mmol/L
K	4.5 mmol/L
Urea	8.5 mmol/L
Creatinine	170 μmol/L
Albumin	28 g/L
Bilirubin	25 μmol/L
ALT	60 U/L
ALP	300 U/L
γ-GT	200 U/L
PT	20 s
APTT	50 s
Fibrinogen	0.5 g/L
D-dimer	Elevated

Blood culture: lactose fermenting coliform
Abdominal ultrasound: common bile duct dilatation of 14 mm

1. *Which of the following would not explain the prolonged prothrombin time (PT)?*
   (a) Vitamin K deficiency
   (b) Disseminated intravascular coagulation (DIC)
   (c) Protein C deficiency
2. *What is the likely diagnosis?*
   (a) Cholecystitis
   (b) Ascending cholangitis
   (c) Pancreatitis
3. *What complication of sepsis has occurred?*
   (a) Liver abscess
   (b) DIC
   (c) Meningitis
4. *Which specialty would you need to make an urgent referral to?*
   (a) Haematologist
   (b) Microbiologist
   (c) Gastrointestinal surgeon

Case 29: A patient with inflamed tonsils

A 20-year-old student presented to A&E with a sore throat, malaise and muscle ache. His symptoms had been ongoing for 1 week. He had been given a 5-day course of amoxicillin by his GP, however his symptoms persisted. A couple of his classmates had also had similar symptoms. On examination he was afebrile and haemodynamically stable. He had inflamed tonsils but no exudates, a moderately enlarged hepatosplenomegaly and cervical lymphadenopathy.

The following results were available to you:

Hb	13 g/dl
WCC	20×10^9/L (75% lymphocytes)
Platelets	150×10^9/L
CRP	120 mg/L
ESR	60 mm/h
U&Es	Normal
Albumin	30 g/L
Bilirubin	50 μmol/L
ALT	980 U/L
ALP	180 U/L
γ-GT	100 U/L

Monospot test: positive
Abdominal ultrasound: diffusely enlarged echogenic liver and spleen

1. *What is a monospot test?*
   (a) Serum antibodies against red blood cells of other species
   (b) Serum antibodies against white blood cells of other species
   (c) Serum antibodies against own red blood cells
2. *What is the most likely diagnosis?*
   (a) Streptococcal pharyngitis
   (b) Glandular fever
   (c) Influenza infection
3. *This student re-presented 5 days later with a maculopapular rash across his trunk; what is the likely cause?*
   (a) Measles
   (b) Amoxicillin
   (c) Syphilis

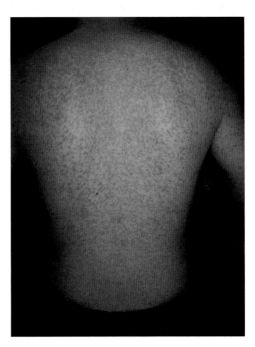

Figure 6.29.1

4. *How is it best to manage this patient?*
   (a) Reassurance
   (b) Antiviral
   (c) Antibiotics

Case 30: A patient with a blistering rash

A 75-year-old man had a 1-week history of a tingling around his right forehead and right eye pain. Two days later he developed a blistering rash on his forehead. The rash became increasingly painful with a yellow, foul-smelling discharge. He became increasingly unwell and feverish. His GP referred him to hospital for an assessment. On examination of his rash you observe crops of vesicles with areas of golden brown crust plus yellow discharge (Fig. 6.30.1). He was alert and orientated. Examination of the central nervous system, chest and heart were normal.

The following results were available to you:

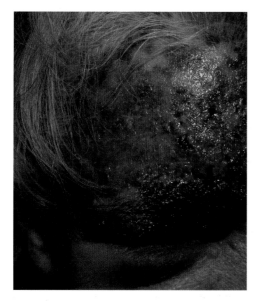

Figure 6.30.1

Hb	13 g/dL
WCC	18×10^9/L (75% neutrophils)
Platelets	150×10^9/L
CRP	120 mg/L
ESR	40 mm/h
U&Es	Normal
LFTs	Normal

1. *What dermatome is involved in this disease process?*
   (a) CI
   (b) V1
   (c) V2
2. *What pathogen is responsible for this disease process?*
   (a) Herpes simplex virus (HSV)
   (b) Varicella-zoster virus (VZV)
   (c) Cytomegalovirus (CMV)
3. *What specialty would this patient need an urgent referral to?*
   (a) Neurologist
   (b) Ophthalmologist
   (c) Dermatologist
4. *Which complication is most likely to have occurred?*
   (a) Secondary bacterial infection
   (b) Post-herpetic neuralgia
   (c) Ramsey Hunt syndrome

Case 31: A breathless homosexual patient

A 27-year-old homosexual man presented with a 6-month history of worsening breathlessness, chest pain and a non-productive cough. He had been unsuccessfully treated in the community with antibiotics. On general inspection he had difficulty in breathing with a respiratory rate of 25 breaths/min, his arterial blood pressure was 130/75 mmHg and he had a heart rate of 100 beats/min. His oxygen saturation was 94% on air. This rapidly declined to 77% on minimal exertion. His hypoxia was confirmed by arterial blood gas; with a PaO_2 of 8.33 kPa. He had a temperature of 38°C.

Examination of his chest revealed fine inspiratory crackles in both his lung bases. He also had a purplish indurated plaque on his palate. You obtained a chest radiograph which showed clear lung fields. The registrar had appropriately arranged for a HIV test, which came back positive, and he had a CD4 count of 45/mm³.

1. *Which of the following is the most useful investigation in establishing the diagnosis?*
   (a) Blood culture
   (b) Induced sputum
   (c) CT of the chest
2. *The chest radiograph shows bilateral perihilar shadowing. Which pathogen is more likely to have caused his illness?*
   (a) *Mycobacterium tuberculosis* pneumonia
   (b) Pneumococcal pneumonia
   (c) *Pneumocystis jirovecii* pneumonia
3. *What other AIDS-defining illness could this man have?*
   (a) Oral *Candida*
   (b) Kaposi's sarcoma
   (c) Pulmonary TB
4. *Given that this man's CD4 count is <200/mm³, which medication would he need to remain on until his CD4 count improves?*
   (a) Amoxicillin
   (b) Fluconazole
   (c) Co-trimoxazole

Case 32: An HIV-positive patient with a right hemiparesis

A 35-year-old sex worker presented with a subacute history of right-sided limb weakness and headache. She was diagnosed with HIV on this presentation. Examination revealed a right hemiparesis without sensory involvement; there were no signs of raised intracranial pressure and she remained afebrile throughout.

The following results were available to you:

CSF

Appearance	Clear
Microscopy	No organisms seen
WCC	2 cells/mm³
RCC	10 cells/mm³

Biochemistry

Protein	0.45 g/L
Glucose	>50%
Cryptococcal antigen	Negative
EBV PCR	Elevated
CMV/VZV/HSV PCR	Not detected
Syphilis serology	Negative

Enhanced CT of the head (ring-enhancing lesion) (Fig. 6.32.1)

1. *She had a trial of anti-Toxoplasma treatment for 1 month but there was no objective improvement. What is the most likely diagnosis?*
   (a) Toxoplasmosis
   (b) Cerebral lymphoma
   (c) Disseminated Cryptococcal disease
2. *What is the most likely range of her CD4 count?*
   (a) <100 mm³
   (b) 200–300 mm³
   (c) >400 mm³
3. *What in the best form of treatment in this instance?*
   (a) Radiotherapy
   (b) Surgical excision
   (c) Chemotherapy

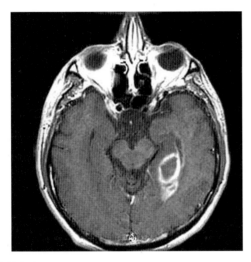

Figure 6.32.1

4. *What next step should you take?*
   (a) Contact tracing of previous sexual partners and offer them an HIV test
   (b) Commence on antibiotics
   (c) Isolate the patient in a side room

Case 33: Recurrent infections in a 49-year-old woman

A 49-year-old woman is referred by her GP with a 5-year history of recurrent chest and sinus infections. She was admitted to hospital the previous year with pneumococcal pneumonia (blood culture positive); at the time of her most recent infection *Haemophilus influenzae* was grown from her sputum. She tends to cough up a small amount of sputum most mornings. She had immune thrombocytopenia (ITP) when she was in her early twenties, but this resolved after a short period on treatment with steroids in modest doses and has not recurred. She currently takes no medication. She has a good appetite and her bowels are regular. Her full blood count shows a normal differential white cell count. A CT scan of her chest shows evidence of bronchiectasis.

1. *Which of the following is the most likely diagnosis?*
   (a) Complement C5 deficiency
   (b) Antibody deficiency secondary to her previous steroid therapy
   (c) Common variable immunodeficiency
   (d) Wiskott–Aldrich syndrome

Case 34: A patient with cough and lymphocytosis

A 72-year-old woman presents acutely with fever and cough productive of green sputum. She is a non-smoker. There is a history of frequent infections over the previous winter requiring antibiotics. Examination of the chest confirms infective signs in the right lower lobe and there are some small axillary lymph nodes.

Results obtained on this admission show a white blood count of 24.3×10^9/L (85% lymphocytes]); IgG is 2.9 g/L (normal range (NR) 6–16), IgA is 0.3 g/L (NR 0.65–3.0), IgM is <0.1 g/L (NR 0.75–2.4); serum electrophoresis shows a faint IgG kappa band and hypogammaglobulinaemia; and urine electrophoresis shows a trace of albumin.

1. *On the basis of these results, which is the most likely underlying diagnosis?*
   (a) IgG myeloma
   (b) Selective IgM deficiency
   (c) Hypogammaglobulinaemia secondary to nephrotic syndrome
   (d) Chronic lymphocytic leukaemia with secondary hypogammaglobulinamia

Infectious Disease: Answers

Case 1: A red, sore venflon site

1. (b) Physical barrier

The skin (a physical barrier) had been breached by the intravenous line allowing the entry of pathogens. Skin integrity is such a key factor in preventing hospital-associated infections, and needless venflon insertion the most common cause of a breach, that the need for any venflon must be very carefully assessed, and weighed against clinical risk. In modern hospital practice it is not considered acceptable to have a 'venflon' inserted as a routine part of the emergency medical admission process. Venflons should *ONLY* be inserted if they are going to be used then and there for intravenous drugs – to insert one because it might be used in the next 24–48 hours is not acceptable practise.

2. (a) Her immune status

The patient has just recovered from a severe infection. Severe infections, whether bacterial or viral, predispose to further infections. It is, for example, well known that patients with flu (influenza A) are particularly predisposed to bacterial pneumonia (e.g. staphylococcal pneumonia), so-called 'double pneumonia'.

3. (a) *Staphylococcus aureus*

Staphylococcus aureus may form part of the skin flora; *S. aureus* and *Streptococcus* typically cause skin infection. Clearly, the fact that she has acquired this infection in hospital does increase the possibility that the *Staphylococcus aureus* is resistant to treatment with multiple antiobiotics, so called methicillin-resistant Staphylococcus aureus MRSA. Though the MRSA form of *Staphylococcus aureus* is no more pathogenic in its natural history than flucloxacillin sensitive *Staphylococcus aureus*, but both forms are highly unpleasant organisms. *Staphylococcus aureus* bacteraemia (positive blood cultures without systemic features of sepsis) is a serious illness, with a significant risk of metastatic infection, particularly in heart valves or joints/bones. *Staphylococcus aureus* septicaemia (positive blood cultures with evidence of sepsis e.g. increased heart rate, lowered blood pressure, fever etc) is a very serious infection, and such patients should be presumed to have metastatic infection, and treated with intravenous antibiotics for a prolonged period.

4. (c) Remove the infected venflon

This is an infected foreign body and should be removed before commencing treatment.

Further reading: Chapter 161 in Medicine at a Glance.

Case 2: A young man with a sore throat and dark urine

1. (a) Current or past infection with group A *Streptococcus*

This is a blood test that looks for antibodies against group A streptococcal antigen. The antibodies can be present for weeks; a high titre is highly suggestive of recent infection.

2. (b) Post-streptococcal glomerulonephritis

Post-streptococcal glomerulonephritis typically presents around 10 days following a group A streptococcal throat infection.

3. (b) Autoimmune phenomena

The glomerulonephritis occurred as an autoimmune response to streptococcal antigens; it may also occur after other streptococcal infections such as scarlet fever.

4. (c) Mesangial proliferation

The typical histology is mesangial proliferation; however, renal is usually not undertaken as, firstly, the diagnosis is usually readily obtained from the clinical context (nephritic pattern renal damage following a streptococcal infection, the latter diagnosed either by a swab or high-titre anti-streptolysin antibodies) and secondly, the prognosis is almost universally benign, with a relatively brief period of symptomatic renal damage followed by total renal recovery. During the period of symptomatic renal damage, decreased urine output, very rarely progressing to complete cessation, oedema, and mild-moderate hypertension can occur. The illness usually resolves spontaneously without any need for renal supportive therapy. Treatment is supportive, and the disease generally resolves in 2–4 weeks.

Further reading: Chapter 140.

Case 3: A patient with flu-like symptoms and a rash

1. (b) Neutrophilia

Raised neutrophil white cell count is the feature most suggestive of bacterial infection in this context. A raised CRP is a good marker of recent inflammation; though in many cases it suggests bacterial infection, and the fact that it is markedly raised here is highly suggestive of bacterial infection, there are many other causes.

2. (a) Haemolytic anaemia

The cause of jaundice are; pre-hepatic, hepatic, and post-hepatic. Though Gilbert's syndrome is possible, there is more evidence in favour of haemolytic anaemia. It is extremely unlikely that his jaundice is due to an intrinsic liver problem, as his liver enzymes are normal, or to post-hepatic bile duct obstruction, as his alkaline phosphatase, a really quite reliable indicator of bile ducts being under pressure, is also quite normal. He has *Mycoplasma* pneumonia which is known to cause haemolytic anaemia and he has a positive Coombs' test.

3. (c) Chest radiograph

A chest radiograph will confirm the diagnosis of pneumonia.

4. (a) Acute and convalescent serology

Mycoplasma serology is definitive. *Mycoplasma* pneumonia is one of a group of organisms that causes atypical pneumonia; atypical in the sense that while the lung is the main site of infection (hence, pneumonia), these infections are all characterised by prominent extra-pulmonary manifestations. Other organisms causing atypical pneumonia include: *legionalla pneumophila* (which results in legionnaires disease), *Chlamydophila pneumoniae* or *psittaci* (the latter resulting in *psittacosis*), and *Coxiella burnetii* (which results in Q fever). In the case of *Mycoplasma* pneumonia, typically, the spread is via infected droplet aerosols, so infection is common in institutions, such as universities, and army barracks, and it most commonly affects those <40 years old. The incubation period is 15–30 days; over this time period there is often a slowly increasingly frequent cough, non-productive, systemic features of infection such as fever and malaise, and a headache. The physical exam is often fairly unremarkable, and the pulmonary signs may be quite unimpressive, even when the chest X-ray shows a fairly florid infection. The extra-pulmonary complications include: cardiac involvement (myocarditis, pericarditis, conduction abnormalities), CNS involvement with encephalitis, Guillain-Barré syndrome, peripheral neuropathy, or transverse myelitis, and haematological involvement with a ccombs positive form of hemolytic anemia. The organism is usually sensitive to macrolide antibiotics, or doxycycline.

Further reading: Chapter 102.

Case 4: A young patient with fever and heart murmur

1. (a) Antistreptolysin O (ASO) titre and echocardiogram

This patient could have rheumatic fever. The diagnosis is made using the modified Duckett Jones' criteria. An ASO titre and cardiac ultrasound (echocardiogram) would help support the diagnosis. The Ducket-Jones' criteria require 2 major, or 1 major and 2 minor criteria to make a diagnosis of rheumatic fever:

Major criteria
- Migratory polyarthritis: this is a migrating arthritis usually starts in the large leg joints and migrates upwards.
- Carditis: the myocardium can be involved, resulting in heart failure, the pericaridium, resulting in a friction rub, or the endocardium resulting in sterile inflammation of a heart valve, resulting in a new murmur.
- Subcutaneous nodules: usually on the extensor surfaces of the elbows or knees, sometimes the back of the wrist.
- Erythema marginatum: a pathognomonic rash starting on the trunk or arms as macules, then spreading outward to form a snake like ring while clearing in the middle. This rash never starts on the face and it is made worse with heat.
- Sydenham's chorea (St. Vitus' dance): a characteristic series of rapid movements without purpose of the face and arms. This can occur very late in the disease, for example, some 6 months after the other manifestations, and is much more common in females.

Minor criteria
- Fever
- Arthralgia
- Raised ESR or CRP
- Leucocytosis
- ECG showing heart block, most typically a long PR interval
- Supportive laboratory data suggesting recent streptococcal infection

2. (a) Previous streptococcal infection

Rheumatic fever is a hypersensitivity reaction to group A *Streptococcus*. His past history of scarlet fever implies that he has had a streptococcal infection.

3. (c) Rheumatic fever

He meets the Jones's criteria, i.e. evidence of streptococcal infection (scarlet fever) and has more than two major criteria: Sydenham's chorea, subcutaneous nodules, arthritis and carditis.

4. (c) Sydenham's chorea

Sydenham's chorea is characterized by involuntary semi purposeful movements. This may be preceded by emotional lability. Not infrequently, families comment that those with Sydenham's chorea are 'fidgety', 'restless', 'never sit still'. They may not comment on the actual choreaform movements.

Further reading: Chapter 91.

Case 5: A patient with presumed infection

1. (b) Ultrasound Doppler scan of her left leg

Although this woman is at risk of a pulmonary embolism (PE), there is no clinical indication for a CTPA. It is more appropriate to diagnose the deep venous thrombosis (DVT) with a Doppler ultrasound.

2. (a) Recent pelvic surgery

Surgery is a major risk factor for DVTs and PEs, especially if the surgery is on the pelvis, or associated with prolonged immobilization. There are many other risk factors for DVT/PE, including malignancy. Indeed, if this woman had active breast cancer, then this would be a more significant risk factor.

3. (a) DVT

Cellulitis is a differential diagnosis and should be excluded but the evidence of sepsis is not convincing. More importantly, the clinical probability of a DVT is high given her recent surgery. This case just emphasizes the point that one can be febrile without having an infection. Indeed, one important cause of *pyrexia of unknown origin* is multiple pulmonary emboli.

4. (a) Activated protein C resistance

She would need a thrombophilia screen, preferentially before commencing on warfarin or after treatment. There are 2 key components to this, firstly tests for genetic abnormalities that increase clotting tendency (e.g. factor V leiden), and secondly, test for acquired causes of a pro-thrombotic state (e.g. anti-phospholipid syndrome etc). The other options are tests to assess bleeding tendency.

Further reading: Chapter 185.

Case 6: A patient with presumed infection and confusion

1. (a) Herpes simplex virus (HSV) infection

The lesions might suggest that she has an HSV viraemia.

2. (b) Viral

A high protein, normal glucose and a raised white cell count that is predominantly lymphocytes all support the diagnosis of an intrathecal viral infection.

3. (c) HSV encephalitis

The subacute history, CSF profile and herpetic lesions all support the diagnosis of HSV encephalitis. Herpes encephalitis is thought to result from retrograde transmission of the herpes virus from the peripheral nerve to the CNS. Typical symptoms include a decreased level of consciousness, and confusion, often with specific temporal lobe abnormalities (this being the commonest site of infection). Diagnosis is made on the clinical picture, CT or preferably MRI findings, and the CSF. The EEG may be suggestive. Untreated, some 70% of infected patients will die, whereas with anti-HS viral treatment (usually aciclovir) the death rate, though still substantial, is reduced to some 20%. Only some 2–5% regain completely normal brain function.

4. (a) CSF HSV polymerase chain reaction (PCR)

There are no diagnostic light or electron microscopy appearances to the virus; growing it is possible, but takes time, whereas polymerase chain reaction amplification and detection is an effective, quick and sensitive means to establish the diagnosis.

Further reading: Chapter 200.

Test	Bacterial	Viral	Fungal	Tubercular
Opening pressure	Elevated	Usually normal	Variable	Variable
White blood cell count	$>= 10^9/L$	$< 10^9/L$	Variable	Variable
Cell differential	Predominance of PMNs	Predominance of lymphocytes	Predominance of lymphocytes	Predominance of lymphocytes
Protein	Mild to marked elevation	Normal to elevated	Elevated	Elevated
CSF-to-serum glucose ratio	Normal to marked decrease	Usually normal	Low	Low

Figure 6.6.1 CSF findings in different forms of meningitis.

Case 7: A patient in hospital with abdominal pain and diarrhoea

1. (c) Stool sample

The stool sample should be examined for *Clostridium difficile* toxin. The history is overwhelmingly suggestive of *Clostridium difficile* toxin associated diarrhoea; an elderly patient, recently in hospital, treated with broad spectrum antibiotics, with typical GI symptoms and findings. Though there is, as always, a differential diagnosis (e.g. ischaemic bowel, etc), *Clostridium difficile* toxin associated diarrhoea is so likely, as to mandate immediate management on this basis.

2. (a) *Clostridium difficile*

This patient has been immunosuppressed following his recent cellulitis and has had a course of antibiotics, both increasing his risk of *Clostridium difficile* toxin associated diarrhoea. The mechanism is usually as follows; broad spectrum antibiotics allow 'protective' colonic bacteria to be replaced by other bacterial species. If the toxogenic form of *Clostridium difficile* is not present, then often antibiotic associated diarrhoea results, usually a nuisance, but rarely dangerous. However, in hospitals, there are large numbers of *Clostridium difficile* toxin producing bacteria around, usually on other patients. Incomplete hygiene allows these bacteria to be passed from one patient, to the environment of another patient, the transmission route being completed when that patient ingests the bacteria. These bacteria then multiply in the large bowel, and symptoms and complications are produced by the toxin.

3. (b) Toxic megacolon

Toxic megacolon is a complication of any colitis and is a surgical emergency. The overall mortality from *Clostridium difficile* toxin associated diarrhoea is probably around 20%, some due to toxic megacolon, some due to the general debilitating effects of prolonged infection on the general health of an already quite frail population, so placing them at risk of falls, and their consequences, pneumonia and renal failure.

4. (a) Isolate in a side room

As part of infection control, this patient should be isolated in a side room.

Further reading: Chapter 25.

Case 8: A man in hospital with a temperature

1. (b) Aspiration

In the late stages of Parkinson's disease, swallowing becomes uncoordinated leading to aspiration pneumonia. The typical location for aspiration pneumonia is the right lower lobe, as the supplying bronchus is the most vertical, so food that has inadvertently entered the bronchial tree finds it most easy to fall straight down, into this bronchus.

2. (b) Make him nil by mouth (NBM)

He would need a formal speech and language therapy assessment, and so should be made NBM in the meantime, the reason being that having made a diagnosis of aspiration pneumonia, one wishes firstly to confirm the mechanism, and secondly prevent further infection.

3. (b) The right main stem bronchus is of a larger calibre and more vertical, therefore the right middle and lower lobes are prone to aspiration pneumonitis

The best oxygenated parts of the lung are the apexes, explaining why the tuberulous organism favours infection there; though Parkinsons disease is associated with poor muscle co-ordination, trembling, it is not particularly associated with respiratory muscle weakness. Most aspiration pneumonia involves the right lower lobe, due to the vertical direction of the supplying bronchus, allowing food to fall directly from the trachea downwards.

4. (c) Tazocin

The aim is to have an antibiotic that is broad spectrum and covers Gram-positive/negative and anaerobic organisms. Local sensitivities to antibiotics vary considerably between hospitals and over time; it is always best to consult either with microbiologists, infectious disease physicians or organ specific specialists as to what the best antibiotics are in any particular situation.

Further reading: Chapter 102.

Case 9: A young man with a fever of unknown origin

1. (b) Vasculitis

He has multiple signs that are anatomically distinct (ear, nerve, lung) and he is cytoplasmic antineutrophil cytoplasmic antibody (c-ANCA) positive. A vasculitic process is more probable, for example Wegeners granulomatosis (by far the most likely, as this vasculitic is very strongly associated with respiratory tract sinus, and ear disease) or another form of microscopic polyangiitis, such as Churg-Strauss. Disseminated infection, for example tuberculosis, could possibly cause this pattern of illness, but he lives in the first world and is HIV negative so making tuberculosis a most unlikely diagnosis. Cancer likewise can cause lesions disseminated in place, but to have multiple cavitating pulmonary lesions is most unlikely.

2. (c) Pulmonary haemorrhage

As this patient is c-ANCA positive he most likely has Wegener's granulomatosis, which causes pulmonary haemorrhages. c-ANCA can be falsely positive, though the higher the titre the less likely this is; however, like any test that isn't perfect, the result should always be interpreted in light of the clinical situation. There are diagnostic criteria for Wegener's granulomatosis, which revolve around finding disseminated inflammation, in the kidneys (microscopic haematuria), lungs (chest X-ray), mouth or nose, and evidence of granulomatus inflammation on a biopsy; 2 out of 4 of these are associated with a fairly high positive predictive accuracy.

3. (c) Glomerulonephritis

This is a vasculitic process that involves the kidney, as a result cyclophosphamide will be part of the treatment plan unless contraindicated.

4. (a) Wegener's granulomatosis

He has mononeuritis multiplex, pulmonary haemorrhages/cavities, evidence of glomerulonephritis and is c-ANCA positive. These are the hallmark of Wegener's granulomatosis. Heart valve infection can give rise to metastatic infection; for example, tricuspid valve endocarditis certainly can give multiple cavitating pulmonary lesions, and renal involvement (microscopic haematuria, progressing all the way to renal failure), however endocarditis is very unlikely to give rise to upper respiratory tract, such as ear involvement, or a mononeuritis multiplex. The clinical context (usually fever and malaise in an IV drug abuser, with a tricuspid regurgitation murmur) makes the diagnosis of tricuspid valve endocarditis.

Further reading: Chapter 213.

Case 10: A patient with respiratory problems and fever

1. (a) Biopsy of liver tissue

The liver is abnormal so the next step would be to get a tissue sample from it. Although an echocardiogram should be done, a liver biopsy is likely to give more answers.

2. (b) Metastatic disease

By far the most likely diagnosis is disseminated malignancy; this would result in exactly this picture. Widely disseminated infection could result in this picture, but if this was due to a typical bacterial pathogen, with this level of infection, he would be extremely sick, and if the diagnosis were disseminated tuberculosis, usually the ethnic and HIV status helps lead to the diagnosis. In this case, the diagnosis is disseminated malignancy, and the likely primary is the oesophagus.

3. (a) Gastroscopy

The origin of the primary cancer needs to be established unequivocally, preferably with a tissue biopsy, to ensure that all treatment options are fully considered. Clearly, if the patient is very unwell, or decides against further investigations for what is likely to be an untreatable condition, investigations should then not be carried out. The CT scan suggests that the primary is in the distal oesophagus, so direct visualization by gastroscopy is preferable to a barium swallow as a tissue sample can also be obtained.

4. (c) Refer to the oncologist

Based on the radiological findings, this man has stage 4 cancer (i.e. distant metastases are present). Treatment is likely to be palliative; however, referral to the oncologist is best both for the multidisciplinary team (MDT) meeting, as occasionally new effective treatments unknown to general physicians become available, and furthermore, oncologists often have very good access to palliative care services.

Further reading: Chapter 191.

Case 11: A patient with a fever and rash

1. (a) Blood culture

A lumbar puncture is contraindicated because of the coagulopathy. Blood cultures should be taken as the antibiotics are being drawn up. The syndrome described is one were immediate antibiotics are crucial – it would have been best if the GP had been able to give them, in the absence of this they should be given by the first hospital clinician they meet. In hospital, it is crucial to obtain blood cultures; however, there is no need for multiple blood cultures spread out over time, the clinical situation will not allow this.

2. (b) Disseminated intravascular coagulation (DIC)

There is overconsumption of platelets and clotting factors, so prolonging the intrinsic and extrinsic clotting cascade, and lowering the fibrinogen level. D-dimers are a breakdown product of the clotting cascade, in this context they are not used to indicate any thromboembolic event. The presence of DIC is clearly a grim prognostic sign.

3. (b) Meningococcal meningitis

A non-blanching purpuric rash is characteristic but only infrequently occurs with other bacterial meningitis.

4. (c) Antistreptolysin O (ASO) titre

This patient has meningococcal meningitis so an ASO titre would be of no benefit. Perhaps surprisingly, organisms can be found in the petechial rash, though skin scrapings are rarely used clinically to establish the diagnosis.

Further reading: Chapter 200.

Case 12: A patient with a fever and rash

1. (b) Erythema nodosum

The description is classic for erythema nodosum; this is a vasculitic eruption, occurring in the deep dermal tissues of the leg, though rarely it can occur on the arms as well. It is often intensively painful. Erythema multiforme usually starts as a symmetrical mildly itchy pink blotchy rash on the extremities, moving to the trunk (centrifugal); the classic lesion in erythema multiforme is the target lesion, which has a pink-red rim with a pale centre, and is almost pathognonomic of the condition. There are multiple causes for erythema multiforme, including: drugs, herpes simplex infection, and mycoplasma. Erythema marginatum consists of pink rings on the trunk and inner aspects of arms and thighs, most typically associated with rheumatic fever.

2. (a) Chest radiograph

In view of her arthralgia + rash + fever, sarcoidosis needs to be considered. There may be evidence of interstitial fibrosis or hilar lymphadenopathy, or both. There is a broad differential of erythema nodosum, which includes: streptococcal infection, mycobacterial infection (both tuberculosis and leprosy), mycoplasma infection, many other infections, sarcoidosis, inflammatory bowel disease, and rarely some of the systemic vasculitides e.g. Behçet's disease. In 30–50% of cases no cause is ever found.

3. (c) Aspirin

Often, erythema nodosum has no aetiology (it is idiopathic).

4. (b) Panniculitis

Panniculitis is characteristic.

Further reading: Chapter 222.

Case 13: An HIV-infected patient with fever

1. (c) Renal biopsy

His renal impairment is probably secondary to the vomiting. Both the bone marrow biopsy and liver biopsy can be sent for histology and TB culture.

2. (b) As the immune system improves on anti-retroviral therapy, previously ignored immune targets are recognized

An *immune reconstitution illness* is a relatively rare syndrome occurring at the start of anti-retroviral treatment. It relates to a sudden increase in the inflammatory reponse, and may result in fever and additional tissue damage. It either relates to increased T cell function detecting subclinical infection (i.e. the unmasking of subclinical infection), or paradoxically, to relapse of a known infection, perhaps as the T cells start to recognize dead and damaged tissue, causing more tissue inflammation. The reaction can be severe, and occasionally steroids are needed to treat it. An important risk factor for the immune reconstitution illness is a drop in the viral load by at least 1 $\log_{10}$.

3. (c) *Mycobacterium avium* complex (MAC)

The presentation of is *Mycobacterium avium* complex infection is usually non-specific; the blood culture is 60–80% sensitive.

4. (c) Marrow infiltration by MAC

A normal lactate dehydrogenase (LDH) makes lymphoma less likely, and severe sepsis would be accompanied by marked clinical signs, including tachycardia and hypotension.

Further reading: Chapter 47.

Case 14: A patient with a fever, sore throat and rash

1. (b) HIV seroconversion

He has risk factors for HIV and the monospot test is negative. An acute hepatitis is excluded by the normal liver function tests.

2. (a) Offer an HIV test and counselling

This patient needs testing for HIV; usually a confirmatory test will be required if the first test is positive.

3. (a) Refer to genitourinary medicine for a sexually transmitted infection (STI) screen and general management of his illness

He should be managed by a specialist.

4. (b) Offer an HIV test to his wife and baby

Both his wife and baby should be tested for HIV. Clearly the patient should be asked his consent to release this sensitive information; there may be considerable ethical problems if he does not agree. Legal and high-level ethical advice may well need to be sought in such a situation.

Further reading: Chapter 163.

Case 15: A traveller with diarrhoea and fever

1. (c) Norovirus

Both *Salmonella typhi* and amoebic dysentery typically cause bloody diarrhoea, whereas norovirus, the causative organism for winter vomiting illness, does not. Furthermore, the incubation time for this viral infection is also a lot shorter.

2. (a) Stool microscopy

In amoebiasis, stool microscopy shows trophozoites, blood and pus cells. Blood cultures may be positive in *Salmonella typhi* infection, but are most unlikely to help establish the diagnosis of amoebic infection.

3. (b) Lactose intolerance

Temporary lactose intolerance is quite common following severe GI infections; typically, food containing lactose provoke cramping abdominal pain, bloating, diarrhoea, within 30 minutes to 2 hours of consumption.

4. (c) Metronidazole

The protracted history of bloody diarrhoea makes *Salmonella* and amoebic dysentery more likely. Amoebic dysentery can be treated with metronidazole and *Salmonella* dysentry with ciprofloxacin. If this fails then a flexi-sigmoidoscopy would be the next step to investigate inflammatory bowel disease.

Further reading: Chapter 48.

Case 16: A traveller with jaundice

1. (b) Hepatitis serology

He has biochemical evidence of hepatitis. Given his recent foreign travel the likely cause is infective. He is relatively well, so a bacterial organism producing bacteraemia or septicaemia is unlikely. Paracetamol needs to be considered in all acute hepatitic illnesses, however the clinical context here makes paracetamol overdose a most unlikely diagnosis.

2. (b) Liver ultrasound scan

This should be done to exclude any abscesses or masses. Abdominal X-ray is unlikely to be abnormal, and even less likely to establish the diagnosis. A liver biopsy is very rarely indicated for an acute hepatitic illness, though is often indicated in chronic hepatitis.

3. (a) Hepatitis A

His self-limiting illness is suggestive of hepatitis A. Hepatitis C does not usually present acutely.

4. (b) Emphasis the importance of malaria prophylaxis

Following his acute infection he should now be immune to hepatitis A. He is lucky that he did not develop a severe form of malaria; prevention is fairly effective and safe with modern chemoprophylaxis.

Further reading: Chapter 127.

Case 17: A patient with fever and joint pain

1. (a) Urethral swab and divided urine sample

A Gram stain should be performed on the slide to look for polymorphs and Gram-negative intracellular diplococci, with the aim of determining whether he has an ongoing gonococcal urethritis.

2. (c) Gastritis

Hepatitis occurs as part of the Fitz–Hugh Curtis syndrome and uveitis as part of Reiter's syndrome. Gastritis is not related to urethritis, or to a syndrome that can be provoked by urethritis.

3. (c) Gonococcal arthritis

Acute monoarthritis in a young man is strongly suspicious of gonococcal arthritis. Reiter's syndrome is a triad of urethritis, arthritis and uveitis. However, the arthritis is sterile, and not usually associated with a pustular rash around the joint – it is this rash that makes the diagnosis of metastatic gonococcal infection the most likely diagnosis.

4. (b) Commence on ciprofloxacin

Gonorrhoea is usually susceptible to the fluoroquinolones. Clearly, in addition to antibiotic treatment, his contacts will need tracing and screening for sexually transmitted infections.
Further reading: Chapter 49.

Case 18: A patient with vaginal discharge

1. (a) Test for a fishy odour with potassium hydroxide (KOH)

Bacterial vaginosis produces a fishy odour and the others do not.

2. (c) *Trichomonas*

A high pH and inflamed vaginal wall is suggestive of *Trichomonas* infection.

3. (c) High vaginal swab for microscopy and culture

About 70–80% of the time you can visualize *Trichomonas* on microscopy; culture can be useful if the microscopy is negative.

4. (b) Metronidazole

This is the treatment of choice for both *Trichomonas* and bacterial vaginosis.
Further reading: Chapter 49.

Case 19: A patient with malaise and fever following a tick bite

1. (b) Lyme disease

The patient has been in an endemic area and has a characteristic rash suggestive of Lyme disease. The lesion is non-tender and does not look cellulitic.

2. (b) Erythema chronicum migrans

The rash usually develops at the site of the tick bite but can develop at other sites.

3. (a) *Borrelia burgdorferi*

The pathogen is transmitted via the tick *Ixodes* sp.

4. (c) Doxycycline

This patient has early disease that should respond to doxycycline.
Further reading: Chapter 165.

Case 20: A farmer with night sweats and a large spleen

1. (c) *Brucella abortus*

The history and examination findings (farmer, malaise, weight loss, neutropenia, hepatosplenomegaly) plus erythema nodosum is suggestive of brucellosis.

2. (b) Blood culture

Diagnosis is based on a positive blood culture or serology.

3. (c) Gram-negative coccobacillus

Brucella is a Gram-negative coccobacillus.

4. (a) Erythema nodosum

Brucella is a rare cause of erythema nodosum. Streptococcal infection is a more important cause in the UK.
Further reading: Chapter 165.

Case 21: A febrile traveller returning from the Gambia

1. (b) Thick and thin blood film

Clearly the working diagnosis is that this lady has malaria, and the concern, given where she went, is that she has falciparum malaria, a potentially rapidly lethal form of malaria. The quickest

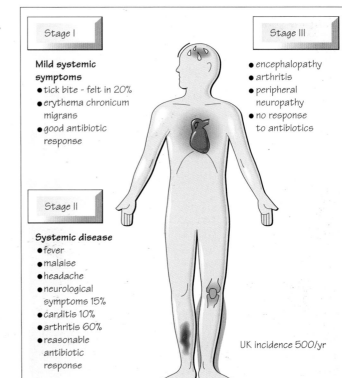

Figure 6.19.1 Features of Lyme disease.

means to establish the diagnosis is to look for forms of the protozoal parasite that infect the red cells. Trophozoites inhabit the red cells, and are identified on the blood film using a Geimsa or Fields stain.

2. (b) Haemolysis

Anaemia is a feature of falciparum malaria. The liver has about 2 or so years of vitamin B_{12} stores, these will clearly not be depleted rapidly. Haemorrhage, particularly from the GI tract, is a cause of anaemia in any sick patient, though usually rapidly becomes apparent; this is not the usual mechanism for anaemia in falciparum malaria.

3. (b) Glucose-6-phosphate dehydrogenase (G6PD) deficiency

People with the other conditions are more likely to have severe malaria. Certain haemoglobin variants, including HbS and HbC also confer protection. Patients heterozygote for HbS, sickle cell carriers, have significant falciparum protection, and few disadvantages, whereas those homozygous for HbS have sickle cell disease, with severe haemolysis, and an illness punctuated by various crises, leading to premature death.

4. (b) 10–14 days

Falciparum malaria usually develops within a week or two of inoculation. The illness develops throughout the incubation period, with increasingly severe symptoms, with fever, malaise, and other systemic symptoms. Though some patients develop the typical fever pattern (fever every 48 hours, coinciding with waves of release of the parasites), most patients do not show such a pattern. Multiple other symptoms may occur, including headache, confusion (cere-

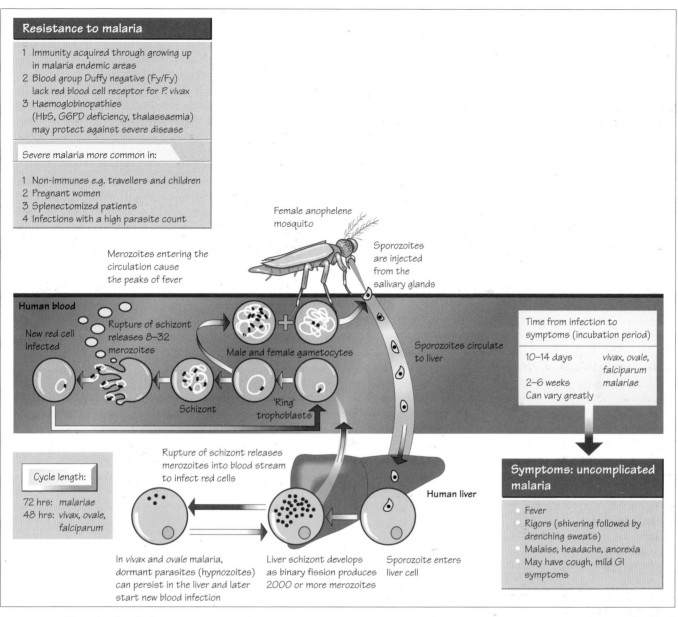

Resistance to malaria

1 Immunity acquired through growing up in malaria endemic areas
2 Blood group Duffy negative (Fy/Fy) lack red blood cell receptor for *P. vivax*
3 Haemoglobinopathies (HbS, G6PD deficiency, thalassaemia) may protect against severe disease

Severe malaria more common in:

1 Non-immunes e.g. travellers and children
2 Pregnant women
3 Splenectomized patients
4 Infections with a high parasite count

Female anophelene mosquito

Sporozoites are injected from the salivary glands

Merozoites entering the circulation cause the peaks of fever

Sporozoites circulate to liver

Human blood

New red cell infected

Rupture of schizont releases 8–32 merozoites

Male and female gametocytes

Schizont

'Ring' trophoblasts

Time from infection to symptoms (incubation period)

10–14 days   vivax, ovale, falciparum
2–6 weeks   malariae
Can vary greatly

Cycle length:

72 hrs: malariae
48 hrs: vivax, ovale, falciparum

Rupture of schizont releases merozoites into blood stream to infect red cells

Human liver

In *vivax* and *ovale* malaria, dormant parasites (hypnozoites) can persist in the liver and later start new blood infection

Liver schizont develops as binary fission produces 2000 or more merozoites

Sporozoite enters liver cell

Symptoms: uncomplicated malaria

• Fever
• Rigors (shivering followed by drenching sweats)
• Malaise, headache, anorexia
• May have cough, mild GI symptoms

Figure 6.21.1 Features of malaria.

bral malaria), respiratory failure and renal failure (sometimes due to the presence of haemoglobin and its breakdown products in the urine, leading to a blackish discolouration, so called 'blackwater fever'). Falciparum malaria is a very common cause of death in sub-Saharan Africa, and also in returning travellers, not only Caucasians, but also those émigrés from sub-Saharan Africa living in Europe and returning to visit their country of origin.
Further reading: Chapter 166.

Case 22: A young man returning from sub-Saharan Africa unwell and drowsy

1. (a) Pain or resistance on passive extension of the knee with a flexed hip and with the patient lying in a supine position

Extending the knee passively in a leg that has been fully flexed at the hip and knee performs Kernig's sign for meningeal irritation: if pain occurs at the base of the back, the sign is said to be

positive. It is a non-specific sign of meningeal irritation, and is positive both in sub-arachnoid haemorrhage as well as many different forms of meningitis. There is an appreciable false negative rate; however, in this case, the implication of the finding is that he is unlikely to have bacterial meningitis, which is part of the differential diagnosis. Woldemar Kernig (1840–1917) was a Russian and Baltic German neurologist who made the original description of his eponymous sign in 1882 (Über ein Krankheitssymptom der acuten Meningitis. *St. Petersburger medicinische Wochenschrift* 1882; VII).

2. (b) *Plasmodium falciparum*

This young man has an illness starting in southern Africa, where he has been for 12 months, characterized by fever, tachycardia, hypotension and splenomegaly. There certainly is a differential diagnosis, including bacterial infection, and other protozoal infections, however malaria due to *Plasmodium falciparum*

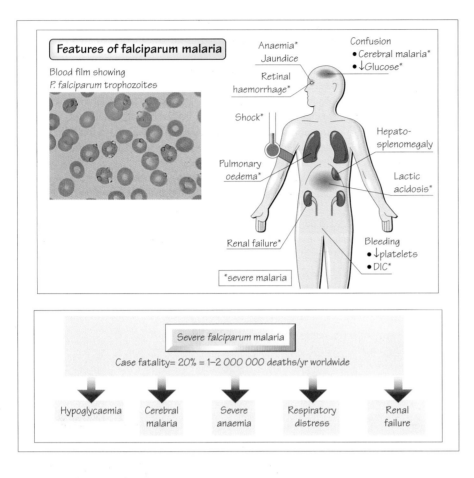

Features of falciparum malaria

Blood film showing
P. falciparum trophozoites

Anaemia*
Jaundice

Confusion
• Cerebral malaria*
• ↓Glucose*

Retinal
haemorrhage*

Shock*

Hepato-
splenomegaly

Pulmonary
oedema*

Lactic
acidosis*

Renal failure*

Bleeding
• ↓platelets
• DIC*

*severe malaria

Severe falciparum malaria

Case fatality= 20% = 1–2 000 000 deaths/yr worldwide

Hypoglycaemia | Cerebral malaria | Severe anaemia | Respiratory distress | Renal failure

Figure 6.22.1 Features of falciparum malaria.

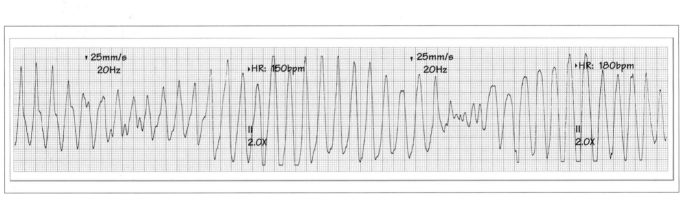

25mm/s 20Hz   ▸HR: 150bpm   25mm/s 20Hz   ▸HR: 180bpm

II 2.0X   II 2.0X

Figure 6.22.2 Torsade de pointes, a possible complication of some antimalarial treatments.

is top of this list. The other malaria species mentioned above (vivax and malariae) do not cause this severity of illness, and are therefore not part of the differential diagnoses.

3. (a) Hypoglycaemia

Splenomegaly occurs in many cases of malaria, and in itself does not imply that the disease is severe. Though one might intuitively feel that thrombocytopenia should be a marker for severe malaria, this is not the case, though disseminated intravascular coagulation certainly is. However, low glucose levels are a marker for severe malaria; this is the result of increased glucose consumption and impaired hepatic gluconeogenesis.

4. (c) Long QT syndrome

Quinine is a cause of long QT syndrome. Long QT syndrome in many cases predisposes to torsade-de-pointes type ventricular tachycardia, and this can be life-threatening.

Further reading: Chapter 166.

Case 23: A patient with asthma and a fever

1. (a) HR 110 + RR > 25 + unable to speak in complete sentences

The British Thoracic Society has issued guidelines defining the severity of asthma and all patients admitted with an acute asthma attack should be severity stratified according to these guidelines, as they determine treatment intensity, and also monitoring.

2. (a) Oxygen + bronchodilators + steroids + antibiotics + anaesthetic/ITU assessment

This man is unwell; he has features of life-threatening asthma (hypotensive) and may well need airway support. The intensive care team should therefore assess him as he may need ITU admission, and he certainly needs high dependency unit (HDU) admission. He must not be allowed to go to a general bed within the hospital medical unit, or worse, an outlying bed.

3. (a) Allergic bronchopulmonary aspergillosis (ABPA)

Though there is a differential diagnosis, by far the most likely underlying diagnosis is that he has allergic bronchopulmonary aspergillosis (ABPA). This is a complication of asthma, due to an allergic response to the aspergillus that has colonised the large airways of the lungs. Typically ABPA presents in patient with previously reasonably well controlled asthma; there are deteriorating symptoms over many months, repeated hospital admissions with low peak flows, chest X-ray shows 'flitting' (transient) infiltrates, and blood tests showing eosinophilia. The diagnosis is made from the clinical picture, and tests showing immune reactivity to aspergillus species (typically precipitating antibodies to aspergillus, aspergillus-specific IgE antibodies; the skin-prick test is almost always positive to Aspergillus fumigatus). Pulmonary vasculitic is an unlikely diagnosis – this usually causes a progressive illness without intermittent spontaneous resolution (so the spontaneously relapsing-remitting nature of the illness is against this diagnosis). Poor compliance can certainly cause repeated admissions; however, this would be unusual in a man previously wellcontrolled, and furthermore would not cause transient pulmonary infiltrates.

4. (a) Type I and III hypersensitivity reaction

The reaction with IgE and *Aspergillus* antigen results in mast cell degranulation with bronchoconstriction (type 1). Immune complexes (type III) and inflammatory cells are then deposited

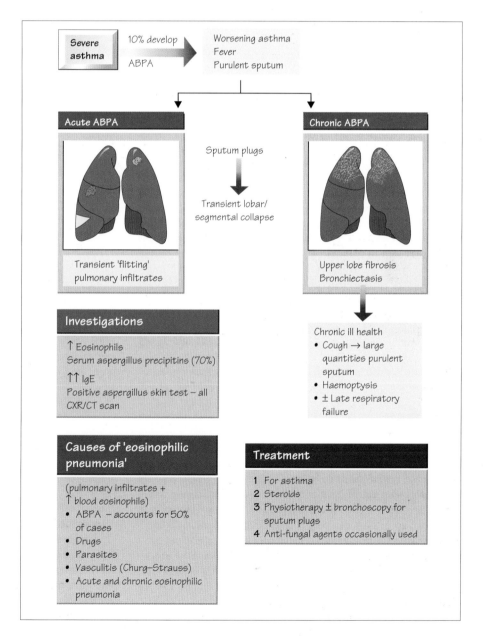

Figure 6.23.1 Clinical features of allergic bronchopulmonary aspergillosis.

within the mucous membranes of the airways, leading to necrosis and an eosinophilic infiltrate.

5. (b) Evidence of bronchiectasis

The tramlines are the radiological sign of bronchiectasis. Bronchiectasis is a complication of ABPA. Bronchiectasis is a condition where the bronchials have dilated as a consequence of the chronic inflammatory process; these damaged bronchi are chronically inflamed and as a consequence become chronically infected with bacterial pathogens, which can result in more inflammation, more symptoms of productive cough, and further bronchiectasis.

Further reading: Chapter 112.

Case 24: An HIV-positive patient with vomiting and fever

1. (c) Indian ink stain

The capsule of the Cryptococcus is very resistant to taking up various commonly used pathology laboratory stains, so that these are not useful to diagnosis. However, the Indian ink method, which produces a negative image, is useful. The principle is that instead of staining the capsule, the background is more intensively stained, so that the cryptococcal capsule becomes visible like a halo around the organism.

2. (b) *Cryptococcus neoformans* var. *neoformans*

This is the most medically important species and causes disease in the immunosuppressed. *Cryptococcus neoformans* var. *gatti* is capable of causing disease in the immunocompetent.

3. (a) Hydrocephalus

Obstructive hydrocephalus is a complication. This occurs when the normal movement of CSF around the brain and spinal cord is disrupted by the infection. DIC is not a feature of cryptococcal meningitis nor is pericardial involvement.

4. (a) Amphotericin B + flucytocine as initial therapy followed by fluconazole

Amphotericin B is used because of its rapid action in killing fungi. It is supplemented with flucytocine for the first 2 weeks or until the patient is afebrile and spinal fluid culture is negative. Then the patient can be placed on maintenance fluconazole.

Further reading: Chapter 164.

Case 25: A refugee with night sweats and haemoptysis

1. (a) Indurated area >5 mm after 48 hours

A positive mantoux is normally considered to be an indurated area of over 5 mm at 48 hours; a strong positive is over 15 mm; interpretation of these results depends upon exposure and immune status. Be aware that what is measured is induration and not redness, for this reason, interpretation is best done by those experienced in reading this test; if required for any of your patients, ask the respiratory nurse or physician both to perform and read the test.

2. (a) Isolate the patient in a negative pressure room

This man has open (sputum smear positive) tuberculosis (TB). He should be isolated ideally in a negative pressure room before commencing on treatment.

3. (a) Inform the Consultant in Communicable Disease Control CCDC

TB is a notifiable disease and as such it is mandatory that the CCDC be informed; his office will carry out contact tracing, which is very necessary.

4. (c) *Haemophilus* influenza

There is a very long list of conditions can result in cavitating lung lesions, and this includes: infection, tumours (especially primary tumours of the lung), vasculitis (especially Wegener's granulomatosis) and pulmonary infarction (not common). The infections at greatest chance of producing lung cavities are the mycobacteria or fungi; however, a number of more typical pneumonia-causing bacterial infections also not infrequently produce lung abscesses, and these include *Staphylococcus aureus* pneumonia. However, *Haemophilus influenza* is not a pathogen that leads to lung cavities.

Further reading: Chapter 102.

Case 26: A patient with abdominal pain and vomiting

1. (a) Cholecystitis

Murphy's sign is the clinical test to detect an inflamed gall bladder – with the patient lying quietly, the examiners hands is placed just under the right rib cage, in the mid costal line, directed upwards. If the gall bladder is inflamed, as the patient breaths in, it hurts more, when the test is said to be positive; for true positivity, it must be negative on the left hand side. It has a high sensitivity for cholecystitis. It was named after the American physician John Benjamin Murphy (1857–1916).

2. (c) Sarcoidosis

Sarcoidosis forms a non-caseating granuloma, i.e. without central necrosis. Indeed, this is the hallmark histologically of sarcoidosis.

3. (a) Culture of a sample from the lymph node

A definitive diagnosis depends upon demonstrating or culturing the organism. It can take up to 8 weeks to culture on a selective

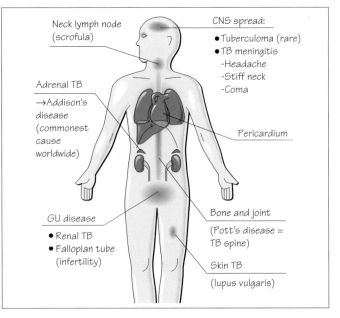

Figure 6.26.1 Features of extra-pulmonary TB.

media. A chest X-ray may provide supportive data, and is certainly indicated, but will not conclusively diagnose the problem.

4. (b) Isoniazid + rifampicin for 6 months with pyrizinamide + ethambutol for the first 2 months

The standard treatment is four drugs for 2 months, followed by a further 4 months' treatment with two drugs; 12 months of therapy is only needed for TB meningitis and bone/joint TB.
Further reading: Chapter 167.

Case 27: A young man with a sore throat

1. (c) Tonsillitis

This patient is febrile and hypotensive and therefore has a bacteraemia (indeed, may well have septicaemia); the source of this is likely to be the tonsils. Glandular fever certainly causes a tonsillitis-type syndrome; however, it does not cause systemic signs of sepsis (tachycardia and low blood pressure). Toxic-shock syndrome causes tachycardia and hypotension, but does not cause a sore throat. It is caused by toxogenic *Staphylococcus aureus* species (more rarely by a *Streptococcus pyogenes* species); the bacteria release a toxin, a superantigen that results in polyclonal T-cell stimulation. This results in fever, hypotension, a widespread rash, and organ failure (including respiratory distress and renal failure). A common site of origin is the tampons of menstruating women, though men can have the illness as well. Tonsillitis is not a feature of the illness, and the rash is usually present, both facts substantially lowering the chance that this illness is toxic shock syndrome.

2. (b) Group A *Streptococcus*

This organism is part of the normal flora of the throat and skin. As mentioned above, this patient is very unlikely to have a viral explanation for their illness, firstly given the low blood pressure and tachycardia, and secondly, given the high polymorph neutrophil count. Listeria would be a very unusual pathogen in an immunocompetent man, it is really an infection either of the immuno-incompetent, or pregnant women. *Staphylococcus aureus* can cause a large number of different infective syndromes, including septicaemia, cellulitis, bone and joint infection, heart valve infection. However, it would be most unusual to find it causing a sore throat.

3. (a) Fluid resuscitation

The patient is shocked therefore fluid resuscitation is a priority; in reality options (a) and (c) probably happen simultaneously.

4. (a) Quinsy

This is also known as a peritonsillar abscess and ENT opinion should be sought.
Further reading: Chapter 161.

Case 28: An elderly woman with fever and right upper quadrant pain

1. (c) Protein C deficiency

Protein C deficiency makes you more prone to forming clots and does not prolong the PT. Warfarin works by opposing the action of vitamin K, so similar clotting abnormalities occur both with warfarin therapy and vitamin K deficiency; their is a decrease in the amount of the vitamin K dependent clotting factors, which are II, VII, IX, and X. This will prolong the PT. DIC consumes many clotting factors, including those of the intrinsic pathway, so prolonging the PT.

2. (b) Ascending cholangitis

She has Charcot's triad – fever, right upper quadrant pain and jaundice. Cholecystitis by itself does not lead to jaundice, and nor does uncomplicated pancreatitis. Ascending cholangitis is the overwhelming most likely clinical diagnosis; this is a very serious illness with an appreciable mortality at any age, but particularly in an 80 year old. Charcot's triad is named after Jean-Martin Charcot (29 November 1825–16 August 1893), a French neurologist and professor of anatomical pathology; if the syndrome includes those of the triad, but also hypotension and altered mental function (common with Gram negative septicaemias in the elderly), it is called Reynolds pentad. Reynolds emphasized the importance of operative relief of the obstructed infection biliary tree, even if patients were moribund, for a successful outcome. From Reynolds BM, Dargan EL (August 1959). "Acute obstructive cholangitis; a distinct clinical syndrome". *Ann. Surg.* **150** (2): 299–303.

3. (b) DIC

There is clinical (purpuric rash) and numerical evidence of clotting and platelet consumption. This is a very serious complication; her projected mortality risk in the absence of DIC was already substantial, the fact that she now has complicating DIC greatly increases her chances of dying.

4. (c) Gastrointestinal surgeon

Her recurrent history of abdominal pain is likely to be biliary colic. She most likely has a stone obstructing her common bile duct and will need endoscopic retrograde cholangiopancreatography (ERCP) for assessment and to relieve any obstruction. A referral to a surgeon or gastroenterologist would be appropriate.
Further reading: Chapter 126.

Case 29: A patient with inflamed tonsils

1. (a) Serum antibodies against red blood cells of other species

The presumptive diagnosis here is infectious mononucleosis due to acute Epstein-Barr virus (EBV) infection. The monospot test depends on the fact that patients infected acutely with the EBV produce heterophile antibodies, that is to say, antibodies that bind to the red cells of other species, such as horses, sheep, etc. When a patient's serum is added to a suspension of horses' red cells, the cells are agglutinated by the heterophile antibody, and collect in a small area in the bottom of the vial. EBV is not the only infection causing a positive monospot test; other infections can do this occasionally, such as toxoplasmosis or rubella, and certain malignancies, particularly lymphomas.

2. (b) Glandular fever

A positive monospot test makes this diagnosis more likely. IgM antibodies to Epstein–Barr virus (EBV) would also support the diagnosis. Furthermore, the demographics and clinical context (age, university attendance, where sexual activity is highly likely, other class mates being similarly affected) all greatly increase the chance that the diagnosis is acute EBV pharyngitis. Influenza usually causes a completely different disease, with systemic upset, indeed prostration, being very likely, severe muscle aches, a great feeling of being unwell, and often very high temperature.

3. (b) Amoxicillin

This is a non-allergic rash; many patients with acute EBV infection develop a rash when given amoxicillin.

4. (a) Reassurance

Treatment is supportive, both for the EBV infection and for the rash. Usually EBV results in a relatively benign self-limiting illness; some patients may be fatigued for some months afterwards. A large proportion of patients have biochemical evidence of liver involvement, though clinical jaundice is rare. Other more serious complications can occur in up to 5%, and include:

- Neurological involvement, including viral meningitis, encephalitis, hemiplegia and transverse myelitis, and Guillain-Barré syndrome
- Blood involvement, a Coombs' positive (autoimmune) haemolytic anaemia, and decreased production of other blood cell lines
- Severe disease course immuno-incompetent patients
- Severe tonsillar hypertrophy and upper airway obstruction
- Splenic rupture, which is the major cause of death in infectious mononucleosi; for this reason, most physicians recommend no contact sports until the illness has clearly settled.
- Cardiac involvement with myo-or peri-carditis

Further reading: Chapter 162.

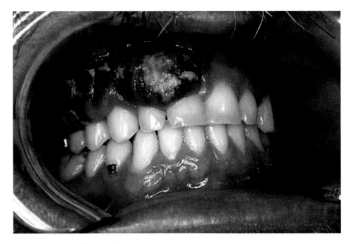

Figure 6.31.1 Kaposi's sarcoma.

Case 30: A patient with a blistering rash

1. (b) V1

The dermatome is the right ophthalmic division of the trigeminal nerve (VI).

2. (b) Varicella-zoster virus (VZV)

The patient has shingles caused by varicella-zoster.

3. (b) Ophthalmologist

He should be seen urgently by the ophthalmologist as this infection could cause complete loss of sight if not dealt with promptly.

4. (a) Secondary bacterial infection

Fever, discharge from the rash and neutrophilia all suggest a secondary bacterial infection. He should be started on appropriate antibiotics.

Further reading: Chapter 162.

Case 31: A breathless homosexual patient

1. (b) Induced sputum

The presumptive diagnosis is pneumocystis pneumonia – years ago, he would have been considered to have *Pneumocystis carinii* pneumonia (PCP), however, the name has of *Pneumocystis carinii* has now been changed to *Pneumocystis jirovecii*. A diagnosis of *Pneumocystis jirovecii* can be definitively confirmed by pathological identification of the causative organism in induced sputum or bronchial washings obtained by bronchoscopy; immunofluorescence assay can be used to show characteristic cysts.

2. (c) *Pneumocystis jirovecii* pneumonia

He has a low CD4 count, desaturates on exercise and has disproportionately low oxygen partial pressure compared with oxygen saturation; these are all feature suggestive of *Pneumocystis jirovecii*. There is an abnormal X-ray in 95% of *Pneumocystis jirovecii* pneumonia cases.

3. (b) Kaposi's sarcoma

The suspicious lesion on his palate is probably Kaposi's sarcoma (Fig. 6.31.1). This malignant tumour, first named after the Hungarian dermatologist Moritz Kaposi (1837–1902), who first described the symptoms in 1872. Previously common in sub-Saharan Africans without HIV, probably due to the endemically high rates of human herpesvirus 8 (HHV-8), the causative agent of Kaposi's sarcoma, also high in immunosuppressed transplant recipients, and gay men with HIV.

4. (c) Co-trimoxazole

All patients with a CD4 count <200 mm³ should be on co-trimoxazole (unless contraindicated) to prevent *Pneumocystis jirovecii* pneumonia. It also confers some protection against other conditions such as pneumococcal pneumonia and malaria.

Further reading: Chapter 162.

Case 32: An HIV-positive patient with a right hemiparesis

1. (b) Cerebral lymphoma

The differential for a ring-enhancing lesion in this case is toxoplasmosis, cerebral abscess or lymphoma. Cerebral lymphoma is the likeliest diagnosis especially with a normal cerebrospinal fluid analysis and failure to clinically improve on anti-*Toxoplasma* treatment. There is some evidence that implicates intrathecal Epstein–Barr virus (EBV) detection with central nervous system lymphoma.

2. (a) <100 mm³

Cerebral lymphoma is an AIDS-defining illness; the CD4 count is usually <100 mm³.

3. (c) Chemotherapy

Cerebral lymphoma carries a poor prognosis. However, the mainstay of treatment is chemotherapy.

4. (a) Contact tracing of previous sexual partners and offer them an HIV test

The patient is unlikely to have any infections that place her at risk to others, unless she starts vomiting blood, she has already had a prolonged trial of the most appropriate antibiotics. Clearly, of crucial important to those she has had sexual contact with and also in the interest of the broader community, it is vital that all her contacts are traced, and those with HIV infection treated early, both for their sake to improve prognosis, as well as to minimize their infectivity to others.

Further reading: Chapter 163.

Case 33: Recurrent infections in a 49-year-old woman

1. (c) Common variable immunodeficiency

Her history is most in keeping with a primary antibody deficiency; ITP often precedes the development of the antibody deficiency. C5 deficiency will predispose to meningitis and atypical lupus-like illness. Her previous steroid therapy is too far in the past to be relevant now. Wiskott–Aldrich syndrome causes a combined defect with small platelets, thrombocytopenia and eczema; it is X-linked.

Further reading: Chapter 170.

Case 34: A patient with cough and lymphocytosis

1. (d) Chronic lymphocytic leukaemia with secondary hypogammaglobulinamia

The very raised lymphocytes count (NR $1.5-4 \times 10^9/L$) is the give away. The presence of small monoclonal bands in the serum is common and secondary antibody deficiency is also common. The lymphocytosis would not be found in myeloma. Selective IgM deficiency is incredibly rare and also would not cause lymphocytosis; The electrophoresis of the urine shows only a trace of albumin, not enough to indicate significant renal protein loss; lymphoctyosis would not occur.

Further reading: Chapter 176.

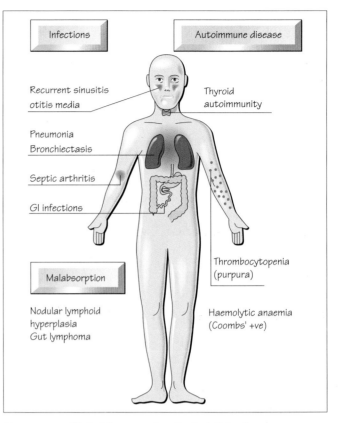

Figure 6.33.1 Clinical features of antibody deficiencies.

7 Haematology: Cases and Questions

Case 1: A patient with shortness of breath

A 51-year-old shop assistant presents to his GP with increasing shortness of breath on exertion. Normally his exercise tolerance when walking is unlimited but more recently he can walk approximately 50 m before having to stop to catch his breath. He also complains of intermittent frontal headaches over the last 2 weeks. On direct questioning, he denies a cough, orthopnoea or haemoptysis. He has not noticed blood in the stool or haematuria. He has never smoked and only drinks occasional alcohol. On examination he had a pulse of 110 beats/min (regular, normal character), BP 115/80 mmHg, pale conjunctivae but no jaundice, and a soft ejection systolic murmur loudest at the aortic area, with no radiation. Abdominal examination was normal.

A full blood count taken 3 years ago showed a haemoglobin of 12.3 g/L with a mean cell volume of 89 fL.

Blood tests showed:

Hb	7.3 g/dL
MCV	72.5 fL
WCC	11.2×10^9/L
Platelets	420×10^9/L

Electrolytes, liver function and inflammatory markers: normal

1. *What is the most likely cause for his systolic murmur?*
   - (a) Aortic sclerosis
   - (b) Flow murmur due to a hyperdynamic circulation
   - (c) Aortic stenosis
   - (d) Mitral regurgitation
2. *Which of the following is the likely cause of his anaemia?*
   - (a) Iron deficiency anaemia
   - (b) Thalassaemia trait
   - (c) Vitamin B_{12} deficiency
   - (d) Anaemia of chronic disease
   - (e) Aplastic anaemia

Case 2: A patient needing a blood transfusion after a road traffic accident

A 31-year-old woman is brought into A&E after a road traffic accident. She has fractured her pelvis and sustained abdominal trauma that requires surgical exploration. In the ambulance, her pulse was 125 beats/min (regular but thready) and BP was 80/30 mmHg. She looks pale and her abdomen is visibly distended. An Hb result from a blood gas analyser shows a level of 6.2 g/dL.

1. *How would you manage her immediate need for a blood transfusion?*
   - (a) She should be cross-matched immediately and only receive blood of the identical blood group
   - (b) She should receive blood of group O, irrespective of rhesus D group
   - (c) She should receive blood of group O which is also rhesus D negative
   - (d) She should receive enough blood to bring her haemoglobin into the normal range before going to theatre

2. *In theatre she requires more blood. The transfusion laboratory reports that her blood group is A positive. Which blood should she not receive?*
   - (a) B positive
   - (b) A positive
   - (c) A negative
   - (d) O positive
   - (e) O negative
3. *After surgery, which successfully stopped the bleeding, the anaesthetist notices that her urine turns very dark in colour. She is also becoming jaundiced. Blood tests show acute renal failure and disseminated intravascular coagulation with a prolonged activated partial thromboplastin time (APTT) and prothrombin time (PT). A full blood count shows her Hb has dropped to 5.9 g/dL. A direct antiglobulin test (Coombs' test) is positive. What is the likely cause for her deterioration?*
   - (a) Sepsis
   - (b) Re-bleeding from the surgical site
   - (c) Acute drug reaction
   - (d) Haemolytic transfusion reaction

Case 3: A patient with an intracranial haemorrhage

A man with a tilting disk aortic valve is on warfarin with a target international normalized ratio (INR) of 2.0–3.0. He presents with an intracranial haemorrhage with an INR of 5.2.

1. *Which factors would be deficient?*
   - (a) II, V, VII, X
   - (b) II, VII, VIII, X
   - (c) II, VII, IX, X
   - (d) VII, IX, X, XI
2. *What treatment should he receive?*
   - (a) Vitamin K and fresh frozen plasma (FFP)
   - (b) Vitamin K and prothrombin complex concentrate
   - (c) FFP only; INR must not fall to less than 2.0
   - (d) Withhold warfarin only
3. *What should his future treatment be?*
   - (a) Restart warfarin when the patient has recovered from the acute event
   - (b) Aspirin
   - (c) Aspirin plus clopidogrel
   - (d) He must not be anticoagulated again
4. *Which of these drugs does not interact with warfarin?*
   - (a) Erythromycin
   - (b) Codeine
   - (c) Valproate
   - (d) Fluconazole

Case 4: A patient on HRT with deep venous thrombosis

A 64-year-old woman taking hormone replacement therapy (HRT) has a proximal deep venous thrombosis (DVT) with no other precipitating factors. She is treated with low molecular weight heparin (LMWH) and warfarin. The heparin is stopped and warfarin continued. Blood is taken for a thrombophilia screen and gives the following results:

INR   2.6
Antithrombin   108%
Protein C   35%
Protein S   37%
Factor V Leiden: present in heterozygous state
Prothrombin mutation: not detected

1. *How many of the five known heritable thrombophilias have been demonstrated?*
   (a) 1
   (b) 2
   (c) 3
   (d) 4
   (e) 5

2. *How long should the warfarin continue for?*
   (a) 6–12 weeks
   (b) 3–6 months
   (c) 6–18 months
   (d) Indefinitely

3. *HRT increases the risk of venous thromboembolism (VTE) by which of the following amounts?*
   (a) 1.2-fold
   (b) 1.5-fold
   (c) 2-fold
   (d) 10-fold

4. *She has three children: two males age 34 and 32 years and a female age 28. The daughter takes the combined oral contraceptive pill. Which of the following statements is true?*
   (a) All the children should have a thrombophilia screen
   (b) The daughter should stop taking the pill
   (c) No family study is indicated
   (d) The daughter should be counselled

Case 5: A pregnant woman with a generalized seizure

A 33-year-old woman who is 12 weeks' pregnant is admitted via A&E with a generalized seizure, reduced conscious level and right-sided weakness. According to her husband, she was perfectly well the day before and there is no history of foreign travel. On examination she has a temperature of 37.8°C, an upper motor neuron weakness affecting the right arm and leg, and a Glasgow Coma Score (GCS) of 10. There is no overt meningism and no rash. A CT of the head was performed which was reported as normal. Results of a lumbar puncture showed that there were no white cells in the cerebrospinal fluid (CSF) and the protein and glucose levels were normal. Blood and CSF cultures have been sent.

Blood results were as follows:

Hb   9.6 g/dL
WCC 12.3×10^9/L
Platelets 35×10^9/L
Urea   16 mmol/L
Creatinine   135 μmol/L
Bilirubin   38 μmol/L
ALT   18 U/L
ALP   185 U/L
Corrected Ca 2.4 mmol/L

1. *Which of the following blood tests would be most helpful in determining the cause of the abnormal full blood count?*

   (a) Coagulation screen (prothrombin time (PT), activated partial thromboplastin time (APTT), fibrinogen and D-dimers)
   (b) Direct antiglobulin test
   (c) Plasma haptoglobins
   (d) Reticulocyte count
   (e) Bone marrow aspirate

2. *A haematologist rings you with the blood film report and says that there are low platelets, polychromasia and numerous red cell fragments. A coagulation screen is normal. What is the significance of numerous red cell fragments and polychromasia?*
   (a) Extravascular haemolysis is likely
   (b) Systemic sepsis is likely
   (c) Bone marrow failure is occurring
   (d) Microangiopathic haemolytic anaemia is present

3. *What is the most likely diagnosis?*
   (a) Idiopathic thrombocytopenic purpura (ITP)
   (b) Thrombotic thrombocytopenic purpura (TTP)
   (c) Warm autoimmune haemolytic anaemia
   (d) Cold autoimmune haemolytic anaemia
   (e) Systemic sepsis with DIC

Case 6: A patient with fatigue and mild jaundice

A 45-year-old woman presents to her GP with a 4-week history of increasing fatigue. She has also noticed that the whites of her eyes have become yellow. On direct questioning, she has had flitting joint pains over the last 6 months, which she has put down to 'growing older'. She is otherwise well and has no relevant past medical history. On examination, she was mildly jaundiced with an erythematous rash over her cheeks and the bridge of her nose. A 2 cm, non-tender spleen could be palpated but there was no lymphadenopathy or hepatomegaly. Her blood results are as follows:

Hb   8.9 g/dL
MCV   105 fL
Platelets 248×10^9/L
Urea   4.6 mmol/L
Creatinine   86 μmol/L
Bilirubin   75 μmol/L
ALT   12 U/L
ALP   115 U/L
Corrected Ca 2.24 mmol/L
Film: polychromasia, spherocytes (Fig.7.6.1)

1. *What is the most likely diagnosis?*
   (a) Pernicious anaemia
   (b) Cold autoimmune haemolytic anaemia (AIHA)
   (c) Warm AIHA
   (d) Paroxysmal cold haemoglobinuria
   (e) Myelodysplasia

2. *What is the most useful additional blood test?*
   (a) Direct antiglobulin test (Coombs' test)
   (b) Reticulocyte count
   (c) Serum vitamin B_{12} and folate levels
   (d) Urinary haemosiderin
   (e) Osmotic fragility assay

3. *What is the best initial management?*
   (a) Folic acid supplementation
   (b) Red cell transfusion

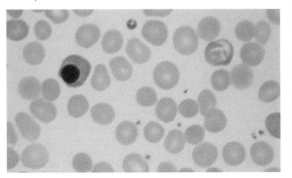

(a) Warm autoimmune haemolytic anaemia: peripheral blood film. There is a circulating nucleated red blood cell (NRBC), polychromasia and microspherocytes.

(b) Direct antiglobulin (Coombs') test (DAT) is a means of detecting immunoglobulin and/or complement coating the red blood cells. Red blood cells are washed and anti-human globulin is added. This may be of broad specificity or specific, e.g. for IgG, IgA, IgM or complement. If agglutination occurs, then the red blood cells must have been coated; if no agglutination occurs, the red blood cells were not coated. In the indirect antiglobulin test, red cells are first incubated with serum at 37°C for 30min; a DAT is then performed, which will be positive if there are antibodies in the serum reacting against the red blood cells.

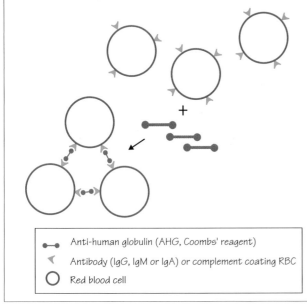

<table>
<tr><td>•—•</td><td>Anti-human globulin (AHG, Coombs' reagent)</td></tr>
<tr><td>⊀</td><td>Antibody (IgG, IgM or IgA) or complement coating RBC</td></tr>
<tr><td>◯</td><td>Red blood cell</td></tr>
</table>

Figure 7.6.1 The peripheral blood film.

   (c) Intravenous immunoglobulin
   (d) Splenectomy
   (e) Prednisolone and folic acid
4. *What further testing is indicated in this patient?*
   (a) Autoimmune screen
   (b) Bone marrow biopsy
   (c) CT scan of the chest, abdomen and pelvis
   (d) *Toxoplasma* serology
   (e) *Mycoplasma* serology

Case 7: A tired patient with lumps

A 29-year-old man originally from Tanzania presents to his GP with lumps under his arms and in his neck and groins. He has also been feeling very run down over the last few months and has lost 12 kg in weight. He works as a porter in the local hospital and he finds the work difficult and stressful. He reports no night sweats or fevers. A review of systems was unremarkable. On examination he had oral candidiasis and widespread, small-volume lymphadenopathy which was non-tender. Cardiovascular, respiratory and abdominal examinations were all normal. In particular, there was no organomegaly.

   Blood tests showed:

Hb	10.5 g/dL
MCV	94 fL
WCC	3.8×10^9/L
Platelets	135×10^9/L

Electrolytes, liver function tests and CRP: normal
1. *What is the most likely diagnosis?*
   (a) Chronic lymphocytic leukaemia (CLL)
   (b) Infectious mononucleosis
   (c) HIV infection
   (d) Disseminated malignancy
   (e) Malaria
2. *Two years after appropriate hospital referral and treatment, the patient presents to his physician with a 5-week history of a rapidly enlarging mass in his neck. On examination, he has a firm, non-tender lymph node mass in the right supraclavicular fossa. The rest of the clinical examination was unremarkable. Routine blood tests were normal. What is the preferred investigation?*
   (a) Open lymph node biopsy
   (b) Fine needle aspirate
   (c) Tru-cut biopsy of the neck mass
   (d) Bone marrow aspirate and trephine
   (e) Sputum cytology

Case 8: A patient with intermittent abdominal pain and mild jaundice

A 25-year-old woman presents to her GP with intermittent abdominal pain over the last few years. The pain is generally localized to the right hypochondrium and is made worse when she eats a fatty meal. Her bowel habits are normal and she has never passed blood in her stools. Her appetite and weight are steady. On examination, she was mildly jaundiced. She had no lymphadenopathy but her spleen was just palpable at 1–2 cm below her left costal margin. On direct questioning, she reports that her mother also has slightly yellow eyes.

   Blood tests showed:

Hb	10.2 g/dL
MCV	102 fL
WCC	6.3×10^9/L
Platelets	275×10^9/L
Electrolytes	Normal
Bilirubin	55 μmol/L (unconjugated)
ALT	25 U/L
ALP	110 U/L

1. *What is the significance of the unconjugated hyperbilirubinaemia?*
   (a) It indicates partial common bile duct obstruction by gallstones
   (b) None – this is a normal finding in a small proportion of the population

(c) It suggests either an increased delivery of bilirubin to the liver or a failure of conjugation by the liver

(d) It indicates chronic alcohol consumption

2. *What is the most likely cause of her splenomegaly?*

   (a) Chronic haemolysis

   (b) Infectious mononucleosis

   (c) Chronic myeloid leukaemia

   (d) Low-grade lymphoma

   (e) Portal hypertension

   (f) Gilbert's syndrome

3. *What is the most helpful investigation to diagnose the cause of her splenomegaly?*

   (a) Splenic biopsy

   (b) Blood film with direct antiglobulin test

   (c) Bone marrow aspirate and trephine

   (d) CT of the chest, abdomen and pelvis

   (e) Doppler ultrasound of the liver and portal vein

Case 9: A patient with lower back pain

A 44-year-old woman presents to her GP with a 3-month history of lower back pain which is particularly worse at the end of the day. The pain is a dull ache, does not radiate anywhere and does not wake her at night. She has recently started taking regular paracetamol. The patient has recently moved to this country from Ghana and works as a secretary. She does not complain of fevers although she has been more tired than usual over the last couple of years. Her appetite and weight are steady.

Recent blood tests showed:

Hb   12.5 g/dL

WCC 3.2×10^9/L (neutrophils 1.1)

Platelets 248×10^9/L

Blood film: neutropenia, otherwise normal

Electrolytes, liver function tests, calcium: normal

1. *What is the most appropriate management of her neutropenia?*

   (a) Stop paracetamol immediately and advise to never take it again

   (b) Request a bone marrow aspirate and trephine

   (c) Start patient on prophylactic antibiotics in case of neutropenic sepsis

   (d) Reassure patient, repeat in 3–6 months' time

Case 10: A patient with shortness of breath and purulent sputum

A 79-year-old man attends A&E with a 4-day history of increasing shortness of breath and purulent sputum. On examination he has right basal crackles extending to the mid-zones and he is centrally cyanosed. Pneumonia is diagnosed and he is commenced on broad-spectrum antibiotics.

Blood tests showed:

Hb   9.7 g/dL

MCV   108 fL

WCC 1.5×10^9/L (neutrophils 0.6)

Platelets 85×10^9/L

CRP   160 mg/L

PT and APTT Normal

Na   138 mmol/L

K   3.8 mmol/L

Creatinine 110 μmol/L

Liver function Normal

Blood film: pancytopenia, dysplastic neutrophils, occasional blast

1. *What is the most likely cause of his leukopenia?*

   (a) Vitamin B_{12} deficiency

   (b) Myelodysplastic syndrome

   (c) Disseminated intravascular coagulation (DIC)

   (d) Myeloma

   (e) Aplastic anaemia

Case 11: A patient with increasing fatigue and mild jaundice

A 53-year-old woman presents to her GP with a 2-month history of gradually increasing fatigue. She does not report any other symptoms. On examination, she is rather pale and mildly jaundiced. She also has vitiligo over her hands. There is no organomegaly.

Blood tests showed:

Hb   7.9 g/dL

MCV   118 fL

WCC 4.5×10^9/L

Platelets 140×10^9/L

Bilirubin   45 μmol/L

ALT   25 U/L

ALP   115 U/L

Electrolytes, calcium and inflammatory markers: normal

1. *What is the most likely diagnosis?*

   (a) Autoimmune haemolytic anaemia

   (b) Pernicious anaemia

   (c) Iron deficiency anaemia

   (d) Anaemia of chronic disease

   (e) Dietary vitamin B_{12} deficiency

Appropriate therapy is initiated. She is reviewed by her GP one month later and although she initially felt an improvement, she is still not back to normal. She is feeling tired again and slightly breathless on exertion.

Repeat blood tests show:

Hb   7.5 g/dL

MCV   75 fL

WCC 5.5×10^9/L

Platelets 220×10^9/L

2. *What is the likely cause of the persistent anaemia?*

   (a) Inadequate vitamin B_{12} replacement

   (b) Coexisting folic acid deficiency

   (c) Iron deficiency

   (d) β-Thalassaemia trait

   (e) Worsening haemolysis

Case 12: A patient with intermittent palpitations

A 74-year-old man attends the general medical outpatient clinic with a 3-month history of intermittent palpitations. He is also complaining of an increasing frequency of frontal headaches and general fatigue. His appetite and weight are steady and bowel habits normal. Physical examination shows pale mucous membranes but is otherwise unremarkable.

Blood tests showed:

Hb   7.9 g/dL

MCV   71 fL

WCC 6.5×10^9/L

PLT 620×10^9/L

Electrolytes   Normal
Bilirubin   12 μmol/L
ALT   15 U/L
ALP   580 U/L
Calcium and inflammatory markers normal

1. *Which of the following would be most useful in coming up with a cause for his anaemia?*
   (a) Serum vitamin B_{12} and folate levels
   (b) Bone marrow aspirate
   (c) Direct antiglobulin test
   (d) Previous blood count results
   (e) Reticulocyte count

2. *The patient is commenced on oral iron replacement therapy. What side effect is most likely to be troublesome to the patient?*
   (a) Constipation
   (b) Diarrhoea
   (c) Rash
   (d) Headache
   (e) Iron overload

3. *What further investigations are indicated?*
   (a) Upper and lower GI imaging
   (b) Upper GI imaging only
   (c) Lower GI imaging only
   (d) *H. pylori* breath test
   (e) Chest X-ray

Case 13: A patient with increasing breathlessness

A 24-year-old student is referred to haematology with a 3-month history of increasing breathlessness on exertion. He is also finding it increasingly difficult to concentrate on his studies due to lethargy. On examination he was pale but not jaundiced. He had a normal cardiovascular, respiratory and abdominal examination.

Blood tests showed:

Hb   7.4 g/dL
MCV   95 fL
WBC 2.6×10^9/L
Platelets 78×10^9/L
Blood film   Unremarkable
Urea   3.5 mmol/L
Creatinine   94 μmol/L
Bilirubin   12 μmol/L
ALT   25 U/L
ALP   168 U/L
Corrected Ca   2.35 mmol/L

Previous blood tests one year ago were normal. A bone marrow aspirate was performed which showed a marked reduction in blood forming cells and no malignant infiltrate.

1. *What is the most likely diagnosis?*
   (a) Idiopathic aplastic anaemia
   (b) Vitamin B_{12} deficiency
   (c) Hypoplastic myelodysplasia
   (d) Peripheral consumption of blood cells
   (e) Folate deficiency

After appropriate treatment, the patient did very well and regained normal blood counts. Five years after the initial diagnosis, he presented to A&E with abdominal pain and bloody diarrhoea. A mesenteric vein thrombosis was diagnosed and he was commenced on anticoagulation.

Blood results at presentation showed:
Hb   9.5 g/dL
MCV   108 fL
WBC 3.8×10^9/L
Platelets 130×10^9/L
Urea   3.6 mmol/L
Creatinine   78 μmol/L
Bilirubin   40 μmol/L
ALT   10 U/L
ALP   135 U/L
Corrected Ca   2.45 mmol/L

2. *Which of the following investigations would be likely to be helpful?*
   (a) Chest X-ray
   (b) Jak2 mutation analysis
   (c) Factor V Leiden assay
   (d) Urinary haemosiderin
   (e) Direct antiglobulin test

Case 14: A patient with a nose bleed and bruising

A 40-year-old man attends A&E with a nose bleed. He has had occasional nose bleeds in the past but this one has lasted for 2 hours. He has also noticed some bruises over his arms and legs and a rash developing over his ankles. On examination, a petechial rash is evident over his legs and there are numerous bruises over his whole body. He has a temperature of 36.9°C. Cardiovascular, respiratory and abdominal examination is normal.

His blood results are as follows:

Hb   8.3 g/dL
WBC 3.2×10^9/L
Platelets 18×10^9/L
CRP   <8 mg/L
PT   32 sec (normal range 12–14)
APTT   55 sec (normal range 22–34)
Fibrinogen   0.4 (normal range 1.5–4)
Biochemistry and liver function tests normal.

1. *What is the significance of the blood film comment?*
   (a) A common finding in septic patients
   (b) Suggestive of acute leukaemia
   (c) Indicative of an appropriate increase in bone marrow output
   (d) Frequently seen in acute viral infections
   (e) Consistent with a diagnosis of idiopathic thrombocytopenic purpura

2. *Which complication has developed in this patient?*
   (a) Disseminated intravascular coagulation (DIC)
   (b) Thrombotic thrombocytopenic purpura
   (c) Neutropenic sepsis
   (d) Acute liver failure
   (e) Idiopathic thrombocytopenic purpura

3. *The patient is treated with cycles of high-dose chemotherapy and discharged with regular follow-up planned. One week after the completion of one of the cycles of chemotherapy, he rings the ward late at night with a temperature of 38°C and feeling shivery. What is the most appropriate advice to give the patient?*
   (a) Take some paracetamol and re-check temperature in 1 hour
   (b) Don't take paracetamol and re-check temperature in 1 hour

(c) Attend the ward immediately for a prescription of oral antibiotics
(d) Attend the ward the in the morning for a medical review
(e) Attend the ward immediately for a medical review

Case 15: A patient with shortness of breath and cough

A 31-year-old man presents to A&E with a 3-week history of increasing shortness of breath and cough when he lies flat. He now has to sleep with six pillows. He has also unintentionally lost 4 kg in weight over the last 2 months and his appetite is poor. He is not complaining of any night sweats or fevers. On examination, he has fixed distended neck veins and respiratory examination reveals stony dullness with reduced breath sounds in the right lung base. Cardiovascular and abdominal examination is unremarkable.

Routine blood tests and an ECG are all normal. Chest X-ray shows a large mediastinal mass measuring 12 cm in transverse diameter.

1. *What is the significance of the fixed distended neck veins?*
   (a) Fluid overload
   (b) Left ventricular failure
   (c) Superior vena cava obstruction (SVCO)
   (d) Right-sided pleural effusion
   (e) Extension of a malignancy along the veins
2. *What is the appropriate immediate management?*
   (a) Arrange immediate biopsy of the mass before steroids are given
   (b) Give high-dose steroids immediately
   (c) Arrange for urgent radiotherapy
   (d) Arrange for surgical resection of the tumour
   (e) Perform a bone marrow biopsy before steroids are given
3. *What is the diagnosis and outlook with appropriate treatment, assuming advanced stage disease?*
   (a) High-grade non-Hodgkin's lymphoma: 50% survival at 5 years
   (b) High-grade non-Hodgkin's lymphoma: 90% survival at 5 years
   (c) Low-grade non-Hodgkin's lymphoma: 50% survival at 9 years
   (d) Hodgkin's lymphoma: 25% survival at 5 years
   (e) Hodgkin's lymphoma: 70% survival at 5 years

Case 16: A patient with a rapidly enlarging neck lump

A 25-year-old man who has recently come to the UK from Zambia presents with a 2-week history of a rapidly enlarging neck lump. He is also feeling tired and run down but with no other specific symptoms. On examination, he has a 5 × 6 cm neck lump in the right anterior triangle of the neck. It is also noticed that he is very thin and has oral *Candidiasis*. Cardiovascular, respiratory and abdominal examination are all normal. CT scan shows that in addition to the neck lump, he has a mass involving the terminal ileum.

Blood results come back as follows:
Hb   11.4 g/dL
MCV   87 fL
WBC   3.8 × 10⁹/L
Platelets   145 × 10⁹/L
Urea and electrolytes, liver function tests, CRP: all normal
A lymphoma is suspected.

1. *What is the most appropriate diagnostic test for lymphoma?*
   (a) CT chest, abdomen, pelvis
   (b) Bone marrow aspirate and trephine
   (c) Fine-needle aspiration (FNA) of the neck lump
   (d) Excision biopsy of the neck lump
   (e) Immunophenotyping of the peripheral blood
2. *What further test is necessary in this patient?*
   (a) HIV antibody test
   (b) Malaria antigen test
   (c) EBV serology
   (d) Hepatitis B serology
   (e) Hepatitis C serology

Case 17: A patient with headache and blurred vision

A 58-year-old accountant presents to A&E with a headache and blurred vision. Over the last few months he has also been feeling very tired and run down, and has lost 12 kg in weight. He is a non-smoker and drinks only occasional glasses of wine with a meal. On examination, he is noted to have a left hemiplegia and fundoscopy shows early papilloedema. Cardiovascular, respiratory and abdominal examination are all normal. Oxygen saturations were 97% on air. A urine dip is positive for blood.

Blood tests show the following:
Hb   18.8 g/dL
MCV   95 fL
WCC   12.5 × 10⁹/L
Platelets   410 × 10⁹/L
Film: normal apart from the high red cell count
U&E, LFT, calcium: all normal
Erythropoietin level: 105 (normal range: 5–35)
CT head: sagittal sinus thrombosis with no space-occupying lesion

1. *What is the significance of the erythropoietin level?*
   (a) Indicates a secondary polycythaemia
   (b) Indicates a primary polycythaemia
   (c) Indicates a relative polycythaemia
   (d) No relevance in distinguishing the causes of a high Hb
   (e) Is only useful in the context of red cell mass studies
2. *What is the most likely underlying cause in this case?*
   (a) Primary polycythaemia due to JAK2 mutation
   (b) Chronic hypoxia
   (c) Gaisbock's syndrome
   (d) Renal cell carcinoma
   (e) Cerebellar haemangioblastoma

Case 18: A patient with burning pains in her fingers

A 75-year-old woman presents to her GP with a 2-month history of burning pains in her fingers and generalized itch. She is otherwise well although not getting much sleep due to her symptoms. She has no history of thrombosis, diabetes or hypertension. She also notes that the itchiness is worse after a bath. Cardiovascular and respiratory examinations were normal. On palapation of the abdomen, a 2-cm spleen could be felt but there was no hepatomegaly.

Blood results came back as follows:
Hb   14.2 g/dL
WCC   13.2 × 10⁹/L
Platelets   1654 × 10⁹/L
Film: variation in platelet size, basophilia
U&E, LFT, calcium, CRP normal

1. *What is the most likely diagnosis?*
   (a) Haemochromatosis
   (b) Cholestasis
   (c) Primary polycythaemia
   (d) Myelofibrosis
   (e) Essential thrombocythaemia (ET)
2. *The JAK2 mutation analysis came back as negative. What is the significance of the JAK2 result?*
   (a) JAK2 mutation is only found in 50% of cases of ET
   (b) JAK2 mutation is found in nearly 100% of ET cases so excludes this diagnosis in her case
   (c) JAK2 mutation is rarely found in ET so is of no relevance here

Case 19: A patient with lower back pain

A 68-year-old woman presents to her GP with a 3-month history of worsening lower back pain. The back pain is localized to the small of her back and has recently been waking her from sleep. Her appetite and weight are steady and she has no other symptoms. She has a history of mild hypertension for which she takes bendroflumethazide. On examination she looks well and has a normal cardiovascular, respiratory and abdominal examination.

Results of investigations are as follows:

Hb	13.4 g/dL
MCV	95 fL
WBC	6.7×10^9/L
Platelets	175×10^9/L
Na	130 mmol/L
K	4.5 mmol/L
Corrected Ca	2.25 mmol/L
Urea	3.5 mmol/l
Creatinine	75 µmol/L
Bilirubin	8 µmol/L
ALT	35 U/L
ALP	640 U/L

Serum electrophoresis: small IgG lambda M band
No immune paresis
Paraprotein level: 6.4 g/L
Skeletal survey: no lytic lesions
Bone scan: An area of increased uptake is seen in L4 vertebra.

1. *Which of the following test results is most consistent with a diagnosis of myeloma?*
   (a) Small IgG lambda M band
   (b) Raised ALP
   (c) Absence of immune paresis (i.e. normal IgM and IgA levels)
   (d) A localized region of increased uptake on the bone scan
   (e) A low sodium level
2. *What is the most likely cause of her back pain?*
   (a) A lytic lesion due to an underlying deposit of myeloma
   (b) Paget's disease
   (c) Metastatic carcinoma
   (d) Simple musculoskeletal lower back pain

Case 20: A patient with increasing nausea

A 45-year-old man presents to his GP with a 3-week history of increasing nausea. Over the last 2 days he has developed a sharp pain in his chest which is worse on lying flat and relieved on sitting forward. He has no other past medical or drug history. On examination, he looks unwell and auscultation of his precordium revealed a rub. Respiratory and abdominal examination were normal.

Blood test results showed:

Hb	9.6 g/dL
MCV	99 fL
WBC	3.3×10^9/L
Platelets	140×10^9/L
Na	138 mmol/L
K	7.3 mmol/L
Corrected Ca	2.5 mmol/L
Urea	35.5 mmol/L
Creatinine	890 µmol/L
Albumin	38 g/L
Bilirubin	9 µmol/L
ALT	23 U/L
ALP	135 U/L

He was admitted to the local renal unit for urgent dialysis. Whilst on the unit, the following results came back:
Serum electrophoresis: immune paresis
No monoclonal band
Skeletal survey: multiple lytic lesions skull and ribs

1. *What is the most likely cause of his electrophoresis result?*
   (a) Nephrotic syndrome with loss of immunoglobulin in the urine
   (b) An underlying low-grade non-Hodgkin's lymphoma
   (c) Common variable immunodeficiency
   (d) Light chain only myeloma
   (e) Monoclonal gammopathy of uncertain significance
2. *Multiple myeloma is diagnosed. What is the median survival for this man?*
   (a) 8–10 years with appropriate therapy
   (b) 1–2 months irrespective of treatment
   (c) Approximately 6–12 months
   (d) Equivalent to age-matched controls

Case 21: A patient with macrocytosis and thrombocytopenia

A 65-year-old publican is seen in haematology outpatients with a macrocytosis and thrombocytopenia. He is feeling well in himself and the abnormal result was picked up incidentally. He has a past history of pancreatitis and hypertension, for which he takes amlodipine. He is a non-smoker and drinks approximately 20 pints of beer per week. On examination, he was overweight and rather pale. There was no jaundice and his cardiovascular, respiratory and abdominal examination were all normal.

His blood results were as follows:

Hb	12.4 g/dL
MCV	108 fL
WBC	5.6×10^9/L
Platelets	138×10^9/L
CRP	<8 mg/L
Na	136 mmol/L
K	4.1 mmol/L
Urea	3.6 mmol/L
Creatinine	75 µmol/L
Bilirubin	12 µmol/L
ALT	25 U/L
ALP	134 U/L

γ-GT	450 U/L
Serum ferritin	250 ng/mL
Serum folate	15 nmol/L
Serum vitamin B$_{12}$	350 pmol/L

1. *What is the most likely cause for his raised MCV?*

   (a) Myelodysplastic syndrome

   (b) Hypothyroidism

   (c) β-Thalassaemia trait

   (d) Alcohol

   (e) Amlodipine

Four years later he is re-referred to haematology outpatients. He has successfully cut down his alcohol consumption to only 1–2 pints of beer per week after having retired. Over the last 6 months he has been increasingly lethargic and has noticed that he bruises more easily than usual. On examination he was pale. Cardiovascular examination revealed a soft ejection systolic murmur over the aortic area which did not radiate. Respiratory and abdominal examination were normal.

Blood tests results now showed:

Hb	8.2 g/dL
MCV	110 fL
WBC	4.8×10^9/L
Platelets	62×10^9/L
CRP	<8 mg/L
Na	143 mmol/L
K	3.8 mmol/l
Urea	4.5 mmol/L
Creatinine	83 μmol/L
Bilirubin	2.6 μmol/L
ALT	35 U/L
AL	150 U/L
γ-GT	120 U/L
TSH	normal

Serum ferritin, folate and vitamin B$_{12}$: all normal

Film: dysplastic neutrophils, variation in red cell size and shape

2. *What is the most likely diagnosis?*

   (a) Myelodysplastic syndrome (MDS)

   (b) Hypothyroidism

   (c) β-Thalassaemia trait

   (d) Alcohol

   (e) Amlodipine

3. *What is the most appropriate treatment?*

   (a) Bone marrow transplantation

   (b) High-dose chemotherapy

   (c) Blood product support

   (d) Aspirin

   (e) Oral steroid therapy

The patient receives regular blood transfusions. Three years later he is reviewed in the haematology out patient clinic with the following blood test results:

Hb	9.8 g/dL
MCV	112 fL
WBC	4.1×10^9/L
Platelets	55×10^9/L
Ferritin	1650 ng/mL

Serum folate and vitamin B$_{12}$: normal

4. *What is the likely cause of his raised ferritin?*

   (a) Chronic infection

   (b) Increased alcohol consumption

   (c) Chronic blood loss from the GI tract

   (d) Hereditary haemochromatosis

   (e) Iron overload due to regular blood transfusions

Case 22: A patient who has suffered a collapse

A 79-year-old man is admitted under the medical take with collapse of unknown cause. He has been feeling unwell for some months with increasing fatigue and back pain. The collapse was preceded by feeling faint and dizzy. He lost consciousness for just a few seconds and was well oriented when he regained consciousness. His back pain has been increasingly severe over the last few weeks, requiring opioid analgesia. He has a past history of hypertension, angina, transient ischaemic attacks and high cholesterol. He is an ex-smoker (having given up 10 years ago) and drinks only occasional alcohol. On examination, he was frail and thin. His BP was 145/90 mmHg and saturations were 96% on air. There was a soft systolic murmur heard over the aortic area which did not radiate. Respiratory examination was normal but on palpation of his abdomen, an enlarged bladder was easily palpable.

Blood tests are as follows:

Hb	8.5 g/dL
MCV	85 fL
WCC	9.2×10^9/L
Platelets	145×10^9/L
CRP	10 mg/L
Na	132 mmol/L
K	3.4 mmol/L
Corrected Ca	2.62 mmol/L
Urea	25.8 mmol/L
Creatinine	350 μmol/L
Bilirubin	12 μmol/L
ALT	15 U/L
ALP	115 U/L
Serum iron	8.9 μmol/L
Serum ferritin	250 ng/mL
Serum folate acid	9.8 nmol/L
Serum B$_{12}$	320 pmol/L

Serum and urine electrophoresis: normal

Chest X-ray: clear

ECG: normal

1. *At this stage, what is the most likely cause of his anaemia?*

   (a) Anaemia of chronic disease

   (b) Bone marrow infiltration

   (c) Myeloma

   (d) Acute myeloid leukaemia

   (e) Renal failure

Over the next few days his renal function improves after a urinary catheter is inserted, but he again becomes anaemic. Blood results at this time show:

Hb	7.8 g/dL
MCV	90 fL
WCC	3.2×10^9/L
Platelets	15×10^9/L

Blood film: leukoerythroblastic with tear drop poikilocytes

2. *What is the significance of a leukoerythroblastic blood film?*

   (a) Indicates acute leukaemia

   (b) Indicates a bone marrow which is recovering from an acute insult

(c) Indicates marrow infiltration or systemic sepsis
(d) Indicates an appropriate marrow response to severe anaemia
(e) Indicates use of granulocyte colony stimulating factor

A bone marrow aspirate is performed. The result comes back 'diffusely infiltrated by malignant cells of non-haemopoietic origin'.

Case 23: A patient with heavy periods

A 36-year-old solicitor presents to her GP with a 5-month history of increasingly heavy periods which now regularly soak through her sanitary towels. She has suffered from the occasional nose bleed since she was a teenager and also complains of intermittent gum bleeding for many years. She has no other symptoms but does have a history of hypertension, for which she was started on lisinopril 3 years ago. On direct questioning, her mother once bled heavily after childbirth, requiring a blood transfusion but the patient herself has never had any children and has never had an operation. Physical examination was entirely unremarkable. A full blood count comes back with the following results:

Hb   11.7 g/dL
WCC 5.8×10^9/L
Platelets 15×10^9/L

APTT, PT, blood film examination, biochemistry and autoantibody screen were all unremarkable.

1. *Which of her symptoms is most suggestive of an underlying platelet disorder?*
   (a) Intermittent gum bleeding
   (b) Occasional nose bleeds
   (c) Increasingly heavy periods
2. *What is the most likely diagnosis?*
   (a) Thrombotic thrombocytopenic purpura
   (b) Idiopathic thrombocytopenic purpura (ITP)
   (c) Familial platelet disorder
3. *What further investigation is required in this patient?*
   (a) Bone marrow aspirate
   (b) Platelet autoantibody assay
   (c) None

Case 24: A patient who has undergone a coronary artery bypass

A 74-year-old man underwent a coronary artery bypass graft 7 days ago. He has a past medical history of type 2 diabetes and hypertension for which he takes gliclazide and ramipril. He also takes regular aspirin (which was stopped prior to surgery) and simvastatin. Since the surgery, he has been unwell on the intensive care unit requiring inotropic support and haemofiltration. Over the last 24 hours, the haemofiltration circuit has been frequently clotting off and the patient has been complaining of a painful left leg. On examination the leg is pale and no peripheral pulses could be identified. His blood counts over the last few days are as follows:

Days post-op:	2	4	5	6
Hb (g/dL)	11.4	11.8	10.9	11.2
WCC ($\times 10^9$/L)	12.6	13.5	13.8	12.9
PLT ($\times 10^9$/L)	250	270	150	75

Three days ago the patient was prescribed broad-spectrum antibiotics for presumed sepsis.

1. *What is the most likely diagnosis?*
   (a) Heparin-induced thrombocytopenia (HIT)
   (b) Post-transfusion purpura
   (c) Idiopathic thrombocytopenic purpura
   (d) Antibiotic-induced thrombocytopenia
2. *What is the most appropriate management?*
   (a) Make sure he is not exposed to any more heparin
   (b) Make sure he is not exposed to any more unfractionated heparin, and use low molecular weight heparin (LMWH) instead
   (c) Make sure he is not exposed to any more heparin and use a non-heparin anticoagulant

Case 25: A patient who has had a total hip replacement

A 56-year-old man has a total hip replacement. He is given low molecular weight heparin (LMWH) as prophylaxis against venous thromboembolism. His regular medication is quinine for night cramps and bendroflumethiazide for hypertension and atorvastatin. Pre-operative full blood count (FBC) is Hb 12.5 g/dL and platelets 305×10^{12}/L. He bleeds more than average and first day post-operatively his Hb is 7.2 g/dL and platelets are 415×10^{12}/L. He has a 3 unit blood transfusion. On day six post-operatively he has a routine FBC showing Hb 11.1 g/dL and platelets 33×10^{12}/L.

1. *Which of his drugs can cause thrombocytopenia?*
   (a) LMWH
   (b) Quinine
   (c) Bendroflumethiazide
   (d) Atorvastatin
   (e) All of these
2. *What is the most likely diagnosis?*
   (a) Heparin-induced thrombocytopenia (HIT)
   (b) Post-transfusion purpura
   (c) Quinine-induced thrombocytopenia
   (d) Disseminated intravascular coagulation (DIC)
3. *Which of the following is not a reasonable part of his immediate management?*
   (a) Stopping LMWH
   (b) Starting warfarin
   (c) Starting an alterative parenteral anticoagulant
   (d) An ultrasound to look for evidence of deep vein thrombosis (DVT)
4. *Which of the following drugs reversibly inhibit platelet function?*
   (a) Aspirin
   (b) Clopidogrel
   (c) Naproxen
   (d) Etoricoxib
   (e) Atorvasatin

Case 26: A patient with severe bruising

A 78-year-old man presents to A&E with severe bruising. Bruising started one month ago. In the past he has had several operations without any problems. His father died of a haemorrhagic stroke at the age of 63 years. He has peripheral claudication for which he takes aspirin 75 mg once a day. There is no other significant past medical history. His PT is 12.0 sec (10–14) and APTT 65 sec (26–34).

1. *What is the most likely diagnosis?*
   (a) Congenital haemophilia A
   (b) Congenital haemophilia B
   (c) Acquired haemophilia A
   (d) Acquired von Willebrand's disease (VWD)
   (e) Warfarin overdose
2. *His plasma (APTT 65 sec) is mixed with normal plasma (50:50 mix) and the APTT repeated immediately and after incubation for one hour. Which of these results are typical of acquired haemophilia?*
   (a) Immediate mix 40 sec, incubated mix 62 sec
   (b) Immediate mix 70 sec, incubated mix 70 sec
   (c) Immediate mix 33 sec, incubated mix 34 sec
3. *For a patient with a severe bleeding history and normal PT and APTT what factor deficiency should be considered?*
   (a) XII
   (b) X
   (c) XIII
   (d) Plasminogen
   (e) Fibrinogen
4. *For a young child with a severe bleeding history and long PT and normal APTT what factor deficiency should be considered?*
   (a) II
   (b) X
   (c) VII
   (d) VIII

Case 27: A patient with easy bruising and heavy periods

A 19-year-old woman presents with easy bruising. Her periods have been heavy since her menarche at age 12. She does not suffer from nose bleeds and has never had an operation or a dental extraction. Her mother had a hysterectomy for heavy periods. The following results are available:

Hb	11.0 g/dL
MCV	72 fL
PT	12 sec (10–14)
APTT	45 sec (26–34)

1. *What investigations would you undertake?*
   (a) II, VII, IX, X
   (b) VIII, IX, XI
   (c) VIII, IX, XI, VWF
   (d) Von Willebrand's factor (VWF)
2. *What is the most likely diagnosis?*
   (a) Von Willebrand's disease
   (b) Haemophilia A
   (c) Haemophilia B
   (d) A platelet disorder
3. *What do her Hb and MCV indicate?*
   (a) They are normal for a woman
   (b) Anaemia of chronic disease
   (c) Iron deficiency anaemia
   (d) Folate deficiency
4. *Which of these are not useful in the treatment of menorrhagia associated with VWD?*
   (a) Desmopressin
   (b) Tranexamic acid
   (c) Contraceptive pill
   (d) Mefenamic acid

Haematology: Answers

Case 1: A patient with shortness of breath

1. (b) Flow murmur due to a hyperdynamic circulation

A flow murmur is common in severe anaemia. Aortic stenosis is unlikely due to the absence of radiation and normal pulse pressure; aortic sclerosis (early aortic valve disease without at the moment a significant gradient) remains a possibility although the patient is rather young for this.

2. (a) Iron deficiency anaemia

Iron deficiency causes a microcytic anaemia. Thalassaemia trait also does this but is unlikely in view of the normal MCV 3 years ago. Vitamin B_{12} deficiency causes a macrocytic anaemia. Anaemia of chronic disease is unlikely in view of the normal inflammatory markers and aplastic anaemia causes a normocytic anaemia, usually with neutropenia and/or thrombocytopenia.
Further reading: Chapter 50 in Medicine at a Glance.

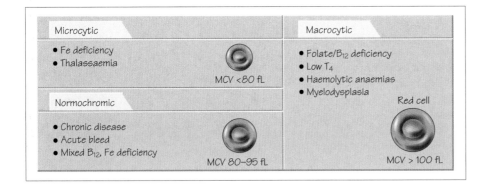

Figure 7.1.1 Classification of anaemia according to red cell size.

Case 2: A patient needing a blood transfusion after a road traffic accident

1. (c) She should receive blood of group O which is also rhesus D negative

She is a woman of childbearing age, and is critically ill from acute blood loss; she needs immediate blood transfusion to save her life. Therefore, in addition to receiving blood with the 'universal donor' ABO group (group O), she should receive rhesus D negative blood in case she is also rhesus D negative thereby avoiding the development of anti-D antibodies that can put subsequent pregnancies at risk. The final option is false – if she is bleeding profusely into her abdomen, a blood transfusion may never raise her Hb to the normal range without surgical intervention.

2. (a) B positive

As she is rhesus D positive, she can receive rhesus D positive or negative blood products. However, as she is group A, she will have circulating anti-B antibodies. She should therefore *not* receive group B or AB red cells.

3. (d) Haemolytic transfusion reaction

The positive antiglobulin test, dark urine, jaundice and falling haemoglobin in spite of successful surgery all indicate acute haemolysis. In someone who has received multiple units of blood, the most likely cause is an acute haemolytic transfusion reaction due to an ABO mismatched unit.
Further reading: Chapter 50.

Case 3: A patient with an intracranial haemorrhage

1. (c) II, VII, IX, X

These are the vitamin K dependent factors; warfarin is a vitamin K antagonist, and therefore he will be deficient in these factors

2. (b) Vitamin K and prothrombin complex concentrate

The INR should be corrected completely using prothrombin complex concentrate (use FFP if this is not available). If not, he is highly likely to sustain further intracranial bleeding, with potentially quite catastrophic results. The chance that his aortic valve prosthesis clots off with a few days or weeks off all warfarin anticoagulation is low (not zero); mitral valve prostheses (which has a larger cross-sectional area, so slower blood flow) are more likely to clot off than aortic valve prostheses. Ball-in-a-cage valves (Starr-Edwards) have a much higher thrombosis potential than tilting disk valves.

3. (a) Restart warfarin when the patient has recovered from the acute event

This will need to be done with a mechanical valve *in situ*. How long he should stay off his warfarin is very unclear, and this decision will need to be based on clinical judgement, incorporating how data on how large the intracranial bleed was, whether he had a re-bleed, etc. His INR will need to be very carefully monitored.

4. (b) Codeine

There are so many drugs that interact with warfarin that it is crucial to look up in the *British National Formulary* (*BNF*) the interaction of every new drug prescribed for patients on warfarin. Drugs particularly likely to interact with warfarin include antibiotics and anti-convulsant drugs.
Further reading: Chapter 184.

Case 4: A patient on HRT with deep venous thrombosis

1. (a) 1

The protein C and S results are compatible with warfarin. Thus the only prothrombotic condition detected is factor V Leiden heterozygosity.

2. (b) 3–6 months

Characteristics of patient*	Risk of recurrence in the year after discontinuation (%)	Duration of therapy
Major transient risk factor	3	3 months
Minor risk factor, no thrombophilia	< 10 if risk factor avoided > 10 if risk factor persistent	6 months Until factor resolves
Idiopathic event; no thrombophilia or low-risk thrombophilia	< 10	6 months†
Idiopathic event; high-risk thrombophilia	> 10	Indefinite
More than one idiopathic event	> 10	Indefinite
Cancer; other ongoing risk factor	> 10	Indefinite

* Examples of major transient risk factors are major surgery a major medical illness, and leg casting
Examples of minor transient risk factors are the use of an oral contraceptive and hormone-replacement therapy
Examples of low-risk thrombophilias are heterozygosity for the factor V Leiden and G20210A prothrombin-gene mutation
Examples of high-risk thrombophilia are antithrombin, protein C, and protein S deficiencies, homozygosity for the factor V Leiden or prothrombin-gene mutation or heterozygosity for both; and the presence of antiphospholipid antibodies
†Therapy may be prolonged if the patient prefers to prolong it or the risk of bleeding is low

Figure 7.4.1 Duration of anticoagulant therapy in DVT.

Factor V Leiden does not alter this. The usual duration of treatment for an uncomplicated proximal deep vein thrombosis is 3–6 months; following discontinuation of warfarin therapy, some 10% of patients per year present with further DVTs/PEs. This is quite a high rate, and is cumulative (i.e. 20% after 2 years etc.); patients must be warned about this risk, so that they present early should they develop relevant symptoms.

3. (c) 2-fold

There are multiple risk factors for VTE hormone replacement therapy increases the risk by about two fold. Recent surgery, increasing age, and cancer are far more powerful risk factors, as are most inherited conditions.

4. (d) The daughter should be counselled

There is no need to test the men. A woman on the oral contraceptive pill without factor V Leiden has about a 4 fold increased risk of VTE, whereas if the daughter has inherited the factor V Leiden gene mutation, her risk of VTE is increased about 35 fold. This is clearly quite a significant risk, and she should be counselled about it, and may wish to either discontinue the contraceptive pill, or be tested for factor V Leiden.

Further reading: Chapter 185.

Case 5: A pregnant woman with a generalized seizure

1. (a) Coagulation screen (prothrombin time (PT), activated partial thromboplastin time (APTT), fibrinogen and D-dimers)

Disseminated intravascular coagulation (DIC) needs to be excluded. In DIC, the PT and APTT would be prolonged, the fibrinogen would be low and the D-dimers raised.

2. (d) Microangiopathic haemolytic anaemia is present

Red cell fragments indicate that haemolysis is occurring within the microvasculature (or in the presence of a prosthetic heart valve). Polychromasia indicates that the bone marrow is responding appropriately by increasing red cell output.

3. (b) Thrombotic thrombocytopenic purpura (TTP)

A microangiopathic haemolytic anaemia and thrombocytopenia with normal coagulation screen suggests TTP until proven otherwise. In this case, the neurological involvement, renal impairment and fever all support the diagnosis.

Further reading: Chapter 182.

Case 6: A patient with fatigue and mild jaundice

1. (c) Warm AIHA

In the absence of herediatary spherocytosis, spherocytes on the blood film suggest an extravascular haemolysis. Polychromasia, splenomegaly and mild jaundice are in keeping with this. Cold AIHA would normally produce red cell agglutination on a blood film.

2. (a) Direct antiglobulin test (Coombs' test)

A reticulocyte would be useful but adds little additional information as the film is known to be polychromatic. A direct antiglobulin test will confirm that there are antibodies coating the red cells. Whilst not diagnostic for AIHA, in this clinical context it is highly suggestive. The osmotic fragility assay is designed to look for hereditary spherocytosis, where cells are more fragile than normal, and a variant of the test, in acid, is designed to look for paroxysmal nocturnal haemoglobinuria.

3. (e) Prednisolone and folic acid

Prednisolone is an effective treatment for idiopathic warm AIHA. Folic acid supplementation should be given as haemolysis can rapidly deplete stores of folic acid.

4. (a) Autoimmune screen

This patient has a butterfly rash and flitting arthralgias. It is possible that the AIHA could be a manifestation of systemic lupus

Risk factor	Estimated relative risk
Inherited conditions[†]	
Antithrombin deficiency	25
Protein C deficiency	10
Protein S deficiency	10
Factor V Leiden mutation	
Heterozygous	5
Homozygous	50
G20210A prothrombin-gene mutation (heterozygous)	2.5
Dysfibrinogenemia	18
Acquired conditions	
Major surgery or major trauma	5–200[#]
History of venous thromboembolism	50
Antiphospholipid antibodies	
Elevated anticardiolipin antibody level	2
Nonspecific inhibitor (e.g. lupus anticoagulant)	10
Cancer	5
Major medical illness with hospitalization	5
Age	
> 50 years	5
> 70 years	10
Pregnancy	7
Estrogen therapy	
Oral contraceptives	5
Hormone-replacement therapy	2
Selective estrogen-receptor modulators	
Tamoxifen	5
Raloxifene	3
Obesity	1–3
Hereditary, environmental, or idiopathic conditions	
Hyperhomocysteinemia[«]	3
Elevated levels of factor VIII (> 90th percentile)	3
Elevated levels of factor IX (> 90th percentile)	2.3
Elevated levels of factor XI (> 90th percentile)	2.2

* Relative risks are for patients with the specified risk factor, as compared with those without the risk factor

† The definition of deficiency of antithrombin, protein C or protein S varies among studies; it is usually defined as a functional or immunologic value that is less than the 5th percentile of values in the general population

\# The risk varies greatly, depending on the type of surgery, the use and type of prophylaxis, and the method of diagnosis

« The definition of hyperhomocysteinemia varies among studies; it is usually defined as a persistent elevation of fasting plasma homocysteine levels or plasma homocysteine levels after methionine loading that are greater than the 95th percentile of the control population or more than 2 SD above the mean for the control population

Figure 7.4.2 Risk factors for venous thromboembolism.

erythematosis. In this case, the antinuclear antibody result was >1/640 and anti-dsDNA titres were raised. *Mycoplasma* infection is associated with cold AIHA.
Further reading: Chapter 172.

Case 7: A tired patient with lumps

1. (c) HIV infection

CLL and disseminated malignancy are unlikely due to his age and absence of a spleen, the history is too chronic for infectious mononucleosis, and malaria usually results in splenomegaly. HIV infection is common in sub-Saharan Africa and persistent, generalized lymphadenopathy is a common feature.

2. (a) Open lymph node biopsy

The presumptive diagnosis is of a lymphoma complicating his HIV infection, though it is also possible that the rapidly enlarging mass is another form of malignancy, or even an infection, e.g. tuberculosis. However, the most likely diagnosis is lymphoma, and investigations should proceed on this basis. For accurate diagnosis, a large amount of material with preserved architecture is desirable. Fine needle aspirate disrupts the lymph node architecture. A Tru-cut biopsy is not always ideal as biopsy samples can be small and crushed. Bone marrow biopsy may be needed to stage a lymphoma but is rarely helpful in the initial diagnosis.
Further reading: Chapter 177.

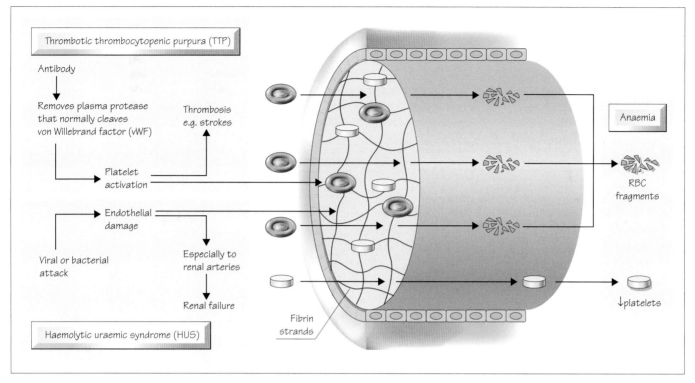

Figure 7.5.1 Anaemia with red cell fragments in the blood.

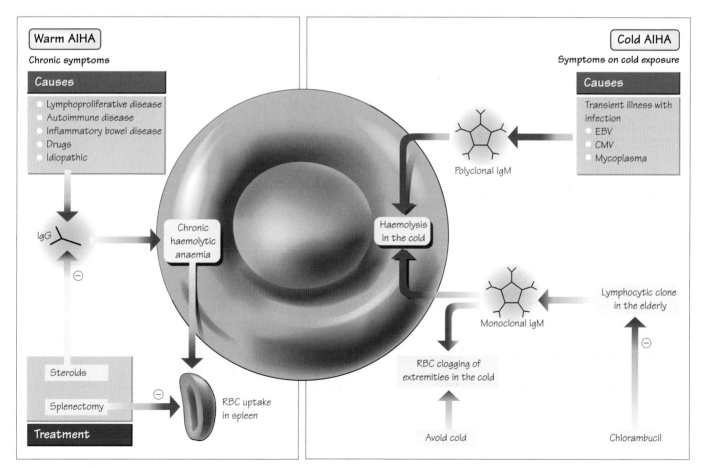

Figure 7.6.2 Different forms of autoimmune haemolytic anaemia.

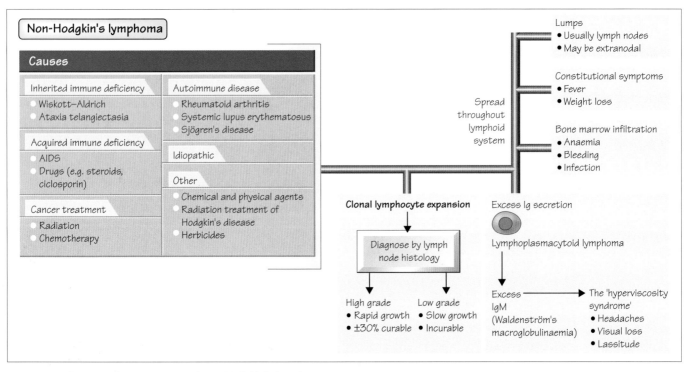

Figure 7.7.1 Causes and consequences of non-Hodgkin's lymphoma.

Case 8: A patient with intermittent abdominal pain and mild jaundice

1. (c) It suggests either an increased delivery of bilirubin to the liver or a failure of conjugation by the liver

Bile duct obstruction would increase the alkaline phosphatase (ALP) and conjugated bilirubin levels. A level of 55 U/L is clearly above the normal range and so indicates pathology.

2. (a) Chronic haemolysis

The mild anaemia with raised mean cell volume (MCV), together with unconjugated hyperbilirubinaemia all suggest haemolysis (Fig.7.8.1). Gilbert's syndrome is a common cause of unconjugated hyperbilirubinaemia but does not cause splenomegaly.

3. (b) Blood film with direct antiglobulin test

Hereditary spherocytosis is the most likely diagnosis. A blood film will show spherocytes (Fig.7.8.2) and a direct antiglobulin test would be negative, indicating that the spherocytes were *not* due to autoimmune haemolysis. The family history of jaundice supports the diagnosis and her abdominal pain is presumably due to pigment gallstones resulting from chronic haemolysis.

Further reading: Chapter 172.

Case 9: A patient with lower back pain

1. (d) Reassure patient, repeat in 3–6 months' time

As this patient has recently moved to the UK from Ghana, she may well be of African ethnic origin where normal range for neutrophils is less than for Caucasians. The count is not sufficiently low enough to worry unduly about an increased infection rate.

Further reading: Chapter 53.

Case 10: A patient with shortness of breath and purulent sputum

1. (b) Myelodysplastic syndrome

Myelodysplastic syndrome causes a reduction in one or more of the peripheral counts and typically raises the MCV. The blood film findings are also suggestive. Vitamin B_{12} deficiency is unlikely as the film would show hypersegmented neutrophils and oval macrocytes. The white count is not affected in DIC and there is nothing to suggest myeloma. In aplastic anaemia, the blood film is usually unremarkable.

Further reading:Chapter 180.

Case 11: A patient with increasing fatigue and mild jaundice

1. (b) Pernicious anaemia

Macrocytic anaemia, mild jaundice and coexisting autoimmune condition (vitiligo) all make pernicious anaemia the most likely diagnosis. In autoimmune haemolysis, the MCV is only slightly raised and splenomegaly is usual. Dietary B_{12} deficiency is rare.

2. (c) Iron deficiency

When vitamin B_{12} replacement is first initiated, the bone marrow demand for iron greatly increases, sometimes precipitating iron deficiency. Simple oral iron supplements should prove effective.

Further reading: Chapter 171.

Case 12: A patient with intermittent palpitations

1. (d) Previous blood count results

The differential of a microcytic anaemia is thalassaemia trait or iron deficiency. If he has had previous, normal blood counts then iron deficiency is likely. A blood film and iron studies would also be useful.

2. (a) Constipation

Oral iron commonly causes constipation.

3. (a) Upper and lower GI imaging

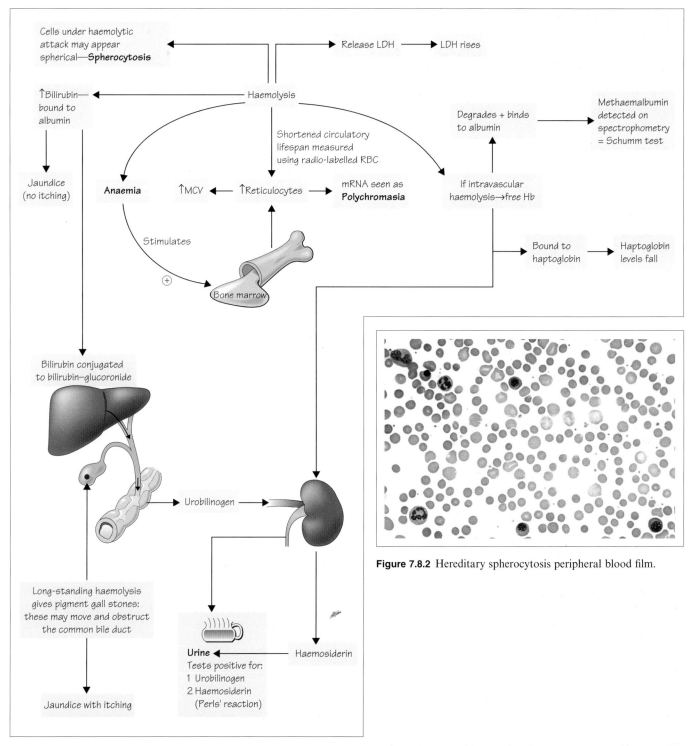

Figure 7.8.1 Consequences of haemolysis.

Figure 7.8.2 Hereditary spherocytosis peripheral blood film.

There is a relatively high incidence of combined upper and lower GI pathology in patients with iron deficiency anaemia, therefore both upper and lower GI imaging should be performed. This means that if an ulcer is found on upper GI imaging, lower GI imaging is still indicated as there may be a fungating colonic cancer.

Further reading: Chapter 171.

Case 13: A patient with increasing breathlessness

1. (a) Idiopathic aplastic anaemia

The main differential diagnosis is between aplastic anaemia and hypoplastic myelodysplastic syndrome (MDS). MDS would be very unusual in this age group.

2. (d) Urinary haemosiderin

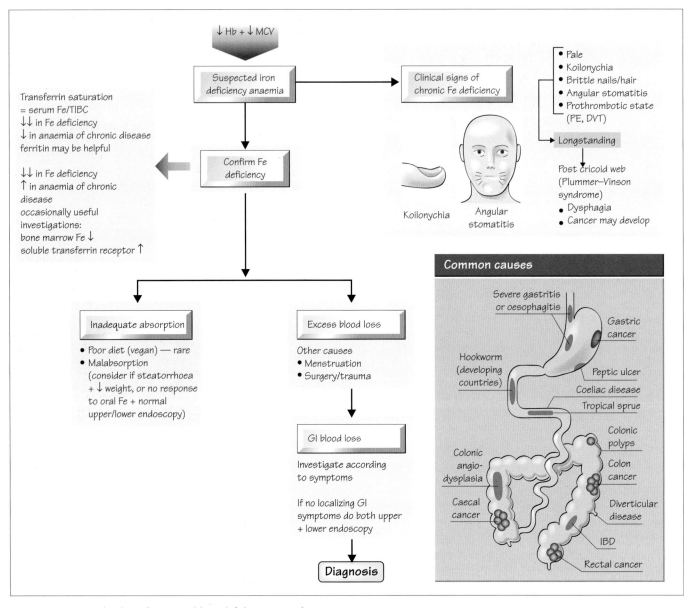

Figure 7.12.1 Investigation of suspected iron deficiency anaemia.

The patient is likely to have developed paroxysmal nocturnal haemoglobinuria which can lead to intravascular haemolysis and thromboses. Pancytopenia with a raised MCV is commonly found. A positive urinary haemosiderin would confirm intravascular haemolysis. The most common diagnostic test for paroxysmal nocturnal haemoglobinuria (PNH) however, would be flow cytometry.

Further reading: Chapter 174.

Case 14: A patient with a nose bleed and bruising

1. (b) Suggestive of acute leukaemia

Blasts are immature, poorly differentiated blood forming cells which are the hallmark of acute leukaemia. In the setting of (a) and (c), more mature precursor cells such as myelocytes and nucleated red cells may be seen. Blasts can be seen but are much less common. In acute viral infections, reactive cells are seen which can sometimes be hard to distinguish from blasts on a blood film.

2. (a) Disseminated intravascular coagulation (DIC)

Low platelets, prolonged PT and APTT with a low fibrinogen all point to DIC which is well known to complicate some cases of acute leukaemia (particularly acute promyelocytic leukaemia, or APL). Although at risk of neutropenic sepsis, the absence of fever and normal CRP suggest this has not yet developed.

3. (e) Attend the ward immediately for a medical review

The patient is highly likely to be neutropenic. Neutropenic sepsis can progress extremely rapidly so he should be admitted to the hospital as soon as possible. He should be medically assessed urgently and intravenous antibiotics should be prescribed and given as soon as possible. Paracetamol may mask a fever and so should not be advised in a neutropenic patient.

Further reading: Chapter 175.

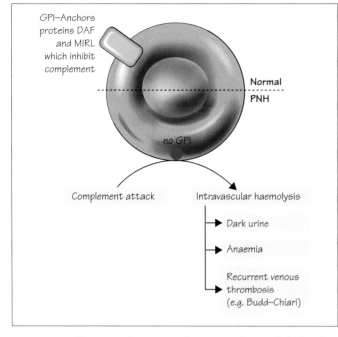

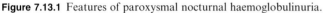

Figure 7.13.1 Features of paroxysmal nocturnal haemoglobulinuria.

Case 15: A patient with shortness of breath and cough

1. (c) Superior vena cava obstruction (SVCO)

SVCO commonly presents with swelling of the face and arms, breathlessness and fixed, distended neck veins. This should not be confused with an elevated jugular venous pressure which has a clear waveform.

2. (a) Arrange immediate biopsy of the mass before steroids are given

Steroids sometimes induce rapid shrinking of the mass, making biopsy and subsequent definitive treatment very difficult. If at all

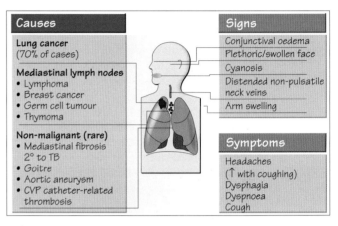

Figure 7.15.1 Superior vena cava obstruction.

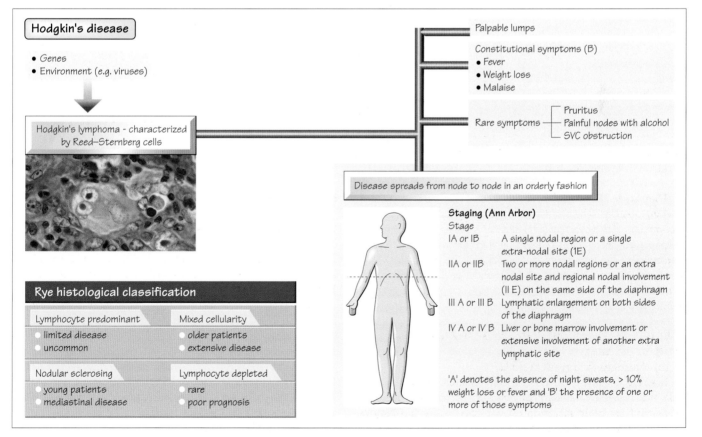

Figure 7.15.2 Features of Hodgkin's disease.

possible, a biopsy should be performed before steroids are given (although this may not always be possible).

The biopsy shows the presence of Reed–Sternberg cells within a background of reactive inflammatory cells.

3. (e) Hodgkin's lymphoma: 70% survival at 5 years

Reed–Sternberg cells are the hallmark of Hodgkin's lymphoma. With modern treatment, advanced stage disease carries an approximately 65–70% cure rate.

Further reading: Chapter 177.

Case 16: A patient with a rapidly enlarging neck lump

1. (d) Excision biopsy of the neck lump

FNA is not a reliable test for the diagnosis of lymphoma. An excision biopsy or core biopsy are needed. Although useful for staging lymphomas, bone marrow biopsies are not as helpful in initial diagnosis as biopsy of an affected lymph node.

A diagnosis of Burkitt's lymphoma is made, the cells having a proliferation index of 100%.

2. (a) HIV antibody test

Burkitt's lymphoma is frequently associated with HIV infection. HIV is also common in sub-Saharan Africa and the oral Candida suggests that he is immunocompromised. Appropriate treatment of HIV significantly improves the outcome of any associated lymphoma.

Further reading: Chapter 177.

Case 17: A patient with headache and blurred vision

1. (a) Indicates a secondary polycythaemia

A high Epo level in the context of a patient with a high Hb indicates secondary polycythaemia.

2. (d) Renal cell carcinoma

Chronic hypoxia is ruled out by his oxygen saturations. Gaisbock's is unlikely as he does not smoke or excessively drink. Renal cell carcinoma is likely in view of his history of lethargy and weight loss, and the urine dipstick being positive for blood. A renal ultrasound confirmed the diagnosis.

Further reading; Chapter 178.

Case 18: A patient with burning pains in her fingers

1. (e) Essential thrombocythaemia (ET)

The patient has the symptoms of aquagenic pruritus and erythromelalgia. She has a high platelet count and the findings of splenomegaly, basophilia and normal CRP suggest that this is due to a primary myeloproliferative condition.

2. (a) JAK2 mutation is only found in 50% of cases of ET

JAK2 mutation is found in nearly 100% of cases of primary polycythaemia but only 50% of cases of ET and myelofibrosis

Further reading: Chapter 178.

Case 19: A patient with lower back pain

1. (a) Small IgG lambda M band

Although in myeloma, an IgG paraprotein is usually higher than that seen here, it is the finding most consistent with the diagnosis of myeloma. Typically in myeloma, the uninvolved immunoglobulin subtypes are reduced (immune paresis). ALP is normal in myeloma (due to suppression of osteoblasts by cytokines

released from the malignant plasma cells) and bone scans are negative for the same reason. The exception is when myeloma has led to a pathological fracture.

2. (c) Metastatic carcinoma

The nature of the back pain is worrying in that it wakes her at night. The raised ALP and area of increased uptake on a bone scan suggest metastatic infiltration, e.g. from primary breast carcinoma. The likely cause of the paraprotein is monoclonal gammopathy of uncertain significance.

Further reading: Chapter 179.

Case 20: A patient with increasing nausea

1. (d) Light chain only myeloma

Renal failure in myeloma is usually caused by light chain precipitation in the renal tubules. A urine electrophoresis would therefore reveal the presence of Bence–Jones protein. Answers (a), (b) and (c) can cause hypogammaglobulinaemia but are not likely causes of lytic lesions. Nephrotic syndrome is ruled out by the normal albumin.

2. (c) Approximately 6–12 months

Myeloma which presents as dialysis dependent renal failure has a very poor outlook irrespective of treatments used.

Further reading: Chapter 179.

Case 21: A patient with macrocytosis and thrombocytopenia

1. (d) Alcohol

Excess alcohol consumption commonly causes a high MCV and mild thrombocytopenia. The raised GGT is also a clue.

2. (a) Myelodysplastic syndrome (MDS)

MDS causes a (usually) macrocytic anaemia and can also cause other cytopenias such as thrombocytopenia. The blood film is also highly suggestive of the diagnosis.

3. (c) Blood product support

The patient is now nearly 70 and in most centres this would be too old for bone marrow transplantation. High-dose chemotherapy is only indicated for MDS transforming to acute myeloid leukaemia, or prior to bone marrow transplantation. Aspirin is contraindicated as it will impair platelet function.

4. (e) Iron overload due to regular blood transfusions

Every unit of blood contains 200 mg of iron which the body is unable to excrete. Regular blood transfusions therefore frequently lead to iron overload, with a high ferritin level. The concern is that the iron may deposit in the heart, liver and/or endocrine organs. High alcohol intake, infections and hereditary haemochromatosis are other causes of a high ferritin but are less likely in this case.

Further reading: Chapter 180.

Case 22: A patient who has suffered a collapse

1. (e) Renal failure

With a creatinine of 350 μmol/L, it is highly likely that the kidneys are failing to produce sufficient erythropoietin to support erythropoiesis. Myeloma is a possibility but a normal serum and urine electrophoresis make this unlikely. Bone marrow infiltration is also possible but less likely with a normal white count.

2. (c) Indicates marrow infiltration or systemic sepsis

A leukoerythroblastic film is always abnormal, and usually indicates bone marrow infiltration by malignancy or fibrosis, or systemic sepsis.

Further reading: Chapter 181.

Case 23: A patient with heavy periods

1. (c) Increasingly heavy periods

Intermittent gum bleeding and occasional nose bleeds are both very common in the general population. Although heavy periods are also common, increasing heaviness is more suggestive of an underlying platelet/coagulation problem.

2. (b) Idiopathic thrombocytopenic purpura (ITP)

The bleeding history is short suggesting an acquired disorder. In a well patient with normal physical examination, general blood tests and blood film, ITP is the most likely diagnosis.

3. (c) None

In a young patient with normal physical examination and isolated low platelets on routine blood tests, a bone marrow aspirate is not advised. Platelet autoantibody assays are notoriously unreliable.

Further reading: Chapter 182.

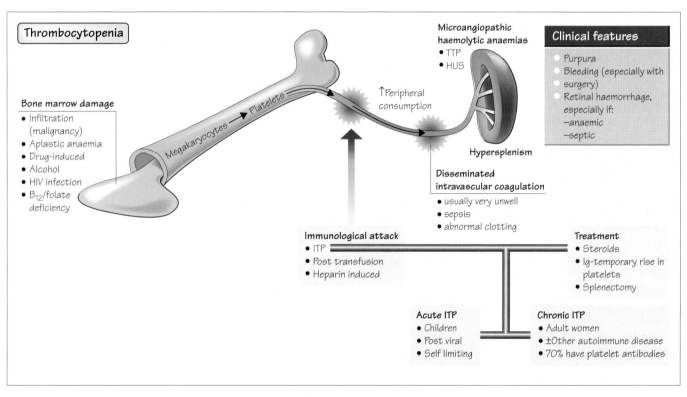

Figure 7.23.1 Causes of thrombocytopenia.

Case 24: A patient who has undergone a coronary artery bypass

1. (a) Heparin-induced thrombocytopenia (HIT)

The combination of a falling platelet count in the context of thrombosis (in this case an acutely ischaemic left leg) suggests HIT. He would have been exposed to heparin during his cardiac bypass and every time he was haemofiltered.

2. (c) Make sure he is not exposed to any more heparin and use a non-heparin anticoagulant

HIT is a pro-thrombotic condition and so anticoagulation must be continued, but LMWH can cross react.

Further reading: Chapter 182.

Case 25: A patient who has had a total hip replacement

1. (e) All of these

There are a large number of drugs that can result in a low platelet count. The underlying mechanism can be very variable and is often unpredictable. The important message is that in any patient with thrombocytopenia an adverse drug reaction may be the cause and should always be considered.

2. (a) Heparin-induced thrombocytopenia (HIT)

The timing (5–10 days after starting LMWH) is classical. Post-transfusion purpura usually occurs 10 days after a blood transfusion.

3. (b) Starting warfarin

This is contraindicated and could precipitate thrombosis in HIT.

4. (c) Naproxen

Aspirin and clopidogrel are irreversible and etoricoxib is a COX-2 inhibitor.

Further reading: Chapter 182.

Case 26: A patient with severe bruising

1. (c) Acquired haemophilia A

This is clearly an acquired disorder with normal PT and long APTT. Acquired haemophilia is more likely then acquired VWD, which is an alternative diagnosis.

2. (a) Immediate mix 40 sec, incubated mix 62 sec

This shows a time-dependent inhibitor. Pattern (b) is seen with immediately acting inhibitors such as a lupus anticoagulant. Pattern (c) is seen with a simple factor deficiency.

3. (c) XIII

Factor XIII deficiency is associated with bleeding and does not affect the coagulation pathways.

4. (c) VII

VII deficiency gives this pattern.

Further reading: Chapter 183.

Case 27: A patient with easy bruising and heavy periods

1. (c) VIII, IX, XI, VWF

The intrinsic pathway needs to be investigated and von Willebrand's disease (VWD) excluded.

2. (a) Von Willebrand's disease

Note the prolonged APTT. Haemophilia A and B are X-linked.

3. (c) Iron deficiency anaemia

Microcytic and known menorrhagia.

4. (d) Mefenamic acid

Mefenamic acid – an NSAID may increase bleeding.

Further reading: Chapter 183.

8 Oncology: Cases and Questions

Case 1: A patient with back pain, cough and breathlessness

A 57-year-old woman presents with worsening health, back pain, cough and breathlessness. She has no significant past medical history. Her mother developed breast cancer in her 60s. She has right-sided, painless axillary lymphadenopathy, and clinical evidence of a right pleural effusion, but no breast mass. A chest radiograph demonstrates a right pleural effusion and lytic bone metastases.

1. *What is the best initial diagnostic strategy?*
   (a) PET/CT scan
   (b) Thoracocentesis or fine-needle biopsy of a palpable node, and immunohistochemical analysis for oestrogen receptor
   (c) Mediastinoscopy
   (d) Excision of axillary node
   (e) Genotyping for BRCA1 and 2

Case 2: A patient with back pain and weight loss

A 32-year-old man presents with a short history of back pain and weight loss. He is ill and in pain. CT scan reveals bulky para-aortic lymphadenopathy. Alpha fetoprotein (α-FP) and beta human chorionic gonadotrophin (β-HCG) are negative, but lactate dehydrogenase (LDH) is elevated.

1. *What is the best management strategy?*
   (a) Testicular ultrasound
   (b) Laparotomy
   (c) Arrange an urgent CT-guided core biopsy, involve an oncologist
   (d) Hydrate, and give allopurinol prior to chemotherapy
   (e) Radiotherapy to the retroperitoneum

Case 3: A patient with worsening back pain and weight loss

A 67-year-old man presents with worsening back pain and weight loss. He has neglected a worsening 'smoker's cough', and had two episodes of haemostysis. He also complains of thirst, constipation and polyuria. He is dehydrated, and appears anaemic, chronically sick and cachectic. There is thoracic spine tender to percussion without long-tract signs, and clinical evidence of a left pleural effusion. A chest radiograph demonstrated a large left hilar mass, with associated pleural effusion and lytic bone metastases.

1. *What is the best unifying diagnosis?*
   (a) Sarcoidosis
   (b) Metastatic colorectal cancer
   (c) Localized lung cancer
   (d) Non-small-cell lung cancer with bone metastases and hypercalcaemia
   (e) Small-cell lung cancer with Cushing's syndrome from ectopic adrenocorticotrophic hormone (ACTH) production
2. *The patient's metabolic issues are best treated with:*
   (a) Demeclocycline
   (b) Bisphosphonate
   (c) Rehydration and bisphosphonate

   (d) Furosemide and prednisone
   (e) Calcitonin

Case 4: A patient who has requested a prostate-specific antigen (PSA) test

A 50-year-old man wants to alter his lifestyle, starts aspirin, gets a colonoscopy, and requests a PSA test. He has a strong family history of cardiac disease and stroke, is hypertensive and obese.

1. *The decision about whether to order a screening PSA depends on:*
   (a) Digital rectal exam
   (b) Estimated lifespan
   (c) Morbidity of curative procedures (radical prostatectomy or radiotherapy)
   (d) Patient-centred decision making
   (e) All of the above

Case 5: An elderly patient with back pain

An 82-year-old man presents with a worsening back pain and debility. He is in failing health and in pain. He is anaemic with an anaemia of chronic disease and an elevated alkaline phosphatase (ALP). Plain films reveal sclerotic bone metastases.

1. *What would be a diagnostic procedure?*
   (a) PSA
   (b) CT scan
   (c) MRI
   (d) Myelogram
   (e) None of the above

Case 6: A man with prostate cancer

A 67-year-old man was admitted to a hospice the preceding night. He has prostate cancer, and complains of pains in his back and legs. He usually gets up early to walk his dog but has not done it for the past few days, and on the day of admission he seemed a little confused. He complains of a dry mouth and has been drinking more than usual recently. The blood tests on admission show Hb 10.0 g/dL, MCV 85 fL, corrected calcium 2.9 mmol/L and glucose 5.9 mmol/L. A doctor had started him on morphine for his back pain a few days ago.

1. *Which of the following is not an explanation for his dry mouth and thirst?*
   (a) Hypercalcaemia
   (b) Diabetes
   (c) Morphine
2. *What is the most likely cause of his confusion?*
   (a) Hypercalcaemia
   (b) Pain
   (c) Drug side effects
   (d) Infection, such as urine or chest
   (e) Metastatic spread of his prostate cancer to his brain
   (f) Any of the above
3. *The patient is given pamidronate to reduce his hypercalcaemia, and seems to be doing well. Initially, his mobility increases considerably, and he gets up and about. However, on the day he*

is due to be discharged he complains of worsening back pain and difficulty passing urine. On examination he has reduced power and reflexes in his legs. He refuses to get out of bed. What should your management be?

(a) Encourage him to get moving so he does not get a deep venous thrombosis (DVT)
(b) Talk to the family about a nursing home admission
(c) Send a midstream urine (MSU) sample to check for a urinary infection
(d) Send him for an emergency MRI scan of his back

4. *What is the significance of his anaemia?*
(a) He needs a blood transfusion
(b) He should be treated with oral iron
(c) This needs no treatment
(d) He should be advised to eat plenty of red meat

Case 7: A distressed woman with shortness of breath

A 75-year-old widow is admitted on a weekend medical take with much worse shortness of breath than usual, which developed in the last 6 hours. She seems very anxious and distressed. Her husband died 10 years ago of asbestosis and she has been recently diagnosed with mesothelioma. She has chest pains and pain in her right calf, which is swollen some 4 cm more than the left. She is taking ibuprofen and paracetamol for the chest pains, which seems to help a bit.

1. *Which of the following is the most likely cause of her increased shortness of breath?*
(a) Heart failure
(b) Mesothelioma
(c) Pleural effusion
(d) Pulmonary embolus (PE)
(e) Panic attack

2. *You are asked to write up some extra analgesia for her. What would be the best choice?*
(a) Diclofenac
(b) Co-codamol
(c) Mefenamic acid
(d) Morphine

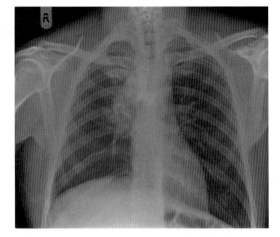

Figure 8.8.1

3. *She is admitted to a hospice some weeks later for terminal care. You are called in the middle of the night to write up some sedation for her as she seems agitated. What should you do?*
(a) Increase the dose of morphine
(b) Start a syringe driver with a benzodiazepine in it
(c) Prescribe haloperidol
(d) Examine her

4. *Which of the following is not an effective treatment for breathlessness in terminal care?*
(a) Oral morphine
(b) Nebulized morphine
(c) Nebulized saline
(d) Benzodiazepines
(e) Blood transfusion for severe anaemia

Case 8: A patient with shortness of breath and swollen face and neck

A 60-year-old man presents to A&E feeling very short of breath. He says that his breathing is worse on lying flat and his family have commented that his face and neck look swollen. Over the last few days his headache has got worse especially when he coughs. He states that the only medical problem he has is a cough which he has attributed to a smoker's cough but he describes haemoptysis is the last month. He does not take any regular medications. On examination he looks plethoric, his face appears swollen and he has dilated veins over his chest wall. His BP is 100/50 mmHg with a pulse rate of 110 beats/min. His oxygen saturations are 92% on room air. Please look at the chest X-ray below (Fig. 8.8.1).

1. *In view of the chest X-ray what major structure in the chest do you think is being compressed to cause this presentation?*
(a) Main bronchus
(b) Superior vena cava (SVC)
(c) Trachea
(d) Aorta

2. *What further investigation would you do to confirm your diagnosis?*
(a) Whole-body bone scan
(b) CT scan of chest
(c) Further chest X-ray
(d) MRI spine

3. *CT scan confirms SVC compression. What treatment would you consider starting immediately in A&E?*
(a) No treatment necessary
(b) Dexamethasone
(c) Heparin
(d) Aspirin

4. *The patient went on to have further treatment. Please look at the X-ray (Fig. 8.8.2); what intervention has he had done?*
(a) Biopsy
(b) Stent insertion
(c) Pneumonectomy
(d) Central venous access

5. *What is the most likely diagnosis?*
(a) Small-cell lung cancer
(b) Lymphoma
(c) Aortic aneurysm
(d) Prostate cancer

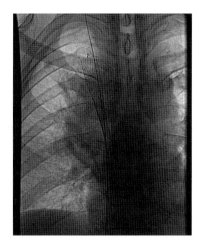

Figure 8.8.2

Case 9: A woman with metastatic breast cancer

A 60-year-old woman has a diagnosis of metastatic breast cancer. You see her in clinic and she tells you that she is feeling more unwell. She describes to you that she feels nauseous, she is constipated and drinking more water that usual. On examination her BP is 110/90 mmHg, pulse 100 beats/min and saturations 99% on room air. She looks clinically dehydrated with reduced skin turgor and dry mucus membranes. Her chest was clear, abdomen was mildly tender but with no rebound or guarding. Blood tests showed:

Na	134 mmol/L
K	4.2 mmol/L
Urea	15 mmol/L
Creatinine	150 μmol/L

1. *What other blood test would you request to explain her symptoms?*
   (a) Autoantibodies
   (b) Serum calcium
   (c) Clotting screen
   (d) Liver function tests
2. *Her calcium comes back at 3.2 mmol/L. What initial treatment do you instigate?*
   (a) Intravenous fluids
   (b) Calcitonin
   (c) Chemotherapy
   (d) Diuretics
3. *She has received 3 L of intravenous fluids; her calcium is still 3.0 mmol/L. What is the next step in your management?*
   (a) Calcitonin
   (b) Measure parathyroid hormone (PTH)
   (c) Intravenous bisphosphonates
   (d) Bone scan
4. *She has a further investigation. Look at the images (Fig. 8.9.1). What type of scan is this?*
   (a) CT scan
   (b) PET scan
   (c) MRI
   (d) Bone scan
5. *Why do you think that this woman has a high calcium?*
   (a) Her tumour secretes calcium
   (b) Hyperparathyroidism

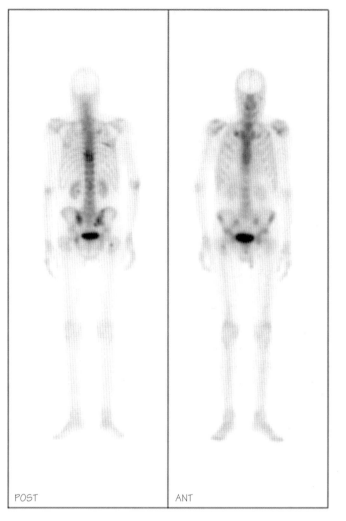

Figure 8.9.1

   (c) Increased osteoclast activity due to bone metastasis
   (d) Increased PTH related peptide released from her tumour

Case 10: A man with prostate cancer

You are asked to see a 60-year-old man with a history of prostate cancer. He is normally fit and active. Over the last few months he has been complaining of back pain that radiates around his chest. Neurological examination reveals spastic legs with brisk reflexes and upgoing planters. Testing sensation showed that he has reduced sensation to light touch to his umbilicus.

1. *What is the likely diagnosis?*
   (a) Cauda equina compression
   (b) Spinal cord compression in the cervical region
   (c) Spinal cord compression in the thoracic spine
   (d) Hypercalcaemia
2. *What initial treatment do you start and which investigation do you organize to confirm your diagnosis?*
   (a) Dexamethasone + organize an urgent CT scan of the spine
   (b) Dexamethasone + bed rest + organize an urgent MRI of the whole spine
   (c) Analgesia + physiotherapy
   (d) Dexamethasone + analgesia and mobilize

3. *His MRI shows a single site of compression at T3. Who would you urgently refer the patient to?*
  (a) Neurosurgeons
  (b) Hospice
  (c) Physiotherapists
  (d) Rehabilitation unit

4. *What is the spinal cord compression likely to be due to?*
  (a) Epidural metastasis
  (b) Intramedullary metastasis
  (c) Posterior extension of vertebral body metastasis
  (d) Paraspinal tumour invasion through intervertebral foramina

Case 11: A woman with advanced ovarian cancer

A 65-year-old woman has advanced ovarian malignancy and all chemotherapy options have been exhausted. Over the past few weeks she has developed abdominal distension and starts vomiting. On examination her pulse is 110 beats/min, BP 100/60 mmHg, respiration rate 22 breaths/min, sats 92% on air. Clinically significant tense ascites is present. She then becomes very uncomfortable and has difficulty breathing. An abdominal X-ray is done which shows no bowel dilatation.

1. *What would you do?*
  (a) Arrange for an ascitic drain to relieve symptoms
  (b) Manage pain with oral opioids and anti-emetics
  (c) Surgical opinion
  (d) Pulmonary embolism is a likely diagnosis and the patient should be anticoagulated

2. *The patient has 8 L of ascitic fluid drained, her breathing improves and vomiting settles. Residual abdominal pain is well controlled on a small dose of opioid. Over the next few days her condition deteriorates and she becomes drowsy but is able to discuss her situation rationally. Biochemistry including serum calcium is normal. There appears to be no reversible cause for her deterioration. What should you do next?*
  (a) The family should be informed that she is likely to die
  (b) Give naloxone, drowsiness is likely to be opioid induced
  (c) An open discussion should take place with the patient about her deterioration
  (d) Sepsis is the most likely diagnosis

3. *The woman understands that she is in the terminal phase of her illness and has asked to be kept as comfortable as possible. Currently her symptoms are well controlled. The following should be considered*
  (a) Review DNAR/CPR (do not attempt resuscitation/ cardiopulmonary resuscitation) status
  (b) If not drinking start intravenous fluids
  (c) Increase dose of opioids
  (d) Ensure that oral morphine and anti-emetics are prescribed

4. *Her condition has deteriorated and she is clearly in the last 24 hours of her illness. She is unconscious but her ascites has once again occurred and her breathing appears noisy. What is the most appropriate?*
  (a) Further ascitic tap
  (b) Opioids, antisecretory and sedatives prescribed subcutaneously

---

  (c) Chest X-ray
  (d) Ensure the nursing staff use suction as initial intervention

Case 12: A man with cancer and constant back pain

A 64-year-old man with a diagnosis of prostate cancer has known bony metastasis which have been recently investigated with an MRI and bone scan. His main problem is of back pain. He currently takes regular paracetamol, diclofenac and codeine. You have decided to commence oral morphine for his pain control. His family is concerned as they have heard that morphine is dangerous.

1. *Which one of the following statements about morphine is true?*
  (a) If morphine is titrated against the patient's pain, clinically significant respiratory depression is uncommon
  (b) Morphine hastens death
  (c) Morphine is always addictive
  (d) Morphine has significant sedatative and hallucinogenic effects

2. *He starts on oral morphine. What side effects do you anticipate?*
  (a) Drowsiness often occurs, progresses and often leads to hallucinations
  (b) Drowsiness can occur, but is mild and wears off on a stable dose after approximately 10 days
  (c) Always co-prescribe an anti-emetic when starting morphine
  (d) Laxatives are needed in 50% of cases

3. *His disease progresses and his prostate specific antigen (PSA) is rising. He develops pain in his mid-right femur that does not respond to an increasing dose of morphine. His pain is increased on weight bearing and he is therefore immobile. Which of the following is true?*
  (a) Since an opioid is most likely to help his pain, the morphine should be further increased
  (b) There is no need for further investigations in view of the progressive disease
  (c) Pain in a long bone on mobility suggests bony deposit and needs to be X-rayed
  (d) The most likely diagnosis is cord compression

4. *X-ray demonstrates a lytic lesion mid-femur with cortical erosion. What would be the optimal way forward in this situation?*
  (a) Due to the patient's advancing disease no further active intervention is indicated
  (b) Radiotherapy is the modality of choice
  (c) Add in anti-inflammatory drugs to the existing regime and mobilize
  (d) Refer to orthopaedics despite advancing disease

Case 13: A man with painless haematuria

A 42-year-old man presents with painless haematuria. He visits his GP who refers him to a urologist. Cystoscopy confirms bladder carcinoma.

1. *What factor is not likely to be the cause of his cancer?*
  (a) Smoking
  (b) Working in clothing factory

(c) Previous history of living in Africa

(d) High alcohol intake

2. *Which organism is associated with chronic bladder infection and the development of bladder cancer?*

   (a) *Schistosoma haematobium*

   (b) Human papilloma virus (HPV)

   (c) Hepatitis C

   (d) Epstein–Barr virus

3. *Which drug is known to be associated with haemorrhagic cystitis and an increased risk of bladder cancer?*

   (a) Aspirin

   (b) Ciclosporin

   (c) Mycophenolate

   (d) Cyclophosphamide

4. *The patient's father has recently been diagnosed with gastric cancer. He is keen to know if there is anything that has caused the cancer. Which of the following factors is NOT associated with the development of gastric cancer?*

   (a) Blood group A

   (b) *Helicobacter pylori* infection

   (c) Previous gastric surgery

   (d) Alcohol

Case 14: A woman with a familial history of cancer

A 32-year-old woman visits her GP as she is anxious about her family history. Her mother died at age 50 from breast cancer and was diagnosed at age 45. Her maternal aunt has ovarian cancer which was diagnosed last year aged 48. Her sister has recently had surgery for a breast lump.

1. *A mutation in which gene is likely to cause this familial cancer syndrome?*

   (a) BRCA1

   (b) FAP

   (c) p53

   (d) c-myc

2. *What is the mechanism underlying carcinogenesis for this gene?*

   (a) Tumour suppressor gene

   (b) Oncogene

   (c) Gene that regulates apoptosis

   (d) Gene that regulates DNA repair

3. *Three months later she presents with metastatic disease. Which of the following factors is unlikely to have contributed to metastasis from the primary site?*

   (a) Invasion of local lymphatic channels

   (b) Raised vascular endothelium growth factor (VEGF) level causing an increase in angiogenesis

   (c) Raised VEGF causing a host immune response

   (d) Increased expression of telomerase

Oncology: Answers

Case 1: A patient with back pain, cough and breathlessness
1. (b) Thoracocentesis or fine-needle biopsy of a palpable node, and immunohistochemical analysis for oestrogen receptor

Oestrogen receptor-positive metastatic breast cancer often presents with bone, pleural, and nodal metastases compared with oestrogen receptor-negative tumours that more commonly have visceral metastases (liver, lung, brain). Mediastinoscopy is only used to confirm operability of potentially curable lung cancer. Excision nodal biopsy is only needed to evaluate the architecture of lymphoma.

Further reading: Chapter 187 in Medicine at a Glance.

Case 2: A patient with back pain and weight loss
1. (c) Arrange an urgent CT-guided core biopsy, involve an oncologist

Although seminoma is associated with an elevated LDH, the diagnosis is much more likely high-grade non-Hodgkin's lymphoma, or Burkitt's lymphoma. While urgent treatment may be life threatening, a tissue diagnosis is essential before deciding on a definitive treatment plan.

Further reading: Chapter 187.

Case 3: A patient with worsening back pain and weight loss
1. (d) Non-small-cell lung cancer with bone metastases and hypercalcaemia

Lung and breast cancer are the commonest causes of malignancy-related hypercalcaemia.

2. (c) Rehydration and bisphosphonate

Tumour-induced hypercalcaemia cases significant dehydration because of a poor oral intake, osmotic diuresis, and calcium-induced diabetes insipidus. After correcting volume depletion bisphosphonates reverse the osteoclast-driven loss of calcium from the skeleton.

Further reading: Chapters 116 and 157.

Case 4: A patient who has requested a prostate-specific antigen (PSA) test
1. (e) All of the above

Screening remains controversial with no proven survival advantage for early intervention in what is often an incurable disease, with considerable morbidity from surgery and radiotherapy, competing co-morbidities, and poorly defined subsets who may be cured with acceptable toxicity.

Further reading: Chapter 188.

Case 5: An elderly patient with back pain
1. (c) MRI

The combination of an elevated PSA and sclerotic bone metastases is pathognomonic for metastatic prostatic cancer.

Further reading: Chapter 190.

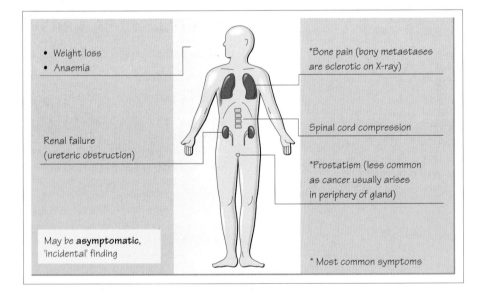

Figure 8.5.1 Features of prostate cancer.

Case 6: A man with prostate cancer
1. (b) Diabetes

Hypercalcaemia causes dry mouth and thirst, as can morphine. Though uncontrolled diabetes certainly causes dehydration, and so may cause a dry mouth, the finding of a normal blood glucose in him excludes this diagnosis.

2. (d) Infection, such as urine or chest

Any of these things can cause confusion, and all need to be addressed. However, in practical terms, brain secondaries with prostate cancer are so rare as to almost be discounted. Confusion with hypercalcaemia relates mainly to the absolute level, though the rate of increase is also relevant. Corrected calcium levels

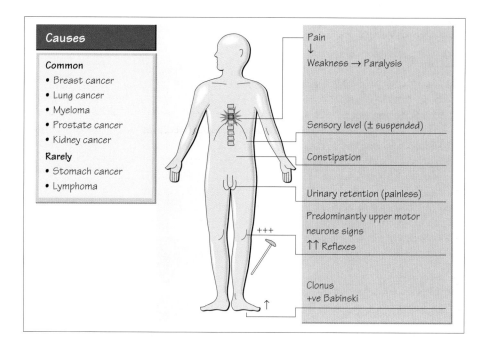

Figure 8.6.1 Causes and consequences of spinal cord compression.

below 3 mmol/L are rarely associated with significant confusion, unless they are rising rapidly, or are associated with a number of other factors that also promote confusion. Many drugs can have confusion as a side effect, particularly the opiates and other painkillers. Relatively minor infections in the elderly, especially if there are other illnesses, such as cancer, can provoke surprisingly major confusion; accordingly, unless there are very clear-cut causes of confusion, chest and urine infection should be looked for.

3. (d) Send him for an emergency MRI scan of his back

This is the clinical picture of spinal cord compression. Although a UTI could cause acute retention, as could prostate disease, it would not explain the neurological signs in his legs. Whether an MRI scan is appropriate depends on his wishes and the stage of his cancer; it may be that this is a pre-terminal event, in which case empathy and palliation are appropriate. Equally, given his relatively good pre-hospice condition ('walking the dog regularly') it may well be that immediate diagnosis and treatment (likely to be neurosurgical decompression) will lead to a long period of good quality life. If one is proceeding down such a treatment line, a realistic discussion needs to be had with the patient and family, and *immediate* MRI scan *must* be performed; while waiting the 60 or so minutes this should take in a modern hospital, it would be appropriate to inform the local neurosurgical/back surgeon that an immediate spinal cord decompression is likely to be required within the next 3 hours.

4. (c) This needs no treatment

This needs no treatment. It is unlikely an iron deficient picture as most such anaemias have an MCV below 80 fL; it would be prudent to send off haematinics (iron, TIBC and ferritin, along with vitamin B_{12} and folate) to confirm this. A haemoglobin level above 10 g/dL does not require a blood transfusion, as it is not low enough to cause any symptoms.

Further reading: Chapter 190.

Case 7: A distressed woman with shortness of breath

1. (d) Pulmonary embolus (PE)

She has signs suggestive of a deep vein thrombosis and the short history of increased breathlessness suggests a PE. However, be aware that this is only the leading diagnosis, not the only possible one. Heart failure is common in the elderly, and may relate to a myocardial infarction (MI), which could cause breathlessness with chest pain (a chest X-ray and ECG are necessary). Her mesothelioma is unlikely to have progressed so rapidly to cause such an increase in breathlessness over a few days, but again the chest X-ray will clarify this, and also help assess the presence and size of a pleural effusion. In taking forward the diagnosis of a PE, be aware that D-dimers will be useless in this situation (malignancy commonly causes them to be raised), and likewise a ventilation–perfusion nuclear scan will be inaccurate (substantial pleural disease); it is likely that the best investigation is a CT pulmonary angiogram.

2. (d) Morphine

She is already taking an NSAID and paracetamol, so diclofenac, mefenamic acid and co-codamol are not suitable. An opiate such as morphine will also help with her subjective feeling of dyspnoea and ease her anxiety.

3. (d) Examine her

There are many reasons she could be agitated – she needs a proper assessment to look for reversible causes such as constipation, pain or infection before changing her treatments.

4. (b) Nebulized morphine

Nebulized morphine is not effective. All the other treatments may help in some circumstances.

Further reading: Chapter 19.

Case 8: A patient with shortness of breath and swollen face and neck

1. (b) Superior vena cava (SVC)

This is a typical presentation of SVC compression; this is an oncological emergency and requires urgent investigations.

2. (b) CT scan of chest

He requires a CT scan of his chest to see whether the SVC is compressed, the extent of the disease and whether intervention would be possible.

3. (b) Dexamethasone

He should be commenced on dexamethasone. He will require further investigations in order to gain a histological diagnosis and guide further treatment. He should also be discussed with the interventional radiologists to see if a stent is possible.

4. (b) Stent insertion

The X-ray shows a superior vena caval stent *in situ*.

5. (a) Small-cell lung cancer

The most likely diagnosis in this case is small-cell lung cancer. Lung cancer accounts for about 70% of the causes for SVC obstruction. The patient is a smoker and gives a history of haemoptysis, making lung cancer the most likely diagnosis.

Further reading: Chapter 54.

Case 9: A woman with metastatic breast cancer

1. (b) Serum calcium

Hypercalcaemia would explain her symptoms of nausea, constipation and polydipsia.

2. (a) Intravenous fluids

The initial treatment for high calcium would be rehydration with intravenous fluids.

3. (c) Intravenous bisphosphonates

Intravenous bisphosphonates are the next step in the management to lower calcium.

4. (d) Bone scan

This is a bone scan, which is a radionuclear scan. The dark spots on the scan or 'hot spots' highlight increased bone activity.

5. (c) Increased osteoclast activity due to bone metastasis

Bony metastases are the most likely cause for hypercalcaemia in metastatic breast cancer.

Further reading: Chapter 157.

Case 10: A man with prostate cancer

1. (c) Spinal cord compression in the thoracic spine

Clinical examination suggests cord compression at the level of the thoracic spine.

2. (b) Dexamethasone + bed rest + organize an urgent MRI of the whole spine

The best investigation for imaging the spine if you suspect cord compression is an MRI scan. The patient should be commenced on high-dose steroids as these may improve symptoms and outcome. He should be kept on best rest as his spine may be unstable and at risk of further damage.

3. (a) Neurosurgeons

His images should be discussed with the neurosurgeons, he is generally fit and his scans show a single site of compression, therefore he may be a candidate for spinal surgery. If he is not felt to be suitable for surgery he should proceed to have radiotherapy.

4. (c) Posterior extension of vertebral body metastasis

The spinal cord and its nerve roots are most commonly compressed anteriorly by posterior extension of haematogenously spread metastasis in the vertebral body, extending into the epidural.

Further reading: Chapter 54.

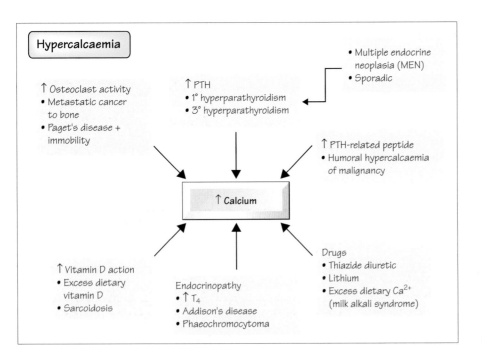

Figure 8.9.2 Features of hypercalcaemia.

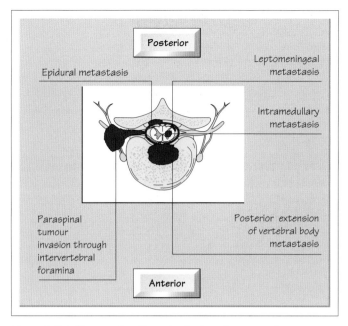

Figure 8.10.1 Causes of malignant spinal cord compression.

Case 11: A woman with advanced ovarian cancer

1. (a) Arrange for an ascitic drain to relieve symptoms

The cause of the patient's symptoms is tense ascites, this is splinting her diaphragm and causing shortness of breath. The abdominal X-ray does not show any dilated bowel loops, making bowel obstruction unlikely. To relieve her symptoms she requires an ascitic drain.

2. (c) An open discussion should take place with the patient about her deterioration

An open discussion should take place with the patient first about her deterioration. Once consent has been gained to talk to the family they can also be involved. The patient has a right to know all the information that she wants about her condition.

3. (a) Review DNAR/CPR (do not attempt resuscitation/cardiopulmonary resuscitation) status

This patient is in the terminal phase of her illness, and the priority is symptom management. All unnecessary and potentially distressing treatments should be discontinued. Her resuscitation status should be reviewed as a priority. Intravenous fluids in this situation are therefore not appropriate. Her symptoms need to be managed and the route of administration of her medication should be appropriate. She has previously been vomiting and is therefore unlikely to absorb oral medications. These should be prescribed subcutaneously.]

4. (b) Opioids, antisecretory and sedatives prescribed subcutaneously

The aim of management at this stage is to keep the patient comfortable. A further ascitic drain is likely to be distressing and is not appropriate. All medication should be prescribed subcutaneously and an antisecretory drug (e.g. anticholinergic) should be administered for noisy breathing secondary to secretions.

Further reading: Chapter 193.

Case 12: A man with cancer and constant back pain

1. (a) If morphine is titrated against the patient's pain, clinically significant respiratory depression is uncommon

Professional and lay fears about the use of opioids have always been a barrier to their effective use. Pain appears to be a physiological antagonist of the depressant effects of opioids on respiration and therefore clinically significant respiratory depression does not occur. Addiction in the sense of 'psychological dependence and craving' does not occur. Morphine is often not started until the patient is virtually moribund, hence the erroneous assumption that morphine hastens death, because these two events are coincident rather than causative. In the past morphine was often prescribed in the form of a cocktail. As the dose of morphine was titrated upwards, the toxic effects of the other drugs emerged – sedation and hallucinations. Hence, the common misconception that morphine has significant sedative and hallucinogenic properties.

2. (b) Drowsiness can occur, but is mild and wears off on a stable dose after approximately 10 days

Laxatives should always be co-prescribed; anti-emetics are not always necessary. Drowsiness tends to wear off after 7–10 days.

3. (c) Pain in a long bone on mobility suggests bony deposit and needs to be X-rayed

His pain is not responding to increasing morphine doses. His leg needs to be X-rayed to look for bony deposits.

4. (d) Refer to orthopaedics despite advancing disease

If the patient has a prognosis of greater than 6 weeks, then orthopaedic referral is appropriate. If significant cortical erosion is seen the risk of fracture is high, this would render the patient immobile with pain that is difficult to control. If stabilization by the othopaedic surgeons is not possible then radiotherapy should be considered.

Further reading: Chapter 134.

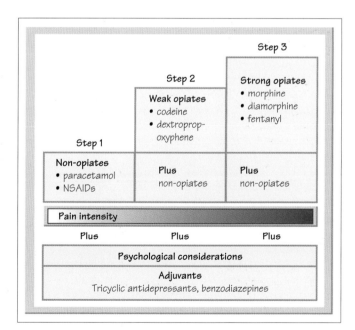

Figure 8.12.1 The analgesic ladder.

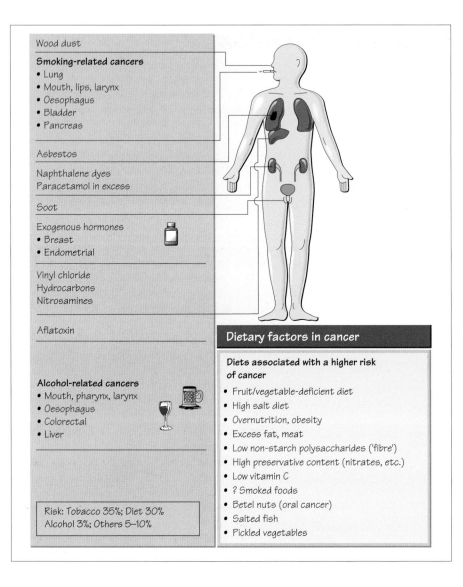

Wood dust

Smoking-related cancers
• Lung
• Mouth, lips, larynx
• Oesophagus
• Bladder
• Pancreas

Asbestos

Naphthalene dyes
Paracetamol in excess

Soot

Exogenous hormones
• Breast
• Endometrial

Vinyl chloride
Hydrocarbons
Nitrosamines

Aflatoxin

Alcohol-related cancers
• Mouth, pharynx, larynx
• Oesophagus
• Colorectal
• Liver

Risk: Tobacco 35%; Diet 30%
Alcohol 3%; Others 5–10%

Dietary factors in cancer

Diets associated with a higher risk of cancer
• Fruit/vegetable-deficient diet
• High salt diet
• Overnutrition, obesity
• Excess fat, meat
• Low non-starch polysaccharides ('fibre')
• High preservative content (nitrates, etc.)
• Low vitamin C
• ? Smoked foods
• Betel nuts (oral cancer)
• Salted fish
• Pickled vegetables

Figure 8.13.1 Chemical factors in carcinogenesis.

Case 13: A man with painless haematuria

1. (b) Working in clothing factory

The relationship between occupational exposure and bladder cancer was first described in 1800. Most bladder carcinogens are aromatic amines. Exposure to chemicals used in the aluminium, dye, paints, petroleum, rubber and textile industries are estimated to account for 20% of bladder cancers. Many studies have demonstrated that smoking accounts for a 2–3-fold increase in bladder cancer (heavy smokers have a 6–10-fold increase). Parasitic infection endemic in certain parts of the world (Africa, Middle East, south-east Asia) causes chronic bladder infection and increased bladder cancer (see Question 2). A link with alcohol has currently not been established.

2. (a) *Schistosoma haematobium*

Infection with *S. haematobium* (also known as bilharzial bladder disease) has been linked to hyperplasia, metaplasia, dysplasia and overt carcinoma of the bladder. In endemic regions, bladder cancer is the most common solid tumour.

3. (d) Cyclophosphamide

The cyclophosphamide metabolite acrolein is a recognized urinary toxin and is responsible for haemorrhagic cystitis and an increased risk of bladder cancer. The uroprotectant mesna inactivates urinary acrolein, concomitant use of mesna and cyclcophosphamide can lower the subsequent risk of developing bladder cancer.

4. (d) Alcohol

A consistent association between alcohol consumption and the risk of gastric cancer has not been demonstrated.
Further reading: Chapter 186.

Case 14: A woman with a familial history of cancer

1. (a) BRCA1

5–6% of all breast cancers are associated with an inherited gene mutation. BRCA1 and BRCA2 are thought to account for the majority of inherited breast cancers.

2. (d) Gene that regulates DNA repair

BRCA1 and 2 genes function as an essential part of the normal mechanisms that repair double-stranded DNA breaks.

3. (c) Raised VEGF causing a host immune response

There is currently no evidence to suggest that a host immune response contributes to the development of metastatic breast cancer.
Further reading: Chapter 186.

9 Neurology: Cases and Questions

Case 1: An elderly patient who has had a fall in the night

A 73-year-old woman presents to A&E because of a fall leading to a scalp laceration that requires suturing. The history is that she fell in the dark while getting up in the night to pass water. The astute attending doctor notices that she is unsteady and walks with a high stepping gait. On examination Romberg's test is positive and she has increased tone in the lower limbs.

1. *The most likely neuroanatomical basis for her problem is:*
   (a) The frontal lobes
   (b) The peripheral nerves
   (c) The spinal cord
   (d) The cerebellum

Case 2: A patient with speech disturbance and difficulty walking

A 54-year-old builder gives a history of 6 months of progressive speech disturbance and difficulty walking.

1. *Which of the following is in favour of a cerebellar cause for his problem?*
   (a) Swallowing disturbance
   (b) A positive Romberg's test
   (c) Extensor plantar responses
   (d) Abnormal saccadic eye movements
2. *Which of the following symptoms is unlikely to arise from lesions of the brainstem?*
   (a) Deafness
   (b) Dysarthria
   (c) Diplopia
   (d) Dysphasia
3. *Hemiplegia may be caused by lesions in:*
   (a) Cerebellum
   (b) Internal capsule
   (c) Conus medullaris
   (d) Thalamus

Case 3: A patient with double vision

A 40-year-old teacher complains of double vision over a 10-day period. On examination he has partial ptosis of the right eye and bilateral failure of eye abduction. The left eye also fails to adduct but this is variable.

1. *What is the most likely explanation for these findings?*
   (a) A brainstem stroke
   (b) A paraneoplastic syndrome
   (c) Multiple sclerosis
   (d) Myasthenia gravis

Case 4: A young woman with facial pain

A young woman is referred with an episode of facial pain which has the features of trigeminal neuralgia. Her GP has started her on carbamazepine. During the examination you note that she has significant bilateral gaze-evoked nystagmus but does not seem to be aware of any visual disturbance.

1. *What is the most likely cause of the nystagmus?*
   (a) Viral infection of the inner ear
   (b) Demyelinating disease
   (c) Congenital nystagmus
   (d) Drugs used to treat facial pain

Case 5: A patient with loss of leg control

A 55-year-old lorry driver notices that during a long journey he is having difficulty with the foot controls on his vehicle. At a convenient moment he stops and gets out of his cab and immediately his legs give way. He is aware of a sharp ache in the back. On admission to hospital he is found to have a flaccid paralysis of the legs, absent tendon reflexes and loss of sensation to the lower abdomen. However, joint position sense and vibration sense are preserved.

1. *What is the anatomical explanation for the preservation of joint position and vibration senses?*
   (a) These are characteristically preserved in Guillain–Barré syndrome, which is the most likely diagnosis given the absent reflexes and flaccid paralysis
   (b) The dorsal columns are usually spared in transverse myelitis, which, given the back pain, is the most likely diagnosis
   (c) The dorsal columns have a different blood supply to the anterior part of the spinal cord
   (d) A prolapsed intervertebral disc often spares the dorsal columns

Case 6: A patient with weakness of the hands and arms

A 36-year-old pianist notices that his hands feel odd and describes it 'as if they are wrapped up in bandages'. Ten days earlier he had felt unwell with symptoms suggestive of an upper respiratory tract infection and this had resolved within 3 days. Within 2–3 days the odd feeling in his hands subsides but he notices that he has difficulty rising from an armchair after watching TV all evening. The next morning he feels very 'shaky on his feet' and visits his GP who admits him to hospital. Within 24 hours after admission he can no longer walk and is noticed to have weakness of the upper limbs and weakness of eye closure.

1. *The anatomical basis of this problem is most likely to be:*
   (a) In the spinal cord
   (b) In the brainstem in the region of the pons
   (c) The neuromuscular junction
   (d) The peripheral nerves

Case 7: A patient suffering from dizziness

A 54-year-old man with a history of poorly controlled diabetes and hypertension goes to his GP complaining that he awoke that morning with severe dizziness. He has vomited several times and is only comfortable if he keeps his head completely still. There are few physical signs except nystagmus on looking to either side. The GP diagnoses 'acute viral labyrinthitis'. Two days later the patient complains of double vision and slurred speech and is sent to hospital for investigation. While waiting to be admitted by the acute medical team the patient suddenly collapses, lapses into a coma and displays an irregular breathing pattern with periods of apnoea. He is intubated and ventilated. Examination without sedation or muscle relaxants shows a complete flaccid tetraparesis.

1. *Where is the lesion?*
   (a) The basilar artery
   (b) The middle cerebral artery
   (c) The cerebellum
   (d) The basal ganglia

Case 8: A patient with acute-onset shoulder pain

A 45-year-old builder presents with acute onset pain in the right shoulder 5 days after an inoculation against yellow fever. There is nothing to find on examination and he is treated with analgesics. The pain subsides over a couple of weeks. Four weeks later he becomes aware that he is having difficulty using a screwdriver and that some of the muscles in his right hand appear to have thinned.

1. *What is the investigation of choice here?*
   (a) CT scan of the brain
   (b) Nerve conduction studies and electromyography (EMG)
   (c) MRI of the spinal cord
   (d) Lumbar puncture

Case 9: A patient with weakness and wasting of the hand

A 60-year-old man presents with progressive weakness and wasting of his right hand over a 6-month period. On examination he has a diminished biceps reflex but a positive Hoffman's sign (flexion of the terminal phalanx of the thumb in response to tapping the fingers). There is marked wasting of the first dorsal interosseous muscle. Although he has no leg symptoms the tone is mildly increased and the plantars are extensor.

1. *Which of the following statements are correct?*
   (a) The combination of upper and lower motor neuron signs in the arm is pathognomonic of motor neuron disease (MND)
   (b) An MRI of the cervical spine is mandatory to exclude compressive myeloradiculopathy
   (c) The most likely explanation for this combination of symptoms and signs is multiple sclerosis
   (d) Extensor plantars are a normal finding over the age of 60

Case 10: A patient with double vision

A 63-year-old man with a history of angina pectoris is admitted to hospital with double vision in all directions and pain looking to the right. On examination he has an almost complete right ptosis.

1. *The most likely explanation for his double vision is:*
   (a) A brainstem stroke affecting the voluntary gaze centres
   (b) A sixth nerve palsy
   (c) An internuclear ophthalmoplegia
   (d) A third nerve palsy

2. *The most likely diagnosis is:*
   (a) Myasthenia gravis
   (b) Multiple sclerosis
   (c) A posterior communicating artery aneurysm
   (d) An ischaemic (microvascular) third nerve palsy

3. *Monocular visual loss can arise due to lesions of:*

(a) The optic nerve
(b) The optic radiation
(c) The optic chiasm
(d) The visual cortex

4. *In a sixth nerve palsy:*
   (a) Objects are separated in an oblique plane
   (b) There is partial ptosis
   (c) The pupil is normal
   (d) There is monocular diplopia

Case 11: A patient with a worsening tremor

An elderly patient is referred with a tentative diagnosis of Parkinson's disease (PD) because of a progressively worsening tremor.

1. *Which of the following features make the diagnosis of PD less likely?*
   (a) Tremor involving the leg
   (b) Tremor that worsens with anxiety
   (c) A history of isolated tremor for over a year without the development of any other features of PD
   (d) Tremor of the head

2. *Essential tremor:*
   (a) Always responds to alcohol
   (b) Is often familial
   (c) Is never disabling
   (d) Is associated with a higher risk of subsequently developing PD

Case 12: A patient with possible depression

You are asked to see a bus driver to consider whether he has developed a major depression. There is a history of increasingly erratic behaviour at work including several incidents of 'road rage' in which passenger safety was at risk. Things came to a head when he turned up for work smelling of alcohol and was suspended. There have been several 'life events' in the preceding year including separation from his wife and the death of his mother from dementia, for which she had been in a long-term nursing home for 5 years. You notice that his gait is slightly erratic and he is very fidgety throughout the consultation. He does indeed score highly on the Beck depression inventory and is drinking excessively, though there is no evidence that he is intoxicated at the time of the consultation.

1. *What is the most likely diagnosis of his mother's dementia?*
   (a) Alzheimer's disease
   (b) Cortical Lewy body disease
   (c) Huntington's disease
   (d) Alcoholic brain disease

Case 13: A pregnant patient with a stiff neck

You are called to see a 24-year-old woman on the obstetric ward who has been admitted with hyperemesis gravidarum in the first trimester. Shortly after admission she complains that she has a stiff neck and on examination her eyes are held fixed in upgaze.

1. *What is the most likely diagnosis?*
   (a) An occulogyric crisis
   (b) Meningitis

(c) A cerebral haemorrhage

(d) Hysteria

Case 14: A patient who has had an episode of altered awareness

A 70-year-old man, who is a life-long smoker, presents with an episode of altered awareness. He describes 'feeling peculiar' while watching TV and then next remembers his wife standing over him asking him if he is OK. His wife reports that she noticed that he became slightly pale, his head turned to the left and his right arm jerked for about 10–20 seconds. He was vague and disorientated for the next couple of hours.

1. *What is the appropriate course of action?*
   (a) An MRI or CT brain should be performed within a week
   (b) Urgent carotid Doppler studies
   (c) Start anticonvulsants and review in 3 months with an EEG
   (d) Aspirin

Case 15: A patient with possible epilepsy

A 22-year-old woman is referred for investigation of possible epilepsy. There have been three episodes in total in which she has collapsed, on each occasion in a night club. She is able to remember feeling 'spaced out' and as if she is 'not there', she has a warm tingling feeling around her mouth. She next remembers a crowd of people around her and being helped to the ground and outside to get some fresh air which makes her feel better.

1. *The following features of this case are consistent with a diagnosis of primary generalized epilepsy:*
   (a) The nightclub location
   (b) The prodrome of a feeling of dissociation
   (c) Her age
   (d) Sensory symptoms in the face

Case 16: A patient with right hemiplegia

A 64-year-old man presents 1 hour after the sudden onset of right hemiplegia.

1. *The following are contraindications to thrombolysis:*
   (a) Atrial fibrillation
   (b) Rapidly improving symptoms before institution of therapy
   (c) Diabetes
   (d) Two ischaemic lesions on imaging

Case 17: A patient with a thunderclap headache

A 48-year-old woman presents 3 hours after a thunderclap headache. She is drowsy but there are no focal neurological signs. A CT scan of the brain is normal.

1. *Which of the following are true?*
   (a) A normal CT in a drowsy patient rules out subarachnoid haemorrhage (SAH)
   (b) Given the high probability of SAH in this case it is best to proceed straight to angiography
   (c) A lumbar puncture (LP) should be delayed until approximately 12 hours as xanthochromia takes some time to form
   (d) An LP should be performed immediately

Case 18: A man with sudden-onset left-sided paralysis

A 75-year-old man presents with a sudden-onset left-sided paralysis, diagnosed as being due to a middle cerebral artery infarct. His blood pressure is 180/100 mmHg.

1. *Concerning the management of his blood pressure after acute stroke, which of the following is true?*
   (a) Systolic blood pressure (BP) should be maintained below 140 mmHg in the first few days
   (b) In the secondary prevention of stroke patients with carotid stenosis of greater than 70% should only be treated with antihypertensives if the systolic BP is greater than 160 mmHg
   (c) Acute reduction of BP may expand the area of infarction
   (d) After tissue plasminogen activator (tPA) BP should be lowered if it rises above 210 mmHg

2. *Although he had an infarct, if he had had a spontaneous intracerebral haemorrhage (ICH), which of the following would be true:*
   (a) Has the highest mortality of any kind of cerebrovascular accident
   (b) Most survivors have a good outcome
   (c) Is always associated with headache
   (d) Can be distinguished from cerebral infarction using MRI in the first 12 hours

3. *The risk of subarachnoid haemorrhage (SAH) is increased in:*
   (a) Smokers
   (b) Patients with diabetes
   (c) Those taking regular vigorous exercise
   (d) Males

Case 19: A patient who has collapsed after an occipital headache

A 46-year-old woman collapses soon after a sudden occipital headache. A CT scan on admission to hospital shows subarachnoid blood and she is commenced on nimodipine.

1. *Over the next 2 weeks what is the most life-threatening complication?*
   (a) Hydrocephalus
   (b) Re-bleeding
   (c) Cerebral vasospasm
   (d) Cerebral oedema

2. *Which of the following statements about chronic subdural haematoma is correct?*
   (a) Most patients are taking warfarin
   (b) 80% give a history of antecedant trauma
   (c) Seizures are common
   (d) Focal neurological signs may be absent

3. *Which is the commonest presentation of cerebral venous thrombosis?*
   (a) Subacute encephalopathy
   (b) Idiopathic intracranial hypertension
   (c) Isolated seizures
   (d) Thunderclap headache

Case 20: An elderly patient with a decline in mobility

A 78-year-old man goes into decline after the death of his wife. He is noticed to be generally slowing down and when visiting his daughter was found wandering at night and reported that his brother, who had died 10 years previously, was present in the room with him. During the day he was lucid but there was an obvious decline in his general mobility.

1. *An MRI scan in this patient is likely to show:*
   (a) Frontal and temporal atrophy
   (b) Diffuse ischaemia
   (c) Generalized atrophy with sparing of the hippocampus
   (d) A lesion in the occipital cortex

Case 21: A patient with memory difficulties

A 51-year-old senior solicitor consults a neurologist because he is concerned about his memory. He frequently forgets the names of his junior colleagues and becomes flustered in meetings. His mother died of Alzheimer's disease at the unusually young age of 55 years. On examination there are no physical abnormalities and the mini mental state examination (MMSE) score is 28/30. The patient was highly anxious during the consultation.

1. *What is the most appropriate course of action?*
   (a) Reassure the patient that, since he is clearly functioning well in his job and self-referred, he is most likely suffering from understandable anxiety but that there is no need for further investigation
   (b) Send DNA for analysis of the presenilin-1 and presenilin-2 genes
   (c) Perform an MRI scan
   (d) Ask for formal neuropsychological testing and review in 6 months

Case 22: A patient with rapidly progressive unsteadiness

A 70-year-old woman presents with rapidly progressive unsteadiness and cognitive change such that she goes from normal independence to needing help with dressing in 6 weeks. On examination she has ataxia and brief low-amplitude jerks of her hands. An MRI scan of the brain is said to be normal for her age. Two weeks later she is unable to walk and her speech has reduced to single words.

1. *What is the most useful next investigation?*
   (a) Visual evoked potentials
   (b) EEG
   (c) Lumbar puncture
   (d) Brain biopsy

Case 23: A young woman having grand mal seizures

A 24-year-old woman is brought by ambulance to the A&E department with repeated grand mal seizures; she is not known to have a seizure disorder, and a letter to her boyfriend is found on her, detailing an unhappy end to the relationship and her wish to end her life. After several further seizures, she then starts to fit continuously.

1. *Which of the following drugs in overdose can cause status epilepticus?*
   (a) Aspirin
   (b) Paracetamol
   (c) Amitriptiline
   (d) Heroin

Case 24: A patient with blurred vision in one eye

A young woman presents with painless blurring of vision in her left eye over a week. Examination shows mild swelling of the optic disc and her colour vision is reduced. An MRI scan of the brain is normal.

1. *What is her percentage risk of developing multiple sclerosis (MS)?*
   (a) 50%
   (b) 80%
   (c) 25%
   (d) 100%

Case 25: A patient with unsteadiness following childbirth

A 30-year-old woman of white European origin, with a history of optic neuritis 3 years previously presents with unsteadiness and sensory loss over her trunk one month after giving birth to her first child. She is naturally concerned having read that MS is 'partly genetic' to know if her baby daughter is at risk of developing the disease in later life.

1. *The life-time risk of the child being affected is approximately:*
   (a) 1 in 1000
   (b) 5 in 1000
   (c) 50 in 1000
   (d) 30%

2. *Corticosteroids in MS:*
   (a) Are associated with a high risk of psychiatric complications if given to patients with cognitive involvement
   (b) Decrease the chance of disability at 5 years
   (c) Are a useful adjunctive treatment for secondary progressive disease
   (d) Should always be given intravenously

3. *Which of the following best describes a typical MS relapse?*
   (a) Of acute onset, evolving over hours and improving within 1–2 weeks
   (b) Of insidious onset over weeks to months
   (c) Developing over a few days to a few weeks, reaching a plateau for several weeks and showing recovery over months
   (d) Episodes of paroxysmal symptoms lasting several minutes, increase in frequency, build up and coalesce into a consistent pattern over a few days

Case 26: A patient with weight loss, low-grade fever and headache

A 35-year-old man born in southern Africa but living in Europe for the past 5 years presents with weight loss, low-grade fever, headache and confusion over a 2-week period. An MRI scan of the brain shows dilated ventricles and some enhancement of the basal meninges. A CSF examination shows lymphocytes 80 cells/μL and a raised protein.

1. *The most likely diagnosis is:*
   (a) HIV encephalopathy
   (b) Schistosomiasis
   (c) Tuberculous (TB) meningitis
   (d) Sarcoidosis

Case 27: A patient with drowsiness and confusion

A 50-year-old accountant presents to the emergency department with a 2-day history of drowsiness and confusion. His wife said he went to bed with a headache and has been sleepy ever since. On examination there are no focal signs and no neck stiffness but the patient is febrile. A CT scan is initially reported as normal but a lumbar puncture shows lymphocytes 50 cells/μL.

1. *The diagnosis of herpes simplex encephalitis is established by:*
   (a) Response to aciclovir
   (b) Polymerase chain reaction (PCR)
   (c) EEG
   (d) Viral culture

Case 28: A patient with weight loss, anorexia and fatigue

A 53-year-old farmer presents with a month's history of weight loss, anorexia and fatigue. He is admitted with acute back pain and urinary retention. His ESR is 90 mm/hour.

1. *What unusual organism could explain his symptoms?*
   (a) Listeria
   (b) Legionella
   (c) Brucella
   (d) Herpes zoster

Case 29: A patient with new-onset daily headache

A 50-year-old woman presents with new-onset daily headache over a 3-week period. It is only minimally responsive to simple analgesia. She also complains of neck stiffness. A CT scan of the brain is normal. Her ESR is elevated at 60 mm/hour. A temporal artery biopsy is normal.

1. *The appropriate course of action is:*
   (a) An MRI scan
   (b) Start steroids
   (c) A lumbar puncture
   (d) Prescribe amitriptiline

2. *Gliomas, primary brain tumours arising from glial cells, are:*
   (a) Decreasing in frequency
   (b) Caused in some patients by excessive mobile phone use
   (c) Easily resectable
   (d) Almost never inherited

Case 30: A patient with gait ataxia

A 65-year-old woman with a history of breast cancer treated with local excision and radiotherapy 3 years previously presents with gait ataxia developing over a week. A CT scan shows a solitary lesion with the appearance of a metastasis in the midline of the cerebellum (vermis). A search for evidence of disseminated malignancy (mammogram, chest X-ray, bone scan, etc.) is negative.

1. *Which of the following best describes the appropriate management?*
   (a) Any form of cerebral involvement with breast cancer carries a grave prognosis and the patient should be offered palliative care
   (b) The lesion should be excised followed by radiotherapy
   (c) A period of surveillance with serial MRI scans will allow planning of further treatment
   (d) Intrathecal chemotherapy is the only treatment which has been shown to be effective in this situation

2. *Tumours of the cerebellopontine angle cause:*
   (a) Diplopia
   (b) Wasting of the tongue
   (c) Facial weakness
   (d) Loss of sense of smell

Case 31: A patient who cannot move his legs after an operation

A 48-year-old man undergoes a coronary artery bypass graft procedure. Twenty-four hours post-operatively concerns are raised when he complains he cannot move his legs. On examination he has a symmetrical flaccid paralysis and is areflexic. He has impaired light touch and pinprick below the upper abdomen. Examination of vibration and joint position sense in the feet is normal.

1. *What is the most likely explanation for this man's paralysis?*
   (a) A reaction to epidural analgesia
   (b) Disc prolapse
   (c) Dissection of the thoracic aorta
   (d) Thrombosis of the anterior spinal artery

Case 32: A patient who has unsteady gait after a hip replacement

A 60-year-old woman undergoes a hip replacement under general anaesthetic. During the recovery phase as she is mobilizing she undergoes a deterioration in her gait and complains that her feet, and to a lesser extent her hands, feel 'numb'. On examination she has a bilateral spastic paraparesis with extensor plantars and absent ankle jerks. Proprioception is markedly impaired in the feet and fingers.

1. *What is the likely explanation for these neurological findings?*
   (a) Damage to the spinal cord during surgery
   (b) A complication of halothane anaesthesia
   (c) Neurosyphilis
   (d) Malignant spinal cord compression

Case 33: A patient with gait disturbance and back pain

A 76-year-old man presented with a 3-day history of progressive gait disturbance, back pain and urinary hesitancy. On examination he has increased tone in the lower limbs and bilateral but asymmetrical weakness. His bladder was palpable and he had 800 mL of urine drained on catheterization.

1. *The most appropriate investigation of this problem is:*
   (a) Plain spinal X-ray
   (b) Lumbar puncture
   (c) Urgent MRI of the spine
   (d) Myelogram

Case 34: A patient with diminishing walking distance

A 65-year-old man gives a 6-month history of progressively diminishing walking distance. He describes the build-up of low back pain after about 200 m with numbness of the groin. Symptoms also occur on prolonged standing and are relieved by lying down or bending forward. Neurological examination of the lower limbs is normal.

1. *What is the most likely diagnosis?*

(a) Intermittent claudication due to atheroma of the iliac arteries

(b) Lumbar spinal stenosis

(c) Spinal arteriovenous malformation

(d) Spinal arachnoiditis

Case 35: A patient with double vision

A 55-year-old man presents with a 2-day episode of double vision which occurs 3 days into a episode of flu-like viral symptoms. By the time he is seen in outpatients the double vision has resolved but he feels generally 'run down' and tired. There is nothing to find on examination except mild ptosis of the left eye.

1. *Which of the following statements is true?*

(a) A negative anti-ACh receptor antibody test excludes myasthenia gravis in this patient

(b) Ocular myasthenia patients are more likely to be antibody negative

(c) A tensilon test should be performed to see if the ptosis improves

(d) The condition is likely to be a reaction to a virus

2. *Which of the following conditions typically causes proximal muscle weakness?*

(a) Tuberculosis (TB)

(b) Schizophrenic psychosis

(c) Grave's disease

(d) Hypercholesterolaemia

3. *Which of the following occur as extra-motor manifestations of motor neurone disease (amyotrophic lateral sclerosis)?*

(a) Dementia

(b) Bladder weakness

(c) Loss of proprioception

(d) Loss of visual acuity

4. *Which of the following does not occur in mitochondrial myopathies?*

(a) Diabetes mellitus

(b) Deafness

(c) Retinitis pigmentosa

(d) Motor neuron degeneration

Case 36: A patient with a progressive decline in mobility

A 70-year-old woman is who is normally fit and walks several kilometres per day presents with a progressive decline in mobility over a 3-month period such that her walking distance is limited to 100 metres. She describes that her feet feel 'odd, as if wrapped in bandages' and at night she is kept awake by cramps and general discomfort. On examination there is distal weakness in the lower limbs (ankle dorsiflexion MRC3/5), loss of vibration sense to the pelvis and reduced light touch to the knees. The motor conduction velocity in the lower limbs is reduced at 25 m/sec (normal 45–70 m/sec)

1. *Which of the following statements is correct?*

(a) The most likely cause is diabetes mellitus

(b) Investigation will reveal an underlying malignancy in most patients presenting in this way at this age

(c) The patient should be treated with intravenous immunoglobulin

(d) A peripheral nerve biopsy is required before starting treatment

Case 37: A patient whose leg 'gives way'

A 48-year-old woman presents to her GP with a 2-day history of her right leg 'giving way'. Three months earlier she had been diagnosed with Dukes B colon carcinoma and underwent a hemicolectomy. The postoperative recovery had been complicated by a deep venous thrombosis and she had been warfarinized. On examination she has isolated weakness of knee extension, an absent right knee jerk and was slightly tender on deep abdominal palpation.

1. *Which nerve(s) is involved?*

(a) Obturator

(b) Lumbosacral plexus

(c) L2,3 roots

(d) Femoral

Case 38: A patient with suspected Parkinson's disease

A 70-year-old patient has been diagnosed with Parkinson's disease (PD) by his GP but is referred because he has not responded to L-dopa after 6 months and seems to be getting worse.

1. *Which of the following features would make you question the diagnosis of PD?*

(a) Poor sleep pattern

(b) Restless legs syndrome

(c) Absence of tremor

(d) Early falls

Case 39: A patient with obsessive compulsive disorder and a tremor

A 19-year-old university student fails her first year exams despite having a strong academic record at high school. Over the preceding year she has developed features of obsessive compulsive disorder (OCD) with frequent hand washing and other ritualistic behaviours. She is referred to a neurologist when she is noticed to have a tremor. On examination she has evidence of dystonia around the mouth (intermittent lip curling and snarling and mild drooling of saliva).

1. *What is the most likely diagnosis?*

(a) Wilson's disease

(b) Juvenile-onset Parkinson's disease due to a mutation in the parkin gene

(c) Tourette's syndrome

(d) Huntington's disease

Case 40: A patient with abnormal movements

A 69-year-old man presents with a 2-year history of abnormal movements. Initially he was thought to be 'fidgety' but the movements evolved into frank chorea. In other ways he was functioning normally and there was no evidence of cognitive decline. MRI scanning of the brain does not show significant evidence of atrophy more than would be expected for the patient's age.

1. *What is the most likely diagnosis?*

(a) Senile chorea

(b) Thyrotoxicosis

(c) Huntington's disease (HD)

(d) Antiphospholipid syndrome

2. *Which of the following is a feature of Parkinson's disease (PD)?*

(a) Paralysis of the extraocular muscles
(b) A 20% chance of developing dementia by 10 years
(c) Peripheral neuropathy
(d) Increased risk in smokers

Case 41: A patient with a poorly localized headache

A 67-year-old woman, who has not previously been a headache sufferer, presents with a 4-week history of poorly localized headache. She had been sleeping poorly of late and admitted to feeling low in mood, with generally reduced energy levels and loss of appetite. Physical examination was normal. Her GP treated her with amitriptiline. Two weeks later her headache was slightly worse and she presented to A&E with sudden painless loss of vision in her left eye.

1. *The most appropriate initial investigation is:*

(a) An MRI brain scan
(b) Erythrocyte sedimentation rate (ESR)
(c) Carotid Doppler

Case 42: A patient with increasing headache

A 23-year-old woman complained of increasing headache over a 3-month period. When she bends over or coughs she 'sees stars'. On examination she was overweight but appeared well. Examination of the eyes reveals bilateral swelling of the optic discs and an enlarged blind spot. A non-contrast enhanced CT scan of the brain is reported as normal.

1. *The normal CT scan rules out the following:*

(a) Raised intracranial pressure
(b) Sagittal vein thrombosis
(c) Obstructive hydrocephalus

Neurology: Answers

Case 1: An elderly patient who has had a fall in the night

1. (c) The spinal cord

Proprioceptive loss (Romberg's sign, loss of balance in the dark) could be due to a peripheral neuropathy or a disease of the dorsal columns of the spinal cord. The presence of increased tone in the lower limbs, however, suggests that the spinal cord is the site of disease here. The patient also had extensor plantar responses and the diagnosis was vitamin B_{12} deficiency.

Further reading: Chapter 58 in Medicine at a Glance.

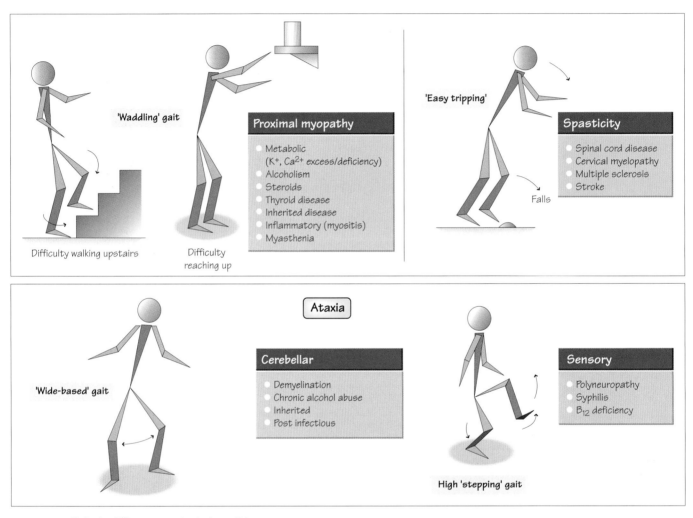

Figure 9.1.1 Gaits in different neurological conditions.

Case 2: A patient with speech disturbance and difficulty walking

1. (d) Abnormal saccadic eye movements

Romberg's test is normal in cerebellar disease. In addition to nystagmus, eye movements in cerebellar disease are characterized by broken saccades with overshoot on lateral gaze. Swallowing dysfunction is only a late feature of cerebellar disease.

2. (d) Dysphasia

Language disorders are cortical in origin and should be distinguished from dysarthria which is commonly a brainstem or cerebellar symptom.

3. (b) Internal capsule

The posterior limb of the internal capsule carries corticospinal tract fibres and lesions lead to mild–moderate hemiplegia with predominant spasticity.

Further reading: Chapter 59.

Case 3: A patient with double vision

1. (d) Myasthenia gravis

The combination of ptosis and variable bilateral weakness of the extraocular muscle suggests that the muscles are the site of pathology. It would be very unusual to have bilateral sixth nerve palsies and a third nerve palsy (which in any case often causes very marked rather than partial ptosis).

Further reading: Chapter 60.

Case 4: A young woman with facial pain

1. (b) Demyelinating disease

Trigeminal neuralgia in young people raises the suspicion of multiple sclerosis, especially if bilateral. It is characteristic of MS that previous 'silent' episodes of demyelination go unnoticed by the patient but leave physical signs. Many patients with central nystagmus (usually cerebellar) have relatively few symptoms.

Further reading: Chapter 63.

Case 5: A patient with loss of leg control

1. (c) The dorsal columns have a different blood supply to the anterior part of the spinal cord

The rapid evolution, interscapular pain and sparing of the dorsal columns are highly suggestive of anterior spinal artery thrombosis. This initially causes a flaccid paralysis with reduced reflexes ('spinal shock') but will evolve in most cases to a severe spastic paraplegia with sphincter involvement.

Further reading: Chapter 202.

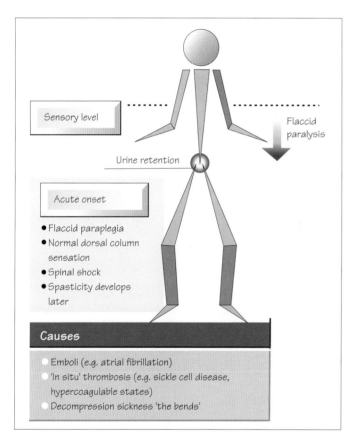

Figure 9.5.1 Clinical features of anterior spinal artery thrombosis.

Case 6: A patient with weakness of the hands and arms

1. (d) The peripheral nerves

The history is typical of Guillain–Barré syndrome, an inflammatory para-infectious peripheral neuropathy with a predilection for affecting nerve roots. The symmetry and the mixture of sensory and motor features should suggest a neuropathy.

Further reading: Chapter 204.

Case 7: A patient suffering from dizziness

1. (a) The basilar artery

The combination of disequilibrium, double vision and nystagmus suggest a brainstem lesion. Basilar artery thrombosis causes catastrophic decline into coma because of the brainstem respiratory and arousal centres are affected.

Further reading: Chapter 194.

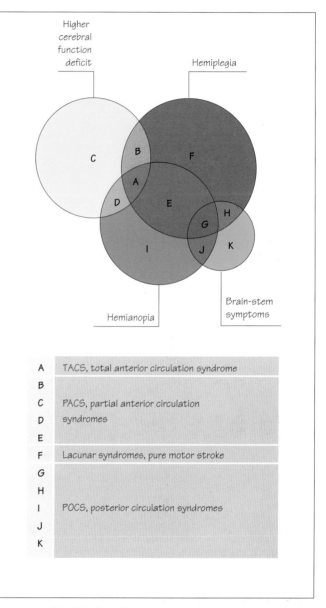

Figure 9.7.1 Classification of stroke.

Case 8: A patient with acute-onset shoulder pain

1. (b) Nerve conduction studies and electromyography (EMG)

The history suggests brachial neuritis, an idiopathic inflammatory plexopathy. The only recognized precipitant is vaccination. The resolution of the pain here makes a structural lesion (such as malignant infiltration) unlikely, so an MRI is unlikely to be informative.

Further reading: Chapter 204.

Case 9: A patient with weakness and wasting of the hand

1. (b) An MRI of the cervical spine is mandatory to exclude compressive myeloradiculopathy

Although the diagnosis in this case was MND, an MRI of the cervical spine is mandatory to rule out a compressive cause, spondylotic myelopradiculopathy, which can occasionally present as a pure motor syndrome.

Further reading: Chapters 202 and 203.

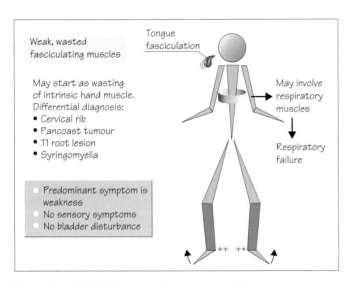

Figure 9.9.1 Clinical features of motor neuron disease.

Labels in figure:
- Weak, wasted fasciculating muscles
- Tongue fasciculation
- May start as wasting of intrinsic hand muscle. Differential diagnosis:
  • Cervical rib
  • Pancoast tumour
  • T1 root lesion
  • Syringomyelia
- May involve respiratory muscles
- Respiratory failure
- • Predominant symptom is weakness
  • No sensory symptoms
  • No bladder disturbance

Case 10: A patient with double vision

1. (d) A third nerve palsy

The signs are very suggestive of a third nerve palsy; if the pupil was dilated and unreactive to light, this would suggest external compression of the nerve, for example, due to an aneurysm of the posterior communicating artery, a 'surgical' third nerve lesion. Further examination reveals that the right pupil reacts normally to light: these are the signs of a 'medical' third nerve palsy.

2. (d) An ischaemic (microvascular) third nerve palsy

As explained above, a third nerve palsy results in most of the affected eyes external ocular muscles being paralysed, the eyeball then is deviated in the direction of the remaining active (tonic) muscles. The major remaining active muscle is the lateral rectus, innervated by cranial nerve VI, pulling the eye laterally. The parasympathetic nerves, which constrict the eye, surround the nerve, and are very vulnerable to external compression. Most external compressive lesions require surgery; hence a third nerve palsy with papillary dilatation is referred to as a 'surgical' third nerve lesion, whereas other causes, such as microvascular damage due to diabetes, are referred to as 'medical' third nerve palsies.

3. (c) The optic chiasm

Monocular visual loss arises anterior to the optic chiasm.

4. (a) Objects are separated in an oblique plane

A sixth nerve palsy results in horizontal separation of the images at a distance, worse on looking to the affected side, with a normal pupil.

Further reading: Chapter 60.

Case 11: A patient with a worsening tremor

1. (d) Tremor of the head

Tremor of the head is not a feature of PD, but does occur in essential tremor and cerebellar disease. All tremors are worse when people are anxious.

2. (b) Is often familial

Essential tremor, although it may appear mild to the observer, can often be socially and even physically disabling for patients. A family history is present in over half of patients. Alcohol responsiveness is not universal.

Further reading: Chapter 62.

Case 12: A patient with possible depression

1. (c) Huntington's disease

The family history and features on examination suggest that this patient has Huntington's disease (HD). HD is associated with considerable social and familial disruption and it is not uncommon for the diagnosis to be concealed within a family and for a label of dementia or 'Alzheimer's disease' to be used.

Further reading: Chapter 197.

Case 13: A pregnant patient with a stiff neck

1. (a) An occulogyric crisis

She has been treated with a dopamine antagonist anti-emetic (e.g. prochlorperzine or metoclopramide). Occulogyric crisis is a rare and idiosyncratic reaction to anti-dopaminergic drugs and is self-limiting but can be treated acutely with procyclidine.

Further reading: Chapter 231.

Case 14: A patient who has had an episode of altered awareness

1. (a) An MRI or CT brain should be performed within a week

Although this apparent seizure may be due to cerebrovascular disease it is very important to exclude a primary or secondary (metastatic) brain tumour.

Further reading: Chapter 64.

Case 15: A patient with possible epilepsy

1. (c) Her age

The most likely diagnosis is this case is hyperventilation, although it would be prudent to perform an EEG. Although it seems plausible that strobe lighting in a nightclub could provoke seizures, this is relatively rare and seizures are also likely to occur outside of this setting. Sleep deprivation is a good trigger for generalized epilepsy and so there is often a history of events occurring the day after late nights out. The clear history of dissociation and facial tingling is typical of hyperventilation attacks which often occur in a stressful social situation.

Further reading: Chapter 64.

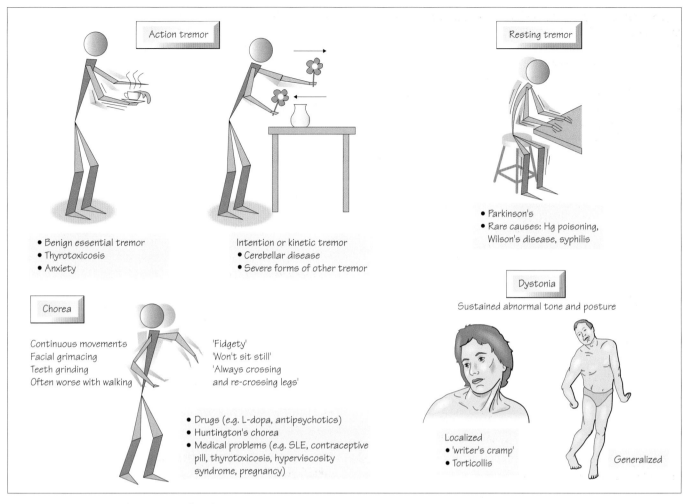

Figure 9.11.1 Tremor and movement disorders.

Case 16: A patient with right hemiplegia

1. (b) Rapidly improving symptoms before institution of therapy

A rapidly improving picture suggests that the presentation may be a prolonged transient ischaemic attack (TIA) and thrombolysis is best avoided. Hypoglycaemia (<2.2) or severe hyperglycaemia are contraindications but not diabetes in itself.

Further reading: Chapter 194.

Case 17: A patient with a thunderclap headache

1. (c) A lumbar puncture (LP) should be delayed until approximately 12 hours as xanthochromia takes some time to form

Current guidelines are that an LP should be delayed until 12 hours after onset in CT-negative thunderclap headache as evidence suggests that bilirubin will be undetectable in the initial few hours. There is no indication for proceeding to angiography without an LP in most cases, though the increasing availability of high-resolution spiral CT angiography means that most patients in specialist units may have a form of angiography as part of their initial investigation.

Further reading: Chapter 196.

Case 18: A man with sudden-onset left-sided paralysis

1. (c) Acute reduction of BP may expand the area of infarction

The management of BP after stroke is a controversial area and the evidence base for most situations is lacking. However, it is clear that too rapid reduction in BP can be harmful and that raised systemic arterial BP is a normal response to maintain cerebral perfusion pressure. Because of collateral circulation it is not clear that patients with major arterial stenosis should be managed differently to others, though critical stenosis with ongoing symptoms in the relevant territory would prompt caution about BP treatment.

2. (a) Has the highest mortality of any kind of cerebrovascular accident

Thirty-day mortality for primary ICH approaches 50%, and only 20% of survivors achieve meaningful functional recovery at 6 months. Headache is a pointer to ICH but can also occur in ischaemic lesions. MRI cannot reliably diagnose haemorrhage in the first 24 hours after onset.

3. (a) Smokers

Good unbiased population-based evidence for the risk factors for SAH is lacking. Smoking (relative risk 1.9), hypertension (relative risk 2.8) and female gender (relative risk 1.6) are consistent associations. A small proportion of SAH occurs in people with specific genetic syndromes including polycystic kidney disease and Ehlers–Danlos. Although the actual rupture leading to SAH may occur in a few patients immediately after physical exertion there is no evidence that this contributes to the overall risk of developing an aneurysm and SAH. A family history of two first-degree relatives with SAH is associated with a relative risk of 4.

Further reading: Chapters 194 and 196.

Case 19: A patient who has collapsed after an occipital headache

1. (b) Re-bleeding

Re-bleeding occurs in 20–30% of patients in the first 2 weeks and carries a high fatality rate. The other complications are manageable and increase the chance of disability rather than death.

2. (d) Focal neurological signs may be absent

About 50% recall a head injury and this may have been very mild and of uncertain relevance. Anticoagulation clearly raises the risk but is responsible for a minority of cases. Seizures can occur but are rare.

3. (a) Subacute encephalopathy

A subacute and generalized encephalopathy with drowsiness, headache, raised intracranial pressure and seizures is the classical and commonest presentation.

Further reading: Chapter 196.

Case 20: An elderly patient with a decline in mobility

1. (c) Generalized atrophy with sparing of the hippocampus

This patient fulfils the diagnostic criteria for dementia with Lewy bodies (DLB). Typical features include Parkinsonism, fluctuating cognition, well formed visual hallucinations and syncopal attacks. Memory is relatively preserved early which can help distinguish this condition from Alzheimer's disease.

Further reading: Chapter 197.

Case 21: A patient with memory difficulties

1. (d) Ask for formal neuropsychological testing and review in 6 months

Most patients who ask to be referred because of memory problems are 'worried well'. At first sight a solicitor who is apparently functioning well at work would seem unlikely to have dementia. However, the family history raises the possibility of an autosomal dominant form of Alzheimer's disease. Early in dementia insight is preserved. Both to get some baseline data in case of further progression and to offer some advice and possibly reassurance if things are normal, formal neuropsychological testing with a further review are indicated. This would be more important than ordering a scan, which although it might also allow some baseline assessment, will not be interpretable in the absence of objective evidence of cognitive decline.

Further reading: Chapter 197.

Case 22: A patient with rapidly progressive unsteadiness

1. (b) EEG

The very rapid decline in this patient and the association of ataxia, cognitive change and myoclonus is characteristic of

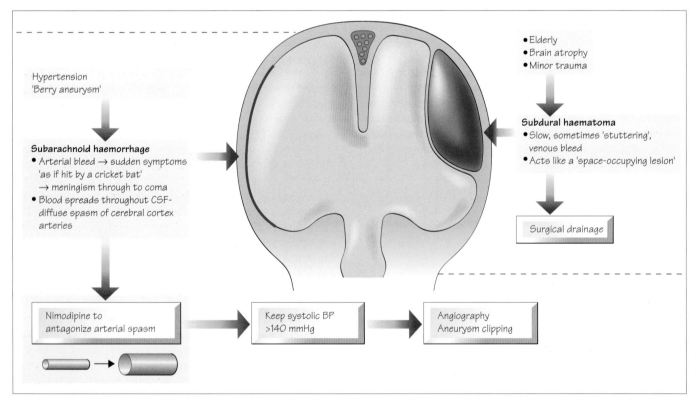

Figure 9.19.1 Unusual causes of intracranial bleeding.

Creutzfeldt–Jakob disease. An EEG showing periodic triphasic sharp wave complexes would make the diagnosis almost certain. If this is not diagnostic a CSF examination (looking for raised 14-3-3 protein) is indicated. Brain biopsy is occasionally performed but as a last resort as the associated infection control measures are onerous.

Further reading: Chapter 197.

Case 23: A young woman having grand mal seizures

1. (c) Amitriptiline

Although the end stage of any severe intoxication with multi-organ failure could be resistant seizure activity, initial presentation with status epilepticus is a recognized feature of overdose with tricyclic antidepressants.

Further reading: Chapter 198.

Case 24: A patient with blurred vision in one eye

1. (c) 25%

The cumulative probability for developing MS after a first episode of optic neuritis is 50%, with the risk highest in the first 5 years. If the MRI is normal at baseline, the risk of MS is 25% at 15 years, and much lower for males and those with atypical presentations of optic neuritis. A single lesion doubles the 15-year risk to 50%. The risk associated with three or more lesions is approximately 80%.

Further reading: Chapter 199.

Case 25: A patient with unsteadiness following childbirth

1. (c) 50 in 1000

Although the exact figure will vary according to the genetic heritage of the mother (there is a north–south European gradient of descending risk), the risk overall is about 1 in 20 for a female with an affected first-degree relative.

2. (a) Are associated with a high risk of psychiatric complications if given to patients with cognitive involvement

Patients with advanced disease are unlikely to benefit from steroid treatment and apparent 'relapses' are often due to intercurrent infections, especially of the bladder. If cognition is affected there is a high risk of inducing confusion, mood changes or even frank psychosis and corticosteroids should be avoided.

3. (c) Developing over a few days to a few weeks, reaching a plateau for several weeks and showing recovery over months

MS relapses can take many forms, but a typical pattern is for the episode to last several months in total with a build up of symptoms over about a week.

Further reading: Chapter 199.

Case 26: A patient with weight loss, low-grade fever and headache

1. (c) Tuberculous (TB) meningitis

This is a typical presentation of TB meningitis, but cerebral TB can also present with a mass lesion (tuberculoma). Establishing the diagnosis can be difficult and treatment should be started while awaiting cultures if acid-fast bacilli cannot be identified from cerebrospinal fluid (CSF).

Further reading: Chapter 200.

Case 27: A patient with drowisness and confusion

1. (b) Polymerase chain reaction (PCR)

PCR is a sensitive (90%) and highly specific (100%) test. The EEG changes are not always classically that of repetitive complexes in the temporal lobes.

Further reading: Chapter 200.

Case 28: A patient with weight loss, anorexia and fatigue

1. (c) Brucella

The history of sub-acute fever and systemic upset in a farmer has a wide differential. The neurological presentation suggests spinal epidural abscess. Brucella is a Gram-negative coccobacilus and occurs in people in close contact with infected cows and sheep. Spinal epidural abscess is a characteristic presentation of neurological brucellosis.

Further reading: Chapter 165.

Case 29: A patient with new-onset daily headache

1. (c) A lumbar puncture

This patient's symptoms (relentless headache with mild–moderate neck stiffness) associated with normal imaging and a raised ESR suggest the possibility of malignant meningitis. Serial lumbar punctures (×3) should be performed, taking 10–20 mL on each occasion which should be sent for cytology. It is often difficult to find tumour cells but there is usually a reactive lymphocytosis. In parallel a search for a primary tumour (chest X-ray, CT abdomen, breast examination and tumour markers) should be carried out.

2. (c) Easily resectable

Primary brain tumours account for about 10% of all deaths from malignancy and the incidence is increasing, though the reason for this is unclear. Resection is very difficult and, although 'debulking' is sometimes carried to relieve pressure, the mainstay of treatment is radiotherapy. In the absence of well-recognized inherited disorders like neurofibromatosis and tuberous sclerosis, gliomas are not typically due to a single gene disorder and the overwhelming majority are sporadic.

Further reading: Chapter 201.

Case 30: A patient with gait ataxia

1. (b) The lesion should be excised followed by radiotherapy

Evidence shows that combined surgery and radiotherapy of a solitary cerebral metastasis can be successful in giving patients like this a good quality of life, even for several years, even though the chance of recurrence and dissemination are high in the long term. The location of this tumour in the posterior fossa is another indication for surgery as it is very likely to cause raised intracranial pressure and coning.

2. (c) Facial weakness

The space between the pons, cerebellum and petrous temporal ridge is traversed by the fifth, seventh and eighth cranial nerves. The usual initial symptom is progressive unilateral deafness and tinnitus which progressed to facial weakness and numbness (fifth nerve, loss of corneal reflex). Common causes are vestibular schwanoma, metastasis or meningioma.

Further reading: Chapter 201.

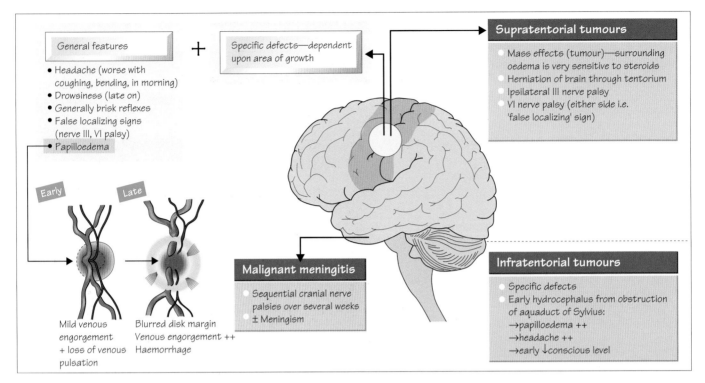

General features

+ Specific defects—dependent upon area of growth

- Headache (worse with coughing, bending, in morning)
- Drowsiness (late on)
- Generally brisk reflexes
- False localizing signs (nerve III, VI palsy)
- Papilloedema

Early   Late

Mild venous engorgement + loss of venous pulsation

Blurred disk margin Venous engorgement ++ Haemorrhage

Supratentorial tumours
- Mass effects (tumour)—surrounding oedema is very sensitive to steroids
- Herniation of brain through tentorium
- Ipsilateral III nerve palsy
- VI nerve palsy (either side i.e. 'false localizing' sign)

Malignant meningitis
- Sequential cranial nerve palsies over several weeks
- ± Meningism

Infratentorial tumours
- Specific defects
- Early hydrocephalus from obstruction of aquaduct of Sylvius:
  →papilloedema ++
  →headache ++
  →early ↓conscious level

Figure 9.30.1 Intracranial neoplasia.

Case 31: A patient who cannot move his legs after an operation

1. (d) Thrombosis of the anterior spinal artery

Spinal artery thrombosis can occur as a complication of thoracic surgery when an embolus travels from the aorta.

Further reading: Chapter 202.

Case 32: A patient who has unsteady gait after a hip replacement

1. (b) A complication of halothane anaesthesia

This patient has sub-acute combined degeneration and her vitamin B_{12} level was found to be low. It is recognized that halothane anaesthesia can precipitate neurological damage when there is occult B_{12} deficiency.

Further reading: Chapter 202.

Case 33: A patient with gait disturbance and back pain

1. (c) Urgent MRI of the spine

The most likely cause of acute cord compression in this age group is malignancy, in this case prostate. Any chance of halting neurological decline requires urgent anatomical diagnosis by MRI and palliative radiotherapy.

Further reading: Chapter 202.

Case 34: A patient with diminishing walking distance

1. (b) Lumbar spinal stenosis

The history is highly suggestive of lumbar spinal stenosis. The combination of congenitally narrow canal and lumbosacral spondylosis which leads to claudication of the cauda equina. Loss of

reflexes in the lower limb are often absent but can sometimes be observed after exercise.

Further reading: Chapter 202.

Case 35: A patient with double vision

1. (b) Ocular myasthenia patients are more likely to be antibody negative

About 10% of patients with myasthenia are negative for the conventional anti-AchR antibody test. This rises to about 40% of patients with isolated ocular myasthenia. A tensilon test is technically difficult to interpret and if the only physical sign is mild ptosis is unlikely to be helpful. Although there are some post-viral syndromes which lead to double vision through a neuropathy (Miller Fisher variant of Guillain–Barré syndrome), in this case the myasthenic symptoms have been precipitated but not directly caused by a viral infection.

2. (c) Grave's disease

Thyroxicosis is frequently associated with a proximal myopathy. Schizophrenia can involve catatonia in which muscles are rigid, CK rises but there is no weakness. Hypercholesterolaemia is occasionally indirectly associated with a myopathy when statins are used in treatment. Myopathy is not a neurological feature of TB.

3. (a) Dementia

About 3–4% develop frank fronto-temporal dementia and about 40% have evidence of loss of executive function on formal psychometric testing. Bladder weakness is not a feature of motor neuron disease (MND) though occasionally patients develop frequency and urgency due to bladder stiffness. Peripheral sensory nerve and dorsal column function is not involved in MND. The intrinsic eye muscles are not affected by MND and therefore visual acuity is normal.

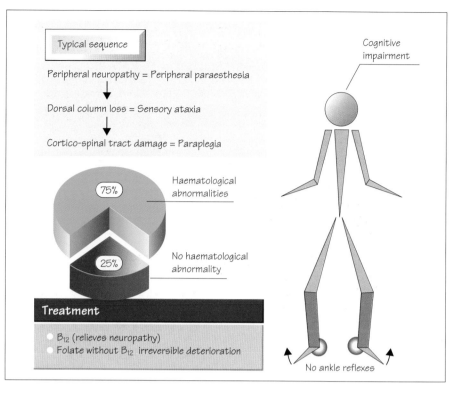

Figure 9.32.1 Clinical features of spinal cord damage due to vitamin B$_{12}$ deficiency.

Syndrome	Clinical features
MELAS syndrome (Mitochondrial encephalomyopathy lactic acidosis and stroke-like episodes)	Seizures Episodes of unconsciousness with lactic acidosis Stroke-like episodes
PEO (Progressive external ophthalmoplegia)	Ptosis, external ophthalmoplegia, limb myopathy Kearns–Sayre syndrome variant; develops age ⩾ 20 years, + pigmentary retinopathy, ataxia and heart block
MERRF (Myoclonic epilepsy with ragged red fibres)	Myoclonic epilepsy Cerebellar ataxia Myopathy
NARP (Neuropathy, ataxia and retinitis pigmentosa)	Proximal muscle weakness, sensory neuropathy, retinal pigmentary degeneration, developmental delay; dementia Ataxia, seizures
LHON (Lebers hereditary optic neuropathy)	Painless subacute visual loss Scotomas Abnormal colour vision
Others, including aminoglycoside induced deafness (AID), maternally inherited Leigh's syndrome (MILS), Pearson's syndrome (PS)	Variable, usually suggested by the title; cardiomyopathy and deafness common in AID, sideroblastic anaemia and pancreatic failure in PS

Figure 9.35.1 Mitochondrial diseases (prevalence is 10–15 per 100 000, i.e. about 6000–9000 in the UK).

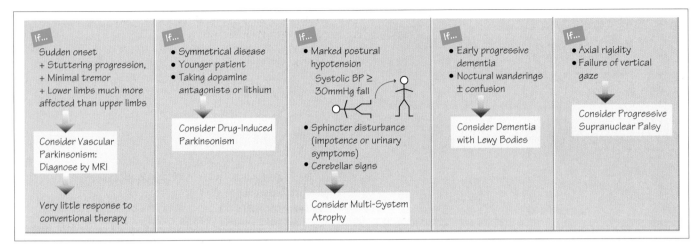

Figure 9.38.1 The different Parkinsonian syndromes.

4. (d) Motor neuron degeneration

Mitochondrial myopathies are complex disorders with a poor genotype phenotype correlation. Diabetes, pigmentary retinopathy, short stature, stroke-like episodes, seizures and deafness are common features. For some reason, motor neuron degeneration does not occur in these diseases, despite the fact that mitochondrial failure is implicated in the pathogenesis of amyostrophic lateral sclerosis.

Further reading: Chapter 203.

Case 36: A patient with a progressive decline in mobility

1. (c) The patient should be treated with intravenous immunoglobulin

The diagnosis is chronic inflammatory demyelinating neuropathy (CIDP) which responds to IVIG (intravenous immunoglobulin) and steroids. This presentation in unlikely to be due to newly diagnosed diabetes as the degree of motor weakness is usually modest in that condition which is dominated by sensory symptoms. Paraneoplastic neuropathy is usually axonal rather than demyelinating. The combination of reduced conduction velocity and sub-acute sensorimotor symptoms is enough to make the diagnosis of CIDP, though a lumbar puncture may also be performed in some cases.

Further reading: Chapter 204.

Case 37: A patient whose leg 'gives way'

1. (d) Femoral

This is a femoral nerve palsy because there is isolated weakness of knee extension (quadriceps) and loss of the knee jerk. It is unlikely to be due to a root lesion as this would have to involve L2,3,4 and other muscle groups would be affected (e.g. internal rotation at the hip). The femoral nerve travels in the psoas muscle. This patient had a spontaneous psoas haematoma as a complication of anticoagulation. The differential includes malignant infiltration from a recurrence of the colon carcinoma, though this would usually cause significant pain.

Further reading: Chapter 56.

Case 38: A patient with suspected Parkinson's disease

1. (d) Early falls

Most patients with PD report a period of several years of poor sleep before the diagnosis is finally apparent. Restless legs syndrome is a common precursor to PD. Tremor is only present in 60–70% of patients with idiopathic PD. Early falling and a failure to respond to L-dopa strongly suggests an alternative diagnosis, probably progressive supranuclear palsy.

Further reading: Chapter 205.

Case 39: A patient with obsessive compulsive disorder and a tremor

1. (a) Wilson's disease

Wilson's disease presents with fulminant liver failure in childhood or with a movement disorder and neuropsychiatric disturbance in young adults. It is one of the only treatable and reversible neurodegenerative disorders and it is critical to identify it early. OCD is increasingly recognized. Diagnosis is by measurement of low caeruloplasmin and copper in serum and increased free urinary copper in a 24-hour urine collection. Treatment is with chelation therapy (penicillamine).

Further reading: Chapter 205.

Case 40: A patient with abnormal movements

1. (c) Huntington's disease (HD)

HD may present in the elderly with predominant chorea and minimal cognitive change. Senile chorea is an obscure entity that may not exist now that molecular tests for HD are available. Antiphospholipid syndrome is less likely to present at this age.

2. (b) A 20% chance of developing dementia by 10 years

Paralysis of the extraocular muscles is not a feature of PD. Dementia is very common in PD patients and increases with age such that if patients survive into their 80's approximately 50% will have frank cognitive impairment. Curiously, smoking has consistently been found in epidemiological studies to be protective.

Further reading: Chapter 205.

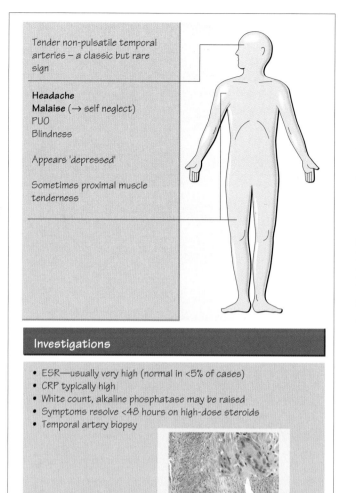

Tender non-pulsatile temporal arteries – a classic but rare sign

Headache
Malaise (→ self neglect)
PUO
Blindness

Appears 'depressed'

Sometimes proximal muscle tenderness

Investigations

- ESR—usually very high (normal in <5% of cases)
- CRP typically high
- White count, alkaline phosphatase may be raised
- Symptoms resolve <48 hours on high-dose steroids
- Temporal artery biopsy

Figure 9.41.1 Clinical features of temporal arteritis.

Case 41: A patient with a poorly localized headache

1. (b) Erythrocyte sedimentation rate (ESR)

The diagnosis is temporal arteritis and an urgent ESR is the most important test. Failure to achieve an initial diagnosis in this case led to irreversible loss of vision. The diagnosis should be suspected in any person over the age of 50 years with new-onset headache.

Further reading: Chapter 215.

Case 42: A patient with increasing headache

1. (c) Obstructive hydrocephalus

In idiopathic intracranial hypertension (the diagnosis in this case), non-contrast CT is normal, though contrast scanning or MRI can reveal venous sinus thrombosis as a cause in some patients. Hydrocephalus means dilatation of all or part of the ventricular system due to obstruction of CSF flow, which can be ruled out by CT.

Further reading: Chapter 63.

10 Ophthalmology: Cases and Questions

Case 1: A patient with a painful, red eye

A 32-year-old man goes to his GP with a painful, red left eye. The pain has increased in intensity over 3 days and is worse looking at bright light. The eye is not sticky, watering or itchy and the vision is only slightly blurred. He has felt tired and has had a cry cough for the past few weeks with aching joints. The eye is globally red around the limbus and the pupil is small; dilating the pupil eases the pain but shows an irregular-shaped pupil.

1. *What is the likely diagnosis?*
   (a) Conjunctivitis
   (b) Iritis
   (c) Corneal ulcer
2. *What systemic disorders might be present?*
   (a) Rheumatoid arthritis
   (b) Ankylosing spondylitis
   (c) Sarcoidosis
3. *What investigations should be undertaken?*
   (a) Serum angiotensin converting enzyme levels, liver function tests (LFTs), calcium
   (b) Chest X-ray
   (c) Examine conjunctival surface
   (d) All of the above
4. *What management is needed that day?*
   (a) Slit-lamp examination to ascertain cells of iritis, measure intraocular pressure, stain cornea
   (b) Corticosteroid and dilating drops, intensive at first then tapering
   (c) Arrange ophthalmic follow up to assess response and review results: refer on if sarcoid diagnosed
   (d) All of the above

Case 2: A patient with a painful red eye, aching joints and nosebleeds

A woman aged 50 years presents with a painful red right eye. The pain had increased over several days, is worse on eye movement and has prevented sleep for the past two nights. The vision is normal. She has been tired, short of breath, with aching joints and has had nosebleeds over the last month with aching over the bridge of her nose. The eye coat is red over several clock-hours with a dark brawny appearance. General examination shows hypertension and bilateral ankle oedema.

1. *What is the likely eye diagnosis?*
   (a) Conjunctivitis
   (b) Dry eye
   (c) Scleritis
   (d) Iritis
2. *Which underlying systemic disorder is most likely?*
   (a) Wegener's
   (b) Sarcoidosis
   (c) Rheumatoid arthritis
   (d) Behçet's syndrome
3. *What immediate investigations are most informative?*
   (a) Urinalysis
   (b) Serum ANCA with anti-MPO and anti-PR3 titres

(c) Chest X-ray for Wegener's especially if cavitation
(d) CT scan of sinuses

Case 3: A patient with a sore red eye and worsening vision

A 28 year-old man had a 4-day history of a sore, red right eye. He complained of slight worsening of vision, dislike of bright lights and a gritty sensation: all in his right eye. He denied any previous similar episodes. He was emmetropic (i.e. no refractive error so he didn't need to wear spectacles or contact lenses).

On examination, right visual acuity was 6/12 and left visual acuity was 6/4. His right eye was injected (that is, red and inflamed) particularly around the limbus (ciliary injection). He disliked light being shone into either eye.

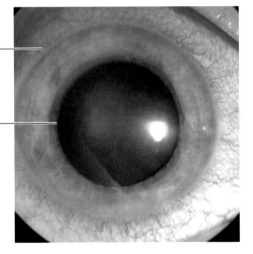

Circumciliary injection

Pupil dilated by cycloplegic drops

Figure 10.3.1

1. *The most likely diagnosis is:*
   (a) Acute bacterial conjunctivitis
   (b) Corneal ulcer
   (c) Cataract
   (d) Acute anterior uveitis
   On slit-lamp examination, he was found to have cells in the right anterior chamber.
2. *Which of the following is usually recommended as the first-line treatment :*
   (a) Daily review, no medication prescribed
   (b) Topical antibiotics, e.g. chloramphenicol and topical steroids, e.g. Maxidex
   (c) Topical cycloplegic, e.g. cyclopentolate, topical steroids, e.g. Maxidex
   (d) Oral steroids, e.g. prednisolone
   On further questioning, he mentioned a recent episode of lower back pain though denied any infections, rashes or ulcers (oral or genital).
3. *What percentage of patients with acute anterior uveitis are HLA-B27 positive?*

(a) 5–10%
(b) 20–30%
(c) 50–60%
(d) 90–100%

4. *Which of the following 'sero-negative arthropathies' (rheumatoid factor negative) is our patient most likely to have?*
   (a) Ankylosing spondylitis
   (b) Reiter's syndrome (reactive arthritis)
   (c) Inflammatory bowel disease
   (d) Psoriatic arthritis

Case 4: An elderly patient with general malaise and headache

An 83-year-old man presented with a week's history of general malaise and headache. He complained of intermittent sharp pains on the left side of his head and in his left eye. He pointed out a couple of itchy blisters over his eyebrow and left upper eyelid, which he noticed that morning.

1. *What is the likely diagnosis?*
   (a) Allergic dermatitis
   (b) Herpes simplex
   (c) Herpes zoster ophthalmicus
   (d) Preseptal cellulitis secondary to insect bites/infected skin lesions

Over the next couple of days, he developed a vesicular rash. This observed the midline and had a dermatomal distribution.

2. *Which of the following suggests a high chance of the eye becoming involved?*
   (a) Itchy blisters over the eyebrow
   (b) History of headache
   (c) His age
   (d) Involvement of the tip of his nose

3. *Which one of the following is false in herpes zoster ophthalmicus?*
   (a) Conjunctivitis is common and always associated with lid margin vesicles
   (b) 50% of patients get dendritic ulcers
   (c) Scleritis is common
   (d) Optic neuritis occurs in about 1 in 400 cases

4. *Treatment is likely to include:*
   (a) Oral (antiviral) aciclovir 800 mg po 5 × a day for 7–10 days, antibiotic (chloramphenicol) ointment and lubricating drops for the conjunctivitis and corneal pseudodendrites
   (b) Antibiotic (chloramphenicol) ointment and lubricating drops for the conjunctivitis and corneal pseudodendrites
   (c) Oral antibiotic (flucloxacillin 400 mg po QDS), lubricating drops for the conjunctivitis and corneal pseudodendrites
   (d) Oral (antiviral) aciclovir 800 mg po 5 × a day for 7–10 days, topical anaesthetic eyedrops for the conjunctivitis and corneal pseudodendrites

Case 5: A patient with deteriorating vision in one eye

A 67-year-old man was rubbing his left eye when he noticed his vision in the right eye was much worse than normal. He denied any eye pain. He wore bifocal spectacles and had been diagnosed with primary open angle glaucoma one year previously. He took eye drops for this ('Xalatan'). He had no history of any eye operations. His type 2 diabetes was a tablet-controlled.

On examination, visual acuities were 6/60 (right eye), 6/6 (left eye). His intraocular pressures (IOP) were 21 mmHg and 18 mmHg in the right and left eyes respectively. Dilated fundal examination of the right eye revealed dilated and tortuous retinal veins, a swollen optic disc, widespread intraretinal haemorrhages and retinal oedema. In the left eye, there was generalized constriction of the retinal arterioles and a couple of intraretinal haemorrhages. His BP was 184/105 mmHg.

1. *What is the likely diagnosis for the right eye?*
   (a) Central retinal artery occlusion
   (b) Anterior ischaemic optic neuropathy
   (c) Diabetic retinopathy
   (d) Central retinal vein occlusion

2. *Which of the following is not associated with an increased risk of retinal vein occlusion?*
   (a) Primary open angle glaucoma/ocular hypertension
   (b) Hypertension
   (c) Senile cataracts
   (d) Diabetes mellitus
   (e) Hypercholesterolaemia

3. *Which of the following suggest a diagnosis of hypertensive retinopathy for the left eye?*
   (a) Arterio-venous narrowing
   (b) Retinal arteriolar narrowing
   (c) Cotton wool spots
   (d) Flame-shaped haemorrhages
   (e) All of the above are true

4. *This man presented to eye casualty 8 weeks later with a very achy throbbing painful and red right eye. What is the suspected diagnosis?*
   (a) Rubeotic glaucoma
   (b) Acute anterior uveitis
   (c) Allergic conjunctivitis
   (d) Anterior scleritis

Case 6: A patient who sees flashes of light in one eye

A myopic (short-sighted) 21-year-old medical student presented to Eye Casualty on Monday morning. She complained of seeing flashes of light (photopsia) in the temporal part of her left eye for the last few days. They were becoming more frequent and yesterday afternoon, she became aware of lots of small black 'floaty bits' 'like flies' in her vision in the left eye and a greyish shadow, which didn't really seem to move and was in the lower part of her vision.

She mentioned falling off her bicycle on Friday night but said she was not hurt in the incident, and she denied any headache. She said that these flashes of light were different to those which accompanied her occasional migraines.

1. *What is your working diagnosis?*
   (a) Ocular migraine
   (b) Posterior vitreous detachment
   (c) Rhegmatogenous retinal detachment
   (d) Occipital lobe tumour

2. *How many risk factors for retinal detachment have been mentioned?*
   (a) 1
   (b) 3

(c) 5

(d) 7

3. *Which of the following systemic conditions is not associated with an increased incidence of retinal detachment?*
   (a) Nelson syndrome
   (b) Marfan's syndrome
   (c) Stickler syndrome
   (d) Ehlers–Danlos syndrome

4. *What percentage of all retinal detachments occur in myopic eyes?*
   (a) 10
   (b) 30
   (c) 40
   (d) 60

Case 7: A child with a headache and swollen eyelids

A 7-year-old boy attends A&E with his mother. He complains of having a 4-day history of headache, and over the last day or so, his right eyelids have become increasingly swollen such that now he is having difficulty opening his right eye. His eye has also become 'more red'. He has no past ocular history.

On examination, his temperature is 38.5°C. His right visual acuity is 6/7.5 and left visual acuity is 6/4. He was found to have restricted eye movements and pain when trying to look in different directions and a mild right proptosis.

1. *What is your working diagnosis?*
   (a) Preseptal cellulitis
   (b) Orbital cellulitis
   (c) Allergic eyelid swelling
   (d) Chalazion

2. *Which of the following is the most likely source of infection in this case?*
   (a) Direct extension from a sinus infection (especially ethmoiditis or dental infection)
   (b) Complication of orbital trauma
   (c) Complication of eye surgery (particularly orbital surgery)
   (d) Vascular extension, e.g. from nearby facial cellulitis

3. *Which of the following is the most suitable management plan?*
   (a) Broad-spectrum oral antibiotics, nasal decongestant and daily review as an outpatient
   (b) Admit for broad-spectrum oral antibiotics and CT scan
   (c) Admit for intravenous broad-spectrum antibiotics, nasal decongestant and CT scan
   (d) Admit for intravenous broad-spectrum antibiotics, nasal decongestant and CT scan and liaise with Paediatrics, ENT, Neuroradiology and Ophthalmologists

4. *Optic nerve function should be monitored frequently in orbital cellulitis. Which of the following is not a test of optic nerve function?*
   (a) Colour vision
   (b) Visual acuity
   (c) Corneal sensation
   (d) Pupillary light reflexes

Case 8: A patient who has vision difficulties while driving at night

A 55-year-old bus driver complained of a 5-month history of increasing difficulty seeing road signs and glare, particularly from oncoming car headlights while driving at night. He wore separate reading and distance glasses and his referring optometrist noted that his prescription had become more myopic (short-sighted). His past medical history included uveitis, asthma and he recalled a right-sided squash-ball ocular injury 15 years earlier.

On examination, right visual acuity was 6/18 correcting to 6/12 with a pin-hole; left visual acuity was 6/9 correcting to 6/7.5 with pin-hole.

1. *Which of the following is unlikely to cause glare?*
   (a) Mydriasis (dilated pupil), e.g. secondary to atropine drops
   (b) Corneal oedema
   (c) Corneal opacity
   (d) Cataract
   (e) Miosis (constricted pupil), e.g. secondary to Pilocarpine eye drops

2. *The examining doctor noted opacification of the normally clear crystalline lens in both eyes and diagnosed bilateral cataracts. Which test do you think he asked for next?*
   (a) Blood pressure
   (b) Blood sugar
   (c) Full blood count
   (d) Ishihara colour vision test

3. *His random blood sugar was 8.0 mmol/L. How many risk factors for cataract does this patient have?*
   (a) 3
   (b) 4
   (c) 5
   (d) 6
   (e) 7

4. *Which of the following statements is false?*
   (a) A perforating or penetrating injury of the lens does not usually cause a cataract
   (b) Patients with diabetes may have transient changes in their spectacle prescription (refraction) because increases in blood sugar cause swelling of the intraocular lens
   (c) A tetanic cataract may occur due to any cause of hypocalcaemia
   (d) A sunflower cataract is a characteristic ocular manifestation in Wilson's disease, an inherited autosomal recessive disorder of copper metabolism

Case 9: A patient who has difficulty seeing out of one eye

A 75-year-old woman was washing her face one morning and after getting soapy water in her right eye, started to rub it. On looking out of the left eye, into the mirror, she could no longer see the tip of her nose, her mouth, her chin or neck. The right vision was normal.

1. *What type of visual field defect did she have?*
   (a) Left homonymous hemianopia
   (b) Left altitudinal field defect
   (c) Right homonymous hemianopia
   (d) Bitemporal hemianopia
   (e) Left arcuate scotoma

2. *She had a headache and found combing her hair uncomfortable. On further questioning, she complained of all of the following symptoms except:*
   (a) Pain on chewing (jaw claudication)
   (b) Recent weight gain

(c) Anorexia

(d) Fever

(e) Proximal muscle and joint aches

On examination, right visual acuity was 6/9, left visual acuity was counting fingers. She had an afferent pupillary defect and a pale, swollen optic disc. Her ESR was 55 mm/hour, and CRP 21 mg/L.

3. *What is your working diagnosis?*

(a) Arteritic anterior ischaemic optic neuropathy (AAION)

(b) Central retinal vein occlusion

(c) Inflammatory optic neuritis

(d) Compressive optic nerve tumour

(e) Central retinal artery occlusion

(f) Non-arteritic anterior ischaemic optic neuropathy (NAAION)

4. *Regarding management, which of the following is advised?*

(a) Immediate systemic steroids

(b) Daily review, start systemic steroids if worsening

(c) Analgesia for headache, temporal artery biopsy and consider giving steroids if headache persists

(d) Formal visual field test followed by temporal artery biopsy and steroids

Case 10: A patient with constant double vision

A 45 year-old woman complained of constant double vision. It resolved when she covered either eye. It was oblique and worse when looking upwards and to the left.

1. *Which of the following statements is false?*

(a) Monocular double vision is usually the result of abnormalities of the refractive media (e.g. astigmatism, keratoconus, corneal, or lens opacities) or retina (e.g. haemorrhage or fluid at the macula)

(b) Monocular double vision is relieved by covering either eye

(c) Binocular double vision can be relieved by covering one eye

(d) Binocular double vision results from misalignment of the visual axes

(e) This patient had binocular double vision

2. *On examination, she had periorbital and lid swelling and retraction of the upper and lower lids. Her left eye showed restriction of upgaze and lateral gaze. What is the most likely diagnosis?*

(a) Myasthenia gravis

(b) Decompensation of an existing phoria

(c) Spectacle problem

(d) Thyroid eye disease

3. *Which of the following extracoular muscles appear to have been affected by fibrosis?*

(a) Superior rectus and inferior rectus

(b) Inferior rectus and medial rectus

(c) Medial rectus and lateral rectus

(d) Medial rectus and superior oblique

(e) Inferior oblique and superior rectus

4. *In thyroid eye disease, which of the following statements is false?*

(a) Proptosis, chemosis, lid retraction and lid lag are other signs of thyroid eye disease

(b) When the medial rectus is involved, the eye typically turns outward (exodeviation)

(c) Orbital CT scan shows thickening of the extraocular muscle bellies with sparing of the tendons

(d) Optic nerve compression may result from compression of the optic nerve at the orbital apex by thickened extraocular muscles

(e) Visual loss from optic neuropathy is an ocular emergency and requires immediate treatment with steroids

Ophthalmology: Answers

Case 1: A patient with a painful, red eye

1. (b) Iritis

Conjunctivitis is not likely because the eye is painful and photophobic. There are characteristic features of iritis, however, including the stuck-down pupil. Corneal ulcer is less likely as the history is several days, there is no watering, vision is not very blurred and the pupil is abnormal.

Idiopathic	50% of cases
Systemic disease	Sarcoidosis Ankylosing spondylitis Inflammatory bowel disease Behçet's syndrome Reiter's disease
Infection	Syphilis Tuberculosis Herpes zoster Herpes simplex Lyme disease
Autoimmune	Juvenile inflammatory arthritis

Figure 10.1.1 Causes of iritis.

2. (c) Sarcoidosis

Rheumatoid arthritis is not associated with iritis. Ankylosing spondylitis is a possible diagnosis, but does not explain all the systemic features. Sarcoidosis is the most likely diagnosis in view of the symptoms.

3. (d) All of the above

All are true. Serum angiotensin converting enzyme levels, LFTs and calcium should be checked for sarcoidosis and chest X-ray for sarcoid. The conjunctival surface should be examined for granuloma to biopsy or a tissue diagnosis should be sought elsewhere.

4. (d) All of the above

All are true. Iritis is a potentially serious disorder, and must be treated as a medical emergency, by the appropriate specialist using appropriate specialist techniques and treatment. Steroid eye drops must only be started (and monitored) by ophthalmologists.

Further reading: Chapter 65 in Medicine at a Glance.

Case 2: A patient with a painful red eye, aching joints and nosebleeds

1. (c) Scleritis

Conjunctivitis is not likely because the eye is painful and not sticky. Dry eye is not likely either because the eye is painful and too red. Scleritis is most likely because of the characteristic pain and appearance of the eye. Iritis is less likely with this pattern of pain.

2. (a) Wegener's

Wegener's syndrome is likely with sinus, chest and renal involvement. Although rheumatoid arthritis can be associated

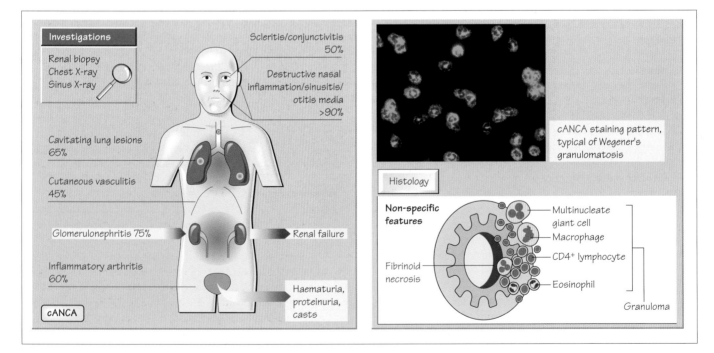

Figure 10.2.1 Features of Wegener's granulomatosis.

with scleritis, the systemic features don't fit. Behçet's syndrome is associated with iritis, not with scleritis.

3. (b) Serum ANCA with anti-MPO and anti-PR3 titres

Urinalysis for protein, blood, casts and plasma creatinine is useful to assess renal involvement (and urgency of referral). Chest X-ray is useful for Wegener's, especially if there is cavitation. CT scan of the sinuses can reveal bone erosion which is typical of upper-airway Wegener's. However, the most informative is likely to be the immunology; this is almost always positive in Wegener's granulomatosis, and false negatives, while possible, are unlikely.

Further reading: Chapter 142.

Case 3: A patient with a sore red eye and worsening vision

1. (d) Acute anterior uveitis

There is no mention of discharge from the eye which rules out bacterial conjunctivitis, he is not a contact lens wearer so corneal ulcer is unlikely, a cataract is uncommon in this age group and does not normally present with a gritty sensation in the eye or photophobia.

2. (c) Topical cycloplegic, e.g. cyclopentolate, topical steroids, e.g. Maxidex

Topical steroids and a cycloplegic, e.g. cyclopentolate, are the mainstay of treatment in acute anterior uveitis (or iritis). A cycloplegic is important to relieve the photophobia which results from ciliary muscle spasm and dilate the pupil to prevent the inflamed iris adhering to the lens behind it. Such adhesions, termed posterior synechiae, give rise to an irregularly-shaped pupil.

3. (c) 50–60%

HLA B27 denotes a genotype on the short arm of chromosome 6. It is present in only 1.4–8% of the general population but in 50–60% of patients with acute anterior uveitis.

4. (a) Ankylosing spondylitis

Acute anterior uveitis occurs in 30% patients with ankylosing spondylitis. The sero-negative arthropathies are autommune diseases. They are strongly associated with acute anterior uveitis and HLA-B27 positivity.

Further reading: Chapter 212.

Case 4: An elderly patient with general malaise and headache

1. (c) Herpes zoster ophthalmicus

Herpes zoster ophthalmicus (Shingles). A flu-like prodrome and pre-herpetic neuralgia usually precede the unilateral vesicular rash.

2. (d) Involvement of the tip of his nose

Involvement of the side of the tip of the nose is called Hutchinson's sign. The external nasal nerve, which supplies the tip of the nose is the terminal branch of the nasociliary nerve (a branch of the ophthalmic division of the trigeminal nerve). The presence of Hutchinson's sign strongly correlates with the likelihood of ocular complications.

3. (c) Scleritis is common

About 50% of patients do tend to develop acute epithelial keratitis within 2 days of getting the rash but typically the lesions are pseudodendritic ulcers. In contrast to the dendritic ulcers seen in herpes simplex infections, the pseudodendrites in herpes zoster ophthalmicus have tapered ends which lack bulbs.

4. (a) Oral (antiviral) aciclovir 800 mg po 5 × a day for 7–10 days, antibiotic (chloramphenicol) ointment and lubricating drops for the conjunctivitis and corneal pseudodendrites

Aciclovir is the most commonly used antiviral for ophthalmic shingles (herpes zoster ophthalmicus). A 200 mg po daily dose of aciclovir is used to treat herpes simplex infections. Infection with the herpes virus can cause reduced or absent corneal sensation, which can predispose to additional corneal disease. Aside from possible use in ocular examination, topical anaesthetic agents would not be recommended in these cases.

Further reading: Chapter 162.

Case 5: A patient with deteriorating vision in one eye

1. (d) Central retinal vein occlusion (Fig.10.5.1)

90% of patients are older than 50 years at the time of diagnosis. It is likely to be ischaemic because of the profound loss of visual acuity.

2. (c) Senile cataracts

All the rest are commonly associated with retinal vein occlusions.

3. (e) All of the above are true

These findings are the cardinal features of hypertensive retinopathy.

4. (a) Rubeotic glaucoma

Poor presenting visual acuity is the most important risk factor for iris neovascularization. Rubeosis iridis develops in about 50% eyes with ischaemic central retinal vein occlusion usually at 2 to 4 months. Vigorous pan-retinal photocoagulation laser treatment is needed to prevent rubeotic glaucoma.

Further reading: Chapter 61.

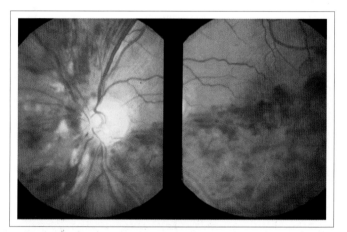

Figure 10.5.1 Central retinal vein occlusion.

Case 6: A patient who sees flashes of light in one eye

1. (c) Rhegmatogenous retinal detachment

Flashes of light in ocular migraine are typically zig-zag-shaped and are not associated with floaters or greyish shadows. In addition, her symptoms are quite different to her usual migraine symptoms and she did not have a headache. An occipital lobe tumour is very unlikely in this age group. With a posterior vitreous detachment, the accompanying shadow tends to be mobile and represents the detached posterior hyaloid face.

2. (c) 5

The risk factors are: myopia, photopsia, floaters, shadow in the vision and trauma. The most common type of retinal detachment is a rhegmatogenous retinal detachment caused by liquefied vitreous passing through a retinal tear and into the potential space between the sensory retina and the retinal pigment epithelium. The Greek word 'rhegma' means break.

3. (a) Nelson syndrome

Nelson syndrome refers to the rapid enlargement of a pituitary adenoma that occurs after the removal of both adrenal glands.

4. (c) 40

Although only 10% of the general population is myopic, more than 40% of retinal detachments occur in myopic eyes.

Further reading: Chapter 61.

Case 7: A child with a headache and swollen eyelids

1. (b) Orbital cellulitis (Fig.10.7.1)

Proptosis and limited eye movements and pain on attempted eye movement suggest orbital involvement. With preseptal cellulitis, there may be tense eyelid oedema and erythema and a mild fever but there is no optic neuropathy (vision is normal, colour vision normal, normal pupillary reflexes), no limitation of eye movement, nor any pain on eye movement and no propotosis. Allergic eye disease is usually bilateral. With a chalazion ('stye') there is usually a well-defined subcutaneous nodule in the eyelid, there may be eyelid swelling and erythema but there is no restriction of eye movement, no proptosis, and no pain on eye movement.

2. (a) Direct extension from a sinus infection (especially ethmoiditis or dental infection)

All are potential sources of infection in orbital cellulitis but (a) is the most likely in this case.

3. (d) Admit for intravenous broad-spectrum antibiotics, nasal decongestant and CT scan and liaise with Paediatrics, ENT, Neuroradiology and Ophthalmologists

Orbital cellulitis is a life-threatening infection of the soft tissues behind the orbital septum. It is more common in children. It requires hospital admission and treatment with intravenous antibiotics and often a multidisciplinary approach. Nasal decongestants are often recommended in children older than 5 years of age.

4. (c) Corneal sensation

This tests the ophthalmic division of the trigeminal nerve (cranial nerve V). (The efferent arm of the blink reflex involves the facial nerve, cranial nerve VII).

Further reading: Chapter 23 in Ophthalmology at a Glance.

Case 8: A patient who has vision difficulties while driving at night

1. (d) Cataract

All the rest are recognized causes of glare.

2. (b) Blood sugar

Once diagnosed, one should determine the aetiology of the cataracts particularly in relatively young patients who are less likely to have age-related cataract.

3. (b) 4

They are: intraocular inflammation (uveitis), asthma (and therefore implied use of inhaled steroids), trauma (squash ball injury is often the cause of asymmetric or unilateral cataracts), and diabetes (his blood sugar was raised).

Patients with diabetes typically develop two types of cataracts. In the juvenile form, the lens opacities are typically anterior or posterior subcapsular and adults may develop age-related cataracts but at an earlier age. It is not unusual for patients to become more myopic due to their cataracts. This is called 'second sight' and it makes distance vision blurry but can improve reading vision temporarily before the cataract develops further.

4. (a) A perforating or penetrating injury of the lens does not usually cause a cataract

A perforating or penetrating injury to the lens usually causes a rapid opacification of the lens (cataract). All the other statements above are true.

Further reading: Chapter 33 in Ophthalmology at a Glance.

Case 9: A patient who has difficulty seeing out of one eye

1. (b) Left altitudinal field defect

Homonymous hemianopias involve the same side of the visual field in both eyes, and likewise a bitemporal hemianopia involves both eyes. An arcuate scotoma is an area of decreased vision extending from the blind spot, arching into the nasal field (following the lines of the retinal nerve fibres). An altitudinal field defect is one where vision is lost above or below the horizontal, which is what she has.

2. (b) Recent weight gain

The most likely diagnosis is blindness due to temporal arteritis; weight gain is not a feature of this, whereas all the others are.

3. (a) Arteritic anterior ischaemic optic neuropathy (AAION)

AAION (giant cell arteritis; GCA) is the correct diagnosis. With NAAION patients tend to be younger with les severe visual loss and usually a normal ESR. With inflammatory optic neuritis, patients tend to be younger without the signs typical of GCA.

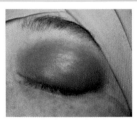
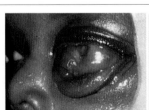

Post-septal orbital cellulitis – pre-drainage

Rhabdomyosarcoma

- Rare malignant orbital tumour of childhood that can metastasize. It may present as orbital cellulitis
- Average age of onset: 7 years
- Grows fast and progresses
- If suspected, urgent referral and biopsy required

Figure 10.7.1 Differential diagnosis of orbital cellulitis.

With a compressive optic nerve tumour, there is progressive visual loss with few symptoms in common with GCA. With central retinal artery occlusion, the optic disc is not swollen, and the retina tends to be pale with a characteristic 'cherry red spot' at the fovea. With central retinal vein occlusion, the retinal shows diffuse retinal haemorrhages.

4. (a) Immediate systemic steroids

Steroids should be given as soon as the patient is suspected of having giant cell arteritis – without delay! Without steroids, the contralateral eye can become involved within 24 hours. Ideally, a temporal artery biopsy should be performed within a week of starting systemic steroids.

Further reading: Chapter 17 in Ophthalmology at a Glance.

Case 10: A patient with constant double vision

1. (b) Monocular double vision is relieved by covering either eye

Binocular double vision can be relieved by covering one eye but if only one eye is causing the diplopia, then only covering that eye will relieve the double vision.

2. (d) Thyroid eye disease

Retraction of the upper and lower lids occurs in about 50% patients with Graves' disease. Up to 50% of patients with thyroid eye disease may develop ophthalmoplegia.

3. (b) Inferior rectus and medial rectus

Whilst any of the extraocular muscles may be involved in thyroid-associated ophthalmoplegia, the inferior and medial recti are most commonly affected.

4. (b) When the medial rectus is involved, the eye typically turns outward (exodeviation)

When the medial rectus is involved, the eye typically turns inward (esodeviation)

Further reading: Chapter 28 in Ophthalmology at a Glance.

11 Rheumatology: Cases and Questions

Case 1: A patient with an unusual red rash

A 35-year-old woman has noted an unusual red rash over her knuckles on her hands and perhaps to a lesser extent on her upper chest and upper back. She is otherwise healthy and has no significant medical or family history. She is on no medications. Her GP reassures her that the rash is of no significance. Over the next few months, she notices that she has much less energy than previously and is concerned that the rash may be spreading to her face. She seems to be puffy around the eyes and everyone seems to comment on it. Her GP agrees and refers her to a dermatologist for a further opinion. The dermatologist is alarmed at the extent of her rash and orders some urgent blood tests. She is started on high-dose prednisolone to clear the rash and the dermatologist explains that she has dermatomyositis.

The rash fades successfully with steroids, but the patient notices after 3 or 4 weeks that she is having difficulty lifting her arms above her head or rising from a chair. She returns to her GP who suggests that she must stop the steroids immediately and performs some urgent blood tests.

1. *Which of the following is true of dermatomyositis?*
   (a) Dermatomyositis is associated with malignancy
   (b) Dermatomyositis occurs predominantly in those over 70 years old
   (c) The skin rash is characteristic
   (d) A specific antibody test confirms the diagnosis
   (e) Intravenous immunoglobulin is useful in severe skin involvement
2. *Steroid therapy:*
   (a) Is associated with an increased risk of osteoporosis
   (b) Is required life-long in this condition
   (c) May result in muscle weakness
   (d) Is useful to treat muscle inflammation in this condition
   (e) Should be commenced at 10 mg/day
3. *Which of the following tests should be included in this woman's work up?*
   (a) Positron emission tomography (PET) scan
   (b) Thyroid function tests
   (c) CPK levels
   (d) Whole-body MRI
   (e) Anti-Jo-1 antibodies

Case 2: An elderly patient with mobility difficulties

A 75-year-old man presents to A&E unable to stand up unaided. He reports an increasing difficulty in general mobility for the last 6 weeks, particularly with activities such as rising from a chair and lifting objects from cupboards above head height. He is otherwise reasonably well, with a background history of hypertension, on diuretic therapy and hyperlipidaemia on a statin.

Initial examination reveals global reduction in motion, which is more pronounced in the proximal muscles of both upper and lower limbs. His muscles are not tender to touch. Neurological examination is normal otherwise with normal reflexes and plantars are downgoing. He is referred to the medicine for the elderly service for further assessment.

1. *Which of the following are true?*
   (a) Proximal muscle weakness may be due to hypothyroidism
   (b) Limb girdle stiffness is commonly of no significance in the elderly
   (c) Full evaluation should include a muscle biopsy
   (d) He needs an urgent CT brain
   (e) The statin should be stopped immediately
2. *Initial blood results reveal an ESR of 95 mm/hour. Renal and liver biochemistry are normal. Which of the following is true?*
   (a) He has myeloma
   (b) He is hypokalaemic
   (c) He should be questioned carefully about scalp tenderness and visual disturbance if this has not been done already
   (d) CPK may not be included on the liver/kidney biochemistry screen and should be checked
   (e) He should commence 60 mg prednisolone immediately
3. *Which of the following are true of polymyalgia rheumatica?*
   (a) It is associated with underlying malignancy which should be aggressively sought
   (b) 15 mg of prednisolone should induce improvement in 48 hours
   (c) Those patients who have difficulty reducing prednisolone due to recurrence of symptoms may benefit form the introduction of an agent such as methotrexate
   (d) Steroid therapy may interfere with blood pressure control
   (e) Up to one fifth may have concurrent temporal arteritis

Case 3: A patient with osteoarthritis in one hip

A 65-year-old woman is admitted via A&E following a slip on a loose carpet at her home. She is an otherwise healthy 65-year-old who is troubled by osteoarthritis of her left hip, the pain of which requires NSAID therapy intermittently. Her medical history is notable only for the birth of three healthy daughters, the eldest of whom is now 32 years old. She lives with her older sister, her husband having died some years ago. Examination reveals her to have a dinner fork deformity at the right wrist, which is tender and bruised. She has an exaggerated thoracic spinal curvature and is tender over her mid thoracic region. Examination is otherwise normal.

1. *Indicate which of the following statements is true in this scenario:*
   (a) She has likely sustained a Colles' facture (fracture distal radius)
   (b) She has sustained an atraumatic/low impact fracture
   (c) Her daily intake of calcium and vitamin D should be reviewed and quantified
   (d) She has osteoporosis
   (e) She should have a DEXA scan
   (f) All of the above
2. *Following surgical fixation of her fracture, she is visited by a fracture liaison nurse. Which of the following are true?*

(a) Her sister's bone health should also be reviewed

(b) She should take regular daily exercise such as swimming

(c) She should aim to ingest 1000–1200 mg elemental calcium per day either via diet or supplementation

(d) She should be prescribed a bisphosphonate without further ado

(e) She should have a thyroid function test and a rheumatoid factor sent

3. *She is prescribed a bisphosphonate drug for treatment of osteoporosis by her GP. Which of the following are true?*

(a) She should have a DEXA scan again in 1 year

(b) She should be advised to take her bisphosphonate at night to avoid side effects

(c) Optimal treatment duration with bisphosphonate is undetermined

(d) Her daughter is at risk of osteoporosis

(e) Hormone replacement therapy (HRT) can be prescribed in addition to a bisphosphonate if the first drug is unsuccessful

Case 4: A young patient with rheumatoid arthritis

A 23-year-old recently qualified dentist has had rheumatoid arthritis for almost five years. He attends a rheumatologist twice yearly and until his recent final exams, has been very well. He was initially commenced on sulphasalazine therapy but when this did not control his arthritis, he was transferred to methotrexate therapy. He presents to his GP feeling rather unwell with a one-week history of a sore throat, which has not cleared, and some gum bleeding. His GP notes that he has low-grade pyrexia and tonsillar enlargement but no other physical abnormality. He carries out some blood tests, which reveal the following:

Hb	9.4 g/dL
WCC	1.2×10^9/L
Neutrophils	0.8×10^9/L
Lymphocytes	0.4×10^9/L
ESR	77 mm/h
Platelets	55×10^9/L

1. *Which of the following are true?*

(a) Methotrexate should be increased as active rheumatoid arthritis may cause marrow suppression

(b) Methotrexate should be stopped as it may cause marrow suppression

(c) Antibiotic cover is not indicated as many 'sore throats' are of viral origin

(d) He needs a blood transfusion

(e) Folinic acid may be useful in reversing his blood counts

The patient is admitted to hospital and with appropriate supportive care and cessation of methotrexate, his condition improves and he is discharged with normal white cell and platelet counts one week later. Six weeks later, his arthritis starts to flare badly and he is unable to use his hands to work, they are so swollen and stiff.

2. *Which of the following are true?*

(a) Steroid therapy should be considered at this point

(b) Methotrexate should be recommenced at a low dose

(c) Anti-tumour necrosis factor (TNF) agents should be considered

(d) Plaquenil is likely to be as efficacious as methotrexate

(e) Rheumatoid factor and CCP antibodies should be measured to guide further therapy decisions

3. *A decision is made to commence an anti-TNF therapy. Which of the following are true?*

(a) He will require screening for latent tuberculosis (TB) infection

(b) He may respond after a single administration of these drugs

(c) If he fails to respond to one drug in this class another of the class may be effective

(d) If he fails to respond to anti TNF medications, there are no further treatment options at this time

(e) The ultimate goal of therapy is to maintain function of his joints

Case 5: A patient with lethargy and weight loss

A 55-year-old male presents to his GP feeling lethargic and having lost weight. He has noted a minor blotchy rash on his lower limbs and some numbness over the ring finger of his left hand. Otherwise he is in good health and requires only a thiazide diuretic for hypertension, which developed about two years ago. He is a non-smoker, non-drinker and lives with his wife and two sons. Physical examination reveals a red raised rash on his lower limbs and decreased light touch sensation over the little finger of the left hand with no detectable weakness.

1. *Which of the following are true?*

(a) He has an ulnar nerve palsy

(b) His renal function and urinalysis should be evaluated

(c) His rash should be biopsied

(d) He may have an underlying malignancy

(e) An NSAID may be prescribed for his generalized symptoms

His GP sends some initial bloods which reveal the following:

Hb	10.1 g/dL
Platelets	220×10^9/L
WCC	Normal but eosinophils = 5% total WCC
ESR	79 mm/h
CRP	55 mg/L
Urea	12.1 mmol/L
Creatinine	114 µmol/L
Urinalysis	+++ blood

2. *Which of the following are true?*

(a) He likely has Wegener's granulomatosis

(b) He has a potentially reversible cause of hypertension

(c) He should be commenced on prednisolone without further ado

(d) Antinuclear antibody (ANA) is likely to be the most useful screening test in this gentleman

(e) A full drug history is necessary

3. *He is referred to a rheumatologist for further investigation and management of likely Churg–Strauss vasculitis. Which of the following are true?*

(a) His ulnar nerve should be biopsied to allow a histological diagnosis to be made

(b) Full investigation should include an ECG

(c) Full history and physical examination should be carried out to determine extent of his disease

(d) He is likely to have strongly positive ANCA

(e) This is a self-limiting condition and steroids have not been proven to alter its course

Case 6: A patient with fatigue and aching joints

A 38-year-old female has noticed recently that she is increasingly fatigued. Additionally she has some pains and aches in her joints and a particularly painful right wrist which she thinks has been swollen on a few occasions over the last year. She presents to her GP who notes that she may be depressed, as she has had difficulty conceiving and has recently been referred for specialist advice. She complains of fatigue, lassitude, generalized pain in both muscles and joints and poor ability to concentrate. Her sister has systemic lupus erythematosus (SLE) and she is concerned that she may be developing it too. There is little to find on examination except a mild swelling of her right wrist.

1. *Which of the following are true?*
   (a) Wrist X-rays may help diagnose SLE
   (b) SLE is more common in first-degree relatives of index cases
   (c) Anti double-stranded DNA antibodies should be ordered as a screening test
   (d) Depression is a recognized feature of SLE
   (e) Antineutrophil cytoplasmic antibody (ANCA) should be ordered as a screening test

   Blood tests reveal the following:

ESR	35 mm/h
Hb	9.2 g/dL
Lymphocytes	1.0×10^9/L
Creatinine	120 μmol/L

   Other routine blood tests are normal
   ANA positive, with a speckled pattern

2. *Which of the following are true?*
   (a) Urinalysis is mandatory
   (b) All her symptoms may be explained by the finding of anaemia
   (c) A positive ANA in this clinical scenario confirms a diagnosis of SLE
   (d) Anaemia is likely to be due to acute haemolysis
   (e) A speckled pattern ANA suggests drug-induced lupus

3. *Following renal assessment a decision is made to carry out a renal biopsy which shows active lupus nephritis. Which of the following are true?*
   (a) A prolonged APTT in the work up for renal biopsy indicates a bleeding tendency which requires full evaluation pre-procedure
   (b) She will require cyclophosphamide therapy
   (c) Her dsDNA titres will guide further treatment
   (d) Renal involvement is associated with pregnancy complications
   (e) Renal involvement is often more severe for those of African or Caribbean origin

Rheumatology: Answers

Case 1: A patient with an unusual red rash

1. (a) Dermatomyositis is associated with malignancy
(c) The skin rash is characteristic
(e) Intravenous immunoglobulin is useful in severe skin involvement

Dermatomyositis has two peaks, one in childhood and the second in the forties–sixties age group. The skin rash is characteristic, but there is no characteristic autoantibody associated with dermatomyositis. Antinuclear antibody (ANA) is positive in 50–70 % but occurs in many other conditions. Anti-Jo-1 antibody may be present and if so defines a subset of this condition which is at risk of interstitial lung disease.

2. (a) Is associated with an increased risk of osteoporosis
(c) May result in muscle weakness

(d) Is useful to treat muscle inflammation in this condition

Steroid therapy is not required life-long; most patients will be able to decrease and stop therapy, perhaps with the addition of a further agent such as azathioprine or methotrexate). It may result in muscle weakness and the possibility of a steroid myopathy must be considered in any patient recently commenced on this drug. Dermatomyositis is, however, associated with clinical myositis and this should be ruled out (CPK, EMG, MRI with or without biopsy). Muscle inflammation should be commenced at 10 mg/day (doses up to 1 mg/kg may be required to treat this condition, particularly in the early stages or during severe flares or where muscle involvement threatens swallowing or ventilatory capability).

3. (b) Thyroid function tests
(c) CPK levels

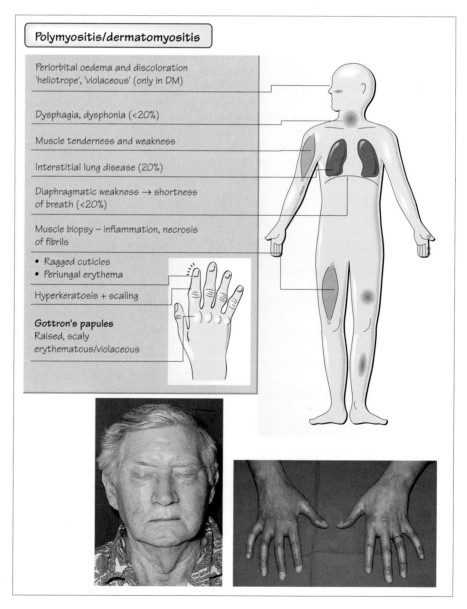

Figure 11.1.1 Features of inflammatory muscle disease.

Medicine at a Glance: Core Cases, 1st edition. Edited by P. Davey. © 2011 Blackwell Publishing Ltd.

Although there is an association with malignancy, a PET scan is not the first-line investigation. Thorough history, examination and targeted tests for neoplasia based on patient age, sex and risk factors should be conducted. Autoimmune diseases cluster and hypothyroidism may result in proximal muscle weakness. CPK levels are diagnostic of muscle inflammation as a feature of dermatomyositis if elevated. A small percentage is normal even with definite muscle inflammation on biopsy, EMG and MRI. Serial measurements are used to tailor treatment. Initial investigations should focus on clinically involved muscle areas to highlight the presence of inflammatory muscle change.

Further reading: Chapter 215 in Medicine at a Glance.

Case 2: An elderly patient with mobility difficulties

1. (a) Proximal muscle weakness may be due to hypothyroidism

Limb girdle stiffness is commonly of no diagnostic significance in the elderly (polymyalgia affects up to 1% of the over 60s and is readily treatable). Polymyalgia rheumatica (PMR) is primarily a clinical diagnosis. Muscles are not inflamed and are therefore non-tender. CPK is normal. Muscle biopsy is an invasive procedure which should only be undertaken if there is diagnostic doubt. The neurological findings do not warrant an urgent brain scan. The statin should not be stopped as the frequency of significant statin myopathy is relatively low; clinical trial data suggest the prevalence of statin-related myalgia or weakness is less than 5%. The spectrum of muscle-related disorders due to statins includes myalgia with normal CPK, myalgia with moderate rise in CPK and myalgia with CPK greater than ten times normal. Overt myopathy and rhabdomyolysis are very rare events with a reported incidence of 0.15 deaths per 1 million prescriptions due to statin-induced rhabdomyolysis. Statins are important drugs in the management of cardiovascular risk in this patient and should be continued as the clinical picture is of limb girdle stiffness and the presence of a raised erythrocyte sedimentation rate (ESR) confirms a diagnosis of PMR.

2. (d) CPK may not be included on the liver/kidney biochemistry screen and should be checked

Myeloma is a cause of raised ESR but does not present in this way. Hypokalaemia is a cause of muscle weakness but renal biochemistry is normal. He should be questioned carefully about scalp tenderness and visual disturbance as up to 20% of those with classical PMR findings will have concurrent temporal arteritis, which may manifest as scalp tenderness, jaw claudication and visual disturbance. The presence of these features warrants a temporal artery biopsy, though this may be negative as vessel wall inflammation is patchy. The distinction between PMR and temporal arteritis is important as temporal arteritis requires much higher doses of steroids than PMR. PMR is treated with 15 mg prednisolone daily and tapering.

3. (c) Those patients who have difficulty reducing prednisolone due to recurrence of symptoms may benefit form the introduction of an agent such as methotrexate

   (d) Steroid therapy may interfere with blood pressure control

   (e) Up to one fifth may have concurrent temporal arteritis

The incidence of malignancy is no higher than in age- and sex-matched controls.

The response to prednisolone is so striking that failure to respond should prompt one to consider alternate diagnoses, e.g.

in this case a statin-induced myopathy. The role of alternate immunosuppression is currently being defined in PMR. It is also important to evaluate the patient thoroughly before deciding to increase steroids in the event of a 'relapse'. Some patient symptoms such as generalized pain, particularly in the absence of a concomitant rise in ESR may be due to non-PMR causes. Blood pressure control is an important consideration in the elderly. Review of blood pressure control is warranted when the patient has been stabilized on steroid therapy. Other considerations regarding steroid therapy include weight gain, hypokalaemia, osteoporosis and cataract formation.

Further reading: Chapter 215.

Case 3: A patient with osteoarthritis in one hip

1. (f) All of the above

The definition of atraumatic is fall from standing height or less. Her daily intake of calcium and vitamin D should be reviewed and quantified (clear guidelines for daily calcium/vitamin D intake are in the text). Lack of dietary sufficiency requires supplementation. This patient has osteoporosis (the WHO definition includes sustaining an atraumatic fracture/ wedge fracture of the spine). Even though she has osteoporosis by definition, a DEXA scan will guide treatment by quantifying response.

2. (a) Her sister's bone health should also be reviewed

   (c) She should aim to ingest 1000–1200 mg elemental calcium per day either via diet or supplementation

First-degree relatives have a higher risk of osteoporosis, so her sister's bone health should be reviewed. Regular daily exercise should be weight-bearing, e.g. walking. There are a number of options for therapy and in general a bisphosphonate is the first option unless there are contraindications such as inability to comply with administration instructions. While hyperthyroidism, coeliac disease and rheumatoid arthritis are secondary causes of osteoporosis, the most significant risk in this patient is her age. Secondary causes should be sought in those with severe or early-onset bone loss – particularly premenopausal women and men. Laboratory screen for secondary causes in all osteoporosis patients is neither clinically indicated nor feasible.

3. (c) Optimal treatment duration with bisphosphonate is undetermined

   (d) Her daughter is at risk of osteoporosis

The recommended follow-up for DEXA scan is 2 years minimum. The most significant risk of bisphosphonate therapy is upper GI ulceration and these medications are taken first thing in the morning on an empty stomach, remaining in an upright posture for a further thirty minutes. Family history is an important risk factor for the development of postmenopausal osteoporosis. HRT is no longer first-line therapy for osteoporosis in postmenopausal women.

Further reading: Chapter 209.

Case 4: A young patient with rheumatoid arthritis

1. (b) Methotrexate should be stopped as it may cause marrow suppression

   (e) Folinic acid may be useful in reversing his blood counts

Methotrexate should not be increased for several reasons. Firstly, no information is given on clinical assessment of joint activity in rheumatoid arthritis: duration of early-morning stiffness, total swollen joint count, total tender joint count and patient assessment of disease activity. Secondly, while rheumatoid arthritis is associated with anaemia this is multifactorial and not due to disease-related marrow suppression. Thirdly, methotrexate is the likely cause of the patient's condition. Methotrexate is a dihydrofolate reductase inhibitor, preventing de novo synthesis of purines and pyrimidines and acts by inhibition of immune cellular proliferation. Accordingly, it has the potential to cause reversible marrow suppression, though in practice this is a rare event. All patients, however, require safety monitoring of full blood count and liver function at 4–6-week intervals. If marrow suppression is suspected, methotrexate should be stopped immediately and appropriate supportive cover offered. This young man is neutropaenic and as he is pyrexial, antibiotic cover will absolutely be required. As sepsis can progress quickly in neutropenia, the patient should be referred immediately to hospital for investigation and management including full sepsis work up (throat swab, blood culture, MSU, etc.) to identify the organism responsible. If there is no evidence of decompensation secondary to anaemia, no evidence of extrinsic blood loss and the drug has been stopped, this young man should regenerate his marrow reasonably quickly providing he has sufficient iron stores available. Blood products remain associated with risk and should not be administered without good clinical indication. Folinic acid bypasses the step in cellular synthesis which is inhibited by methotrexate and should be prescribed to facilitate marrow regeneration. It is not to be confused with folic acid which is prescribed once-weekly for all patients on methotrexate to offset its side effects.

2. (a) Steroid therapy should be considered at this point

(c) Anti-tumour necrosis factor (TNF) agents should be considered

Steroid therapy should be considered as the patient's disease is in flare and he is unable to work. A short course of rescue steroids should be prescribed at low dose (7.5–10 mg) with appropriate bone protection (calcium and Vitamin D supplements). Methotrexate is now contraindicated due to bone marrow toxicity. Anti-TNF agents are generally used when a patient has failed or is intolerant of two DMARDS (disease modifying anti-rheumatic drugs) and requires further therapy. Examples are given in the text. The role of methotrexate as anchor drug is well established. No other DMARD can claim similar efficacy. The role of antibody measurement in rheumatoid arthritis is in diagnosis and prognosis. Neither changes in response to therapy and should not be used to guide therapy beyond noting that those with strongly positive rheumatoid factor or cyclic citrullinated peptide (CCP) antibodies are likely to have an aggressive form of the disease with poorer outcomes and should be treated aggressively from diagnosis onward. Repeated testing is generally unnecessary where the diagnosis is clearly established.

3. (a) He will require screening for latent tuberculosis (TB) infection

(b) He may respond after a single administration of these drugs

(c) If he fails to respond to one drug in this class another of the class may be effective

Certain of the anti-TNF agents are associated with reactivation of latent TB and screening should be performed in all with treatment of latent infection prior to initiation of anti-TNF treatment. Screening varies according to local guidelines and TB prevalence, but generally involves a Mantoux skin test, a chest X-ray and possibly a serological test such as Quantiferon. Patients who test positive for TB require treatment, generally for at least 3 months prior to initiation of anti-TNF therapy.

He may respond after a single administration of these drugs: the majority of patients respond quickly, though after a single dose would be particularly fast. Indeed, those patients not exhibiting a clinical response after 3 months will generally not do so at all and the treatment should be discontinued. Recent trials have shown that failure of one agent does not imply failure of the entire anti-TNF drug class. 'Switching' to an alternate anti-TNF agent may be associated with clinical response. There are also second generation biologic agents available. Even patients with advanced joint disease and deformity can still function reasonably well. The modern goal of therapy is remission.

Further reading: Chapter 211.

Case 5: A patient with lethargy and weight loss

1. (b) His renal function and urinalysis should be evaluated

(c) His rash should be biopsied

(d) He may have an underlying malignancy

The patient has early sensory changes suggestive of a mononeuritis of the ulnar nerve, however motor function is intact. Untreated, this may evolve into an ulnar nerve palsy with classical motor in addition to sensory findings. He is hypertensive and has a vasculitic rash. Renal involvement in vasculitis should be actively investigated and abnormal function or urinalysis followed up by a nephrologist. Biopsy of the rash will allow a tissue diagnosis of vasculitis to be made. An undifferentiated small vessel vasculitis may arise secondary to a number of causes including malignancy. Even if he had pain, which he does not, an NSAID may worsen his hypertension.

2. (b) He has a potentially reversible cause of hypertension

(e) A full drug history is necessary

He clearly has an inflammatory process which is vasculitic in nature but the high eosinophil count suggests that this may be Churg-Strauss syndrome. Other potential causes in a middle-aged male are listed in Fig.11.5.1. He likely has renal involvement, as his renal function is impaired. Renal vasculitis is treatable and his hypertension may improve. He needs a full work up including renal evaluation with biopsy and full immunological tests in order to assess both the extent and activity of his vasculitis. Treatment is planned when all investigations are to hand and aims to induce and subsequently maintain remission of vasculitis with immunosuppression. ANA is very non-specific in the presence of vasculitis. Antineutrophil cytoplasmic antibody (ANCA) are much more likely to be of diagnostic use in a middle-aged man with this constellation of symptoms, signs and results. A number of medications can induce vasculitis, including thiazide diuretics, however these tend to produce a self-limiting rash rather than systemic involvement.

3. (b) Full investigation should include an ECG

(d) He is likely to have strongly positive ANCA

Histological diagnosis is likely to be made by renal biopsy which will need to be undertaken in view of his renal findings.

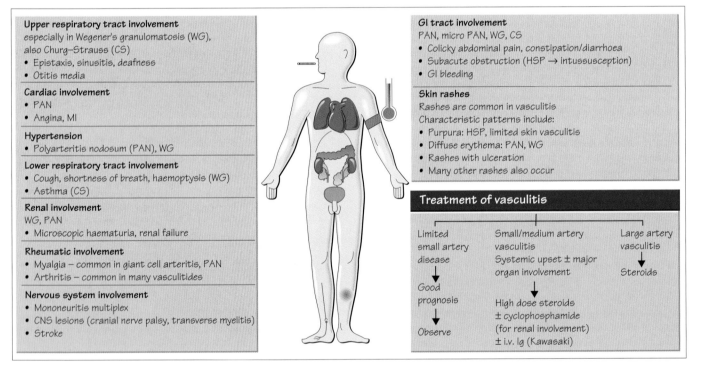

Size of vessel affected	Primary	Secondary
Large arteries	Giant cell artertitis Takayasu's arteritis	Rheumatoid arthritis (aortitis) Anklyosing spondylitis, Behçet's syndrome Infection • Syphilis
Medium arteries	Kawasaki disease Classic polyarteritis nodosa	• Hepatitis B and C
Medium and small arteries	Wegener's granulomatosis* Churg-Strauss syndrome* Microscopic polyangiitis*	RA, SLE, Sjögren's Drugs (see below) Infection, e.g. HIV
Small arteries (leukocytoclastic/hypersensitivity)	Henoch-Schönlein purpura Essential mixed cryoglobulinaemia	• Drugs, e.g. sulphonamides, penicillins, thiazides • Infection, e.g. tuberculosis, group A streptococci • Malignancy, lymphoma • RA, SLE, Sjögren's

*Associated with ANCA antibodies, renal impairment and responsive to immunosuppression with cyclophosphamide
RA, rheumatoid arthritis; SLE, systemic lupus erythematosus

From Scott's Classification of the Vasculitides published in ABC of Rheumatology, BMJ Publishing, 2002

Figure 11.5.1 Classification of the vasculitides.

Upper respiratory tract involvement
especially in Wegener's granulomatosis (WG),
also Churg–Strauss (CS)
• Epistaxis, sinusitis, deafness
• Otitis media

Cardiac involvement
• PAN
• Angina, MI

Hypertension
• Polyarteritis nodosum (PAN), WG

Lower respiratory tract involvement
• Cough, shortness of breath, haemoptysis (WG)
• Asthma (CS)

Renal involvement
WG, PAN
• Microscopic haematuria, renal failure

Rheumatic involvement
• Myalgia – common in giant cell arteritis, PAN
• Arthritis – common in many vasculitides

Nervous system involvement
• Mononeuritis multiplex
• CNS lesions (cranial nerve palsy, transverse myelitis)
• Stroke

GI tract involvement
PAN, micro PAN, WG, CS
• Colicky abdominal pain, constipation/diarrhoea
• Subacute obstruction (HSP → intussusception)
• GI bleeding

Skin rashes
Rashes are common in vasculitis
Characteristic patterns include:
• Purpura: HSP, limited skin vasculitis
• Diffuse erythema: PAN, WG
• Rashes with ulceration
• Many other rashes also occur

Treatment of vasculitis

Limited small artery disease → Good prognosis → Observe

Small/medium artery vasculitis
Systemic upset ± major organ involvement → High dose steroids ± cyclophosphamide (for renal involvement) ± i.v. Ig (Kawasaki)

Large artery vasculitis → Steroids

Figure 11.5.2 Clinical features of vasculitis.

Alternatively skin biopsy would be favourable and diagnostic. Churg–Strauss syndrome can involve the heart and pericardium, in some cases fatally. This is likely to be a peripherally staining p-ANCA if he has Churg–Strauss. The ANCA may return nega-tive following therapy. Life-threatening end-organ disease is not uncommon and the patient must be regularly followed up and a full screening history, exam and lab work up undertaken. The self-limiting vasculitides are those associated with drug ingestion, viral infections and Henoch–Schönlein purpura, which is not common in adults.

Further reading: Chapter 213.

Case 6: A patient with fatigue and aching joints

1. (b) SLE is more common in first-degree relatives of index cases

(d) Depression is a recognized feature of SLE

Even established joint involvement in SLE is rarely associated with radiological abnormality. Jaccoud's arthropathy refers to the finding of clinical features suggestive of a deforming arthritis in the presence of pristine joints on X-ray. The malalignment is correctable by the examiner. SLE is more common in first-degree relatives. ANA is an appropriate screening test. Depression is associated with SLE (Fig.11.6.1) ANCA are associated with vasculitides and this lady has no features which would suggest this to be the case clinically at this point.

2. (a) Urinalysis is mandatory

(c) A positive ANA in this clinical scenario confirms a diagnosis of SLE

Regardless of the presence of any underlying systemic autoimmune disease this lady has a raised creatinine which must be investigated. Bedside testing is indicated and may greatly inform further tests While anaemia may give rise to fatigue and lassitude, she has clear joint swelling which cannot be attributed to anaemia. The combination of positive ANA, anaemia, renal involvement and joint swelling would together fulfill diagnostic criteria (Fig.11.6.2).

While haemolysis is a feature of active SLE, other causes may also be responsible in this case, e.g. menorrhagia, anaemia of chronic disease and renal impairment. A speckled pattern ANA is associated with positivity of antibodies to the extractable nuclear antigens Ro, La, etc. Drug-induced lupus is associated with antihistone antibodies which give homogenous ANA staining.

3. (d) Renal involvement is associated with pregnancy complications

(e) Renal involvement is often more severe for those of African or Caribbean origin

A prolonged APTT (activated partial thromboplastin time) is a screening test for antiphospholipid syndrome which can occur alongside SLE. Although the APTT is prolonged, this is an *in vitro* artefact and the clinical condition is actually that of arterial and venous thromboses. Further investigation is warranted for antiphospholipid syndrome. Treatment of lupus nephritis depends on a number of factors, and while cyclophosphamide remains the cornerstone of therapy, not all patients will require this drug. While dsDNA titres may rise prior to a flare, therapeutic decisions are based on full clinical evaluation of the patient, not an alteration in dsDNA. A patient with a history of lupus nephritis has a higher incidence of pre-term delivery, miscarriage, small for gestational age babies and hypertension. Nonetheless with dedicated expert management many of these patients have successful pregnancies.

Further reading: Chapter 214.

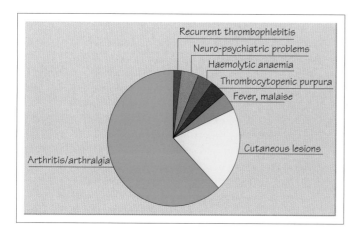

Figure 11.6.1 Presenting features of SLE.

Clinical	Laboratory
Malar rash	Haematological abnormalities
Photosensitive rash	Immunological abnormalities
Discoid lupus rash	ANA positive
Neurological involvement	
Seizures or psychosis	
Renal disease: proteinuria or casts	
Serositis: pleuritis or pericarditis	
Mucosal aphthous ulceration	
Arthritis	

Figure 11.6.2 Diagnostic criteria for SLE. Four out of 11 criteria present at any time is required for a diagnosis of SLE.

12 Dermatology: Cases and Questions

Case 1: A patient with an itchy skin eruption

A 53-year-old married office worker was seen in A&E with a 6-day history of a worsening itchy skin eruption. He had had upper respiratory symptoms for 3 days prior to that for which he had been give a 5-day course of Augmentin by his GP. He still felt vaguely unwell and had become shivery over 3 days. There was a past history of psoriasis (12 years, affecting only his elbows and knees) and hypertension (4 years). For the former he had used a potent topical steroid and for the latter had been on a diuretic for 3 years to which had been added another drug 3 weeks earlier. He only drank at weekends (three or four pints of beer). He had smoked 20 cigarettes a day from age 15 to age 49. There was a family history of psoriasis (mother and aunt) and cardiovascular disease, including hyperlipidaemia, hypertension and myocardial infarction (father and older brother, both smokers). Recently his daughter aged 17 who lived at home had been treated for scabies but his wife was not itching. On examination his temperature was 37.6°C and his pulse was 100 beats/min and regular. There was a widespread erythematous eruption affecting 90% of the body surface including the palms and soles. There were evident psoriatic plaques on the elbows and knees. There was a dusky erythema and diffuse scale involving the scalp. Elsewhere there were areas of more superficial scale and clusters of pustules on the limbs and torso and a few excoriations: around the upper cheek and neck blistering and exfoliation were thought to be present. The nails showed psoriasiform onycholysis and two splinter haemorrhages were seen in one index finger nail. The mucosae were normal. There was pitting oedema of both ankles. Examination of the cardiovascular, respiratory and neurological systems was normal as was examination of the abdomen. Urinalysis was normal. Routine bloods showed a normal haemoglobin, a slightly elevated white cell count, an ESR of 30 mm/hour, a CRP of 37 mg/L, normal urea and electrolytes, normal calcium and phosphate, slightly elevated random glucose, normal liver function tests. The ECG and chest X-ray were normal.

1. *The most important next step to take is:*
   (a) Blood cultures and commencement of intravenous antibiotics
   (b) Admission to hospital
   (c) Phone the GP to find out the name of the new antihypertensive drug
   (d) Echocardiogram
   (e) Urgent dermatology opinion

2. *The most important next investigation is:*
   (a) Skin swab for M, C & S
   (b) Skin biopsy
   (c) Blood cultures
   (d) Skin scrape for scabies
   (e) Fasting glucose and lipids

3. *After hospitalization the next most important management step should be:*
   (a) Intramuscular methotrexate
   (b) Subcutaneous insulin sliding scale
   (c) Very potent topical steroids
   (d) Topical scabicides
   (e) Cessation of all presenting medication

4. *What is the most important imperative for his subsequent management?*
   (a) Low-fat diet
   (b) Absolute life-time ban on alcohol intake
   (c) Regular haemoglobin, blood count, U&Es and liver function tests
   (d) Diet-enriched with omega-3 fish oils
   (e) Long-term prophylactic antistaphylococcal antibiotics

Case 2: A patient with a pigmented lesion on her arm

A 27-year-old national oarswoman attends with a new changing pigmented lesion on her left forearm. She says she is 'moley' but that this lesion is definitely new (6/12) and she thinks she recalls an insect bite. It has grown, become red then slightly brown black then lighter in the centre and bled. She is otherwise well and taking no medication and there is no relevant personal or family history (although she says all of her family are 'moley', especially on her mother's side and she says that an aunt died of a brain tumour).

On examination she is well-built, fair, blue-eyed and tanned where sun exposed (female rowing vest and shorts). There are numerous naevi, of different sizes, shapes and colours, widely distributed including affecting the scalp and scalp margin, buttocks and feet. She had iris lentigines. The presenting lesion is about 4 mm × 5 mm but very irregular of edge and pigment being black at the margins and red in the centre with the hint of erosion towards the centre which is just slightly elevated. There is an infected blister on the left hand and a 1 cm palpable lymph node in the left axilla. There is no organomegaly or other abnormal physical signs.

1. *The patient needs:*
   (a) Immediate excision of suspected melanoma
   (b) Immediate punch biopsy of suspected melanoma
   (c) Elective excision of suspected histiocytoma/ dermatofibroma (insect bite reaction)
   (d) Elective curettage and cautery of suspected basal cell papilloma/seborrheic keratosis
   (e) Measurement of the lesion, clinical photography, oral antibiotics for the hand lesion and review in 3 months

Histology shows a malignant melanoma, Breslow thickness 1.2 mm, ulcerated and narrowly excised. A swab from the hand showed staphylococcus and the lymph node had all but disappeared after oral erythromycin for a week.

2. *She next most needs:*
   (a) Whole-body CT
   (b) Ultrasound of left axilla
   (c) Full blood count, ESR, U&Es, LFTs
   (d) 1-cm wide re-excision of the forearm scar
   (e) Discussion at the skin cancer MDT meeting

She has the wider excision which shows no residual melanoma. An axillary ultrasound is performed which shows no lymphadenopathy.

3. *Her prognosis is:*
   (a) 98% 5-year survival
   (b) 90% 5-year survival
   (c) 80% 5-year survival

(d) 50% 5-year survival

(e) 20% 5-year survival

4. *Which term best summarizes the diagnosis?*

(a) Melanoma

(b) Malignant melanoma

(c) Superficial spreading melanoma/dysplastic nevus syndrome

(d) Sporadic superficial spreading melanoma

(e) Hutchinson's malignant freckle

Case 3: A patient with a pruritic rash

A 40-year-old man visits his GP complaining of a 3-week history of a pruritic rash. He describes an intensive itch, which is worse at night. He has no other co-morbid problems. His wife has also been itchy over this same period. He works as a health care assistant in a nursing home. Examination demonstrates excoriated papules and nodules distributed on his limbs, trunk and genitalia.

1. *During his physical examination, you should pay particular attention to the presence of:*

(a) Pallor

(b) Signs of hyperthyroidism

(c) Generalized lymphadenopathy

(d) Scabetic burrows

(e) Darier's sign

2. *Which of the following is a rapid diagnostic test that can be used by the GP to confirm his clinical suspicion of scabies?*

(a) Isolation and visualization of a mite from infected sites

(b) Lesional skin biopsy

(c) Full blood count

(d) Serological tests for the scabetic mite

(e) Polymerase chain reaction (PCR) to identify scabetic mites from cutaneous scales

3. *The GP demonstrates the presence of mites from infected areas. Which of the choices below may be used for treatment of scabies?*

(a) Permethrin 5% cream

(b) Malathion 0.5% lotion

(c) Oral ivermectin

(d) Sulfur

(e) All of the above

4. *The patient is treated with permethrin 5% cream. Other important management issues that need to be discussed with the patient include:*

(a) The need to treat him and his close personal contacts concurrently

(b) The notion that ongoing pruritus does not necessarily imply treatment failure

(c) The need to wash clothing, linen and towels (used in the week preceding scabetic treatment) in hot water and dry on high heat

(d) The need for treatment repetition after 7 days

(e) All of the above

Case 4: A child with hair loss

A 7-year-old boy is referred to the paediatric dermatology clinic with an 8-month history of focal areas of hair loss on his scalp. He is otherwise fit and well. Physical examination demonstrates the presence of focal scaly plaques, in association with alopecia on his occipital and parietal scalp. Prominent cervical lymph nodes are also present.

1. *The single most important investigation is:*

(a) A scalp biopsy

(b) Full blood count

(c) Examination of scales from scalp by microscopy and culture

(d) Epstein-Barr virus (EBV) serology

(e) HIV test

2. *Microscopy identifies the presence of mycelia elements and the culture grows* Trichophyton tonsurans. *Which of the agents below would be the most appropriate treatment?*

(a) Topical Canesten (clotrimazole)

(b) Oral terbinafine

(c) Topical Daktacort (hydrocortisone/miconazole)

(d) Topical Eumovate (clobetasone butyrate)

(e) Topical terbinafine

3. *What advice can you give to the child's parents in respect of the hair loss?*

(a) The hair loss is permanent with and without treatment

(b) The hair loss is usually reversible following adequate treatment of the child

(c) The longer the infection persists without treatment, the less likely the alopecia will be permanent

(d) The degree of inflammation seen on biopsy correlates with the risk of permanent hair loss

Case 5: A patient with a chronic ulcer

A 60-year-old woman is referred to clinic with a chronic ulcer above the left medial malleolus. Over the last 3 days the ulcer has become increasingly tender and the surrounding skin is erythematous and warm to touch. There is a prior history (more than 10 years ago) of a deep venous thrombosis of that left leg.

1. *The most likely cause of her left medial malleolus ulcer is:*

(a) Arterial ulcer

(b) Pyoderma gangrenosum

(c) Venous ulcer

(d) Squamous cell carcinoma

(e) Vasculitic ulcer

2. *In this setting, the most likely reason(s) for the current deterioration of her leg ulcer is:*

(a) Concurrent cellulitis

(b) Allergic contact dermatitis

(c) Malignant change (Marjolin's ulcer)

(d) Malnutrition

(e) Anaemia

She is febrile (temperature of 38°C) and mildly tachycardic (pulse of 100 beats/min and regular). Blood tests demonstrate a raised white cell count, with neutrophilia, raised ESR and CRP. Her renal and liver function tests are within normal range.

3. *The next single most important investigation which should be undertaken on admission is:*

(a) Patch testing

(b) Doppler venous imaging of the left leg

(c) Nail clippings for mycology

(d) Wound swabs

(e) Blood cultures

4. *The acute management of the patient should include all the following except:*

(a) Rectal examination

(b) Examination of her feet to exclude tinea pedis

(c) Intravenous antibiotics

(d) Potassium permanganate soaks

(e) Topical steroids

Case 6: A patient with blisters on the backs of the hands

A 40-year-old man, known to be hepatitis C positive, is referred to clinic by his gastroenterologists with a 1-month history of blisters on the backs of both hands. These develop with minimal trauma to the skin. He also admits to excessive drinking; his weekly alcohol intake amounts to roughly 25 units per week.

1. *When examining him, an important diagnostic physical finding is the presence of:*
   - (a) Hypertrichosis
   - (b) Gynaecomastia
   - (c) Spider naevi
   - (d) Palmar erythema
   - (e) Testicular atrophy

2. *Which enzyme is deficient in porphyria cutanea tarda?*
   - (a) Protoporphyrinogen oxidase
   - (b) Porphobilinogen deaminase
   - (c) Uroporphyrinogen decarboxylase
   - (d) Uroporphyrinogen III synthase
   - (e) Coproporphyrinogen oxidase

3. *The most important test to confirm the clinical suspicion of PCT is:*
   - (a) Skin biopsy
   - (b) Indirect IMF
   - (c) Hepatitis C serology
   - (d) Liver function tests
   - (e) Uroporphyrin III in urine and faeces

4. *The following are all ways of managing his PCT except:*
   - (a) Venesection
   - (b) Hydroxychloroquine
   - (c) Systemic steroids
   - (d) Avoidance of alcohol
   - (e) Stringent sun protection

Case 7: A patient with atopic dermatitis and worsening itch and rash

A previously fit and well 23-year-old female trainee solicitor known to have atopic dermatitis (AD) is admitted ill with a fever and tachycardia and a 2-day history of worsening itch and rash and actual skin pain. She is on the combined oral contraceptive and has been using the same topical steroids for years. The pulse is 120 beats/min and the BP 95/65 mmHg. She has erythrodermic eczema with multiple small areas of erosion, oozing and impetiginization. There are no other focalizing signs.

1. *The single most important investigation is:*
   - (a) Blood cultures
   - (b) IgE estimation
   - (c) Viral swab for herpes simplex virus (HSV)
   - (d) Microbiology swab
   - (e) HIV test

2. *She is started on intravenous flucloxacillin and benzyl penicillin. What is the next most important component of her management?*
   - (a) Intravenous aciclovir
   - (b) Intravenous gentamicin
   - (c) Intravenous antihistamines
   - (d) Intravenous diamorphine
   - (e) Intravenous methylprednisolone

3. *The patient responds well to treatment. HSV is shown to be present. Blood cultures are negative but several skin swabs grow broadly sensitive staphylococci. When she is discharged which of the following constitutes the least clinically desirable component of her forward management plan?*
   - (a) Medium-term (a few months) oral antibiotics
   - (b) Medium-term (a few months) oral aciclovir
   - (c) Long-term oral antihistamines
   - (d) Long-term oral prednisolone
   - (e) A course of UVB phototherapy

Case 8: A patient with recurrent hives

A 35-year-old woman complains of a 2-year history of recurrent hives. She gets these roughly twice per week, if she is off all treatment. She cannot relate the onset of her symptoms to any triggering factors. She is not on any regular medication and has no other co-morbid problems. She has no family history of any medical problems.

1. *Which of the following from her history and signs will enable you to differentiate between urticarial vasculitis and chronic idiopathic urticaria?*
   - (a) Lesions lasting more than 24 hours and resolving with post-inflammatory hyperpigmentation
   - (b) Erythematous wheals
   - (c) Angioedema
   - (d) Pruritus
   - (e) Relationship to shellfish ingestion

2. *Clinically a diagnosis of urticarial vasculitis is suspected and an early lesion is biopsied. What histological finding if present distinguishes urticaria from urticarial vasculitis?*
   - (a) Leukocytoclastic vasculitis
   - (b) Papillary dermal oedema
   - (c) Eosinophils
   - (d) Basal layer vacuolization
   - (e) A superficial and deep peri-vascular mononuclear cell infiltrate

3. *The histological features and clinical findings are in keeping with urticarial vasculitis. Which of the following investigations is* not *warranted in this setting?*
   - (a) Complement assay
   - (b) Antinuclear antibody (ANA)
   - (c) Hepatitis B serology
   - (d) Hepatitis C serology
   - (e) Total IgE levels

4. *The following drugs may have a therapeutic role in managing urticarial vasculitis except for:*
   - (a) Systemic steroids
   - (b) Colchicine
   - (c) Dapsone
   - (d) Antihistamines
   - (e) Acitretin

Case 9: A patient with hand eczema

A 35-year-old woman is referred to outpatient clinic with hand eczema. She had eczema in her childhood until the age of 7 years. She has been relatively asymptomatic until 6 months ago, following the birth of her first child, when she noticed a recurrence of her eczema, now predominantly affecting her hands. Of note, she does also suffer from hay fever and asthma.

1. *The most likely cause of her hand eczema is:*

(a) An allergic contact dermatitis to rubber gloves

(b) A Type 1 reaction to latex

(c) Irritant contact dermatitis occurring on a background of atopic diathesis

(d) Tinea manuum

(e) Psoriasis

2. *These physical findings are more in keeping with a diagnosis of:*

(a) Allergic contact dermatitis

(b) Atopic eczema

(c) Psoriasis

(d) Irritant contact dermatitis

(e) Tinea manuum

3. *General management of this patient's hand eczema should not include:*

(a) Advice on frequent use of emollients

(b) Advice to minimize house hold duties

(c) Topical steroids

(d) Exclusion diet

(e) Refer for patch testing

Case 10: A patient with a psoriasiform rash

A 26-year-old man presents with a 2-week history of a psoriasiform rash. Prior to onset of his skin rash, he had been feeling lethargic and had a sore throat. He has no other co-morbid problems and is not on any regular medication. He is homosexual and over the last year has had multiple casual sexual partners. He does have a strong family history of psoriasis (both his father and paternal grandfather suffered from this condition). Physical examination demonstrates scattered papules, topped with silvery scales, distributed on his trunk.

1. *In this setting, your differential diagnosis for the cutaneous eruption should include all the following except:*

(a) Guttate psoriasis

(b) Secondary syphilis

(c) HIV seroconversion illness

(d) Pityriasis rosea

(e) Atopic eczema

2. *Both his HIV 1/2 and syphilis serology are negative. What further investigation should be undertaken as part of his acute management?*

(a) A repeat HIV 1/2 serology in 3 months

(b) Antistreptolysin (ASO) titres

(c) Fasting serum glucose

(d) Fasting cholesterol

(e) Thyroid function tests

3. *He has positive ASO titres and based on this, his clinical history and the results of a subsequent throat swab you give him oral antibiotics. You also decide to refer him to an ENT doctor, as he informs you that he has had recurrent sore throat over the last year and you have some concerns about this being a triggering factor for his psoriasis. The most sensible treatment for his psoriasis at this stage is:*

(a) Dithranol (topical)

(b) Crude coal tar (topical)

(c) Methotrexate (oral)

(d) Ciclosporin (oral)

(e) TLO1 phototherapy (narrow band UV-B)

4. *Although most patients with guttate psoriasis have spontaneous resolution of their skin lesions, if he does develop chronic plaque psoriasis, part of his overall management should include:*

(a) Regular prophylactic TLO1 phototherapy

(b) Anti tumour necrosis factor-α (TNF-α) treatments

(c) Advice to stop or reduce his alcohol intake and modify his cardiovascular risk factors

(d) Advice to purchase a home UV machine

(e) Salt-free diet

Case 11: A patient with acne

A 19-year-old female with a 2-year history of acne spots consults you. She has not responded to any topical treatment purchased or prescribed previously. You diagnose acne vulgaris with confidence on the clinical presentation and prescribe an oral antibiotic.

1. *She requires (pick the most likely):*

(a) Pregnancy test

(b) Ovarian ultrasound scan

(c) Serum 17 hydroxy-progesterone

(d) Liver function tests

(e) No investigations

2. *All but one of the following would be suitable first-line oral antibiotics for this patient:*

(a) Oxytetracycline

(b) Erythromycin

(c) Lymecycline

(d) Augmentin

(e) Doxycycline

3. *You prescribe oral erythromycin 500 mg bd and topical clindamycin. After three months she returns with marginal improvement. There is no scarring. Acceptable options include all but one of the following*

(a) Add in a suitable oral contraceptive pill

(b) Switch to oral oxytetracycline

(c) Switch to oral lymecycline

(d) Start oral isotretinoin

(e) Switch to oral trimethoprim

You prescribe oral lymecycline. She has a personal history of migraine and, you discover, a family history of a pill-related deep vein thrombosis (DVT). She presents 3 months later unchanged, perhaps worse and with scarring threatened, on lymecycline. She wants to be treated with oral isotretinoin. The dermatologist agrees that it is clinically indicated.

4. *Only one of the following is true:*

(a) The patient must start on the pill

(b) Isotretinoin can be started immediately

(c) The patient must have a pregnancy test before treatment

(d) The patient must have an ovarian ultrasound

(e) The patient must have a clotting screen

Case 12: A patient with facial redness

A 40-year-old Irish woman is referred to dermatology outpatient clinic with a 3-year history of facial redness.

1. *The differential diagnosis for this woman's red face includes:*

(a) Seborrheic dermatitis

(b) Rosacea

(c) Acne vulgaris

(d) Systemic lupus erythematosus

(e) All of the above

Clinical examination demonstrates telangiectasia on both cheeks in association with papules and pustules. There are no comedones present and there are no scales visible in the nasolabial fold or eyebrows. You suspect this woman has rosacea.

2. *Which aspect of her history will not support you clinical impression of rosacea?*
(a) Worsening of symptoms with alcohol intake
(b) Worsening of symptoms with spicy food
(c) Improvement with topical steroids
(d) Redness of the eye
(e) Worsening of symptoms with coffee

3. *The most appropriate first-line agent for this patient should be:*
(a) Elidel (Pimecrolimus) topical
(b) An oral antibiotic such as doxycycline
(c) Isotretinoin (oral)
(d) Pulse dye laser
(e) Hydroxychloroquine (oral)

4. *The patient enquires about her prognosis. What is the most appropriate response?*
(a) It is likely that she will have complete cure of her rosacea in a few months
(b) It is likely that she will have a complete cure of her rosacea after a few years
(c) She has a chronic disease, and will likely have flares when her systemic therapy is discontinued
(d) It is likely that she will have a persistent and progressive disease despite the use of systemic therapy
(e) She will be cured if she stops drinking altogether

Case 13: A patient with café-au-lait macules

An 11-year-old boy is referred to the paediatric outpatient clinic with 10 café-au-lait macules distributed on his trunk. He was born at 40 weeks gestation and since birth has had an uneventful childhood. His mother has neurofibromatosis (NF) type 1. Physical examination reveals more than two soft nodules on his limbs, which on biopsy are in keeping with neurofibromas.

1. *In what setting can café-au-lait macules be seen?*
(a) Normal neonate
(b) Neurofibromatosis
(c) McCune–Albright syndrome
(d) Tuberous sclerosis
(e) All the above

2. *In this clinical scenario, what other physical signs should be looked for during examination of the young boy?*
(a) Axillary freckling
(b) Mucocutaneous pigmented macules
(c) Cutaneous myxoma
(d) Hypomelanotic macules
(e) Angiokeratoma corporis diffusum

3. *What additional investigation/assessment should be undertaken?*
(a) Full blood count
(b) Ophthalmological assessment
(c) Thyroid function tests
(d) Serum blood glucose
(e) Liver function tests

4. *Other clinical features of NF type 1 include:*
(a) Glaucoma
(b) Plexiform neurofibroma
(c) Learning difficulties
(d) Scoliosis
(e) All the above

Case 14: A patient with de-pigmented patches

A 27-year-old North African man is referred to outpatient clinic with a 2-year history of de-pigmented patches on his face, trunk and limbs. At the onset of his problem he had been seen by a private dermatologist and diagnosed with vitiligo. He was issued with a high potency steroid, however despite the use of this topical steroid, the disease had progressed. He is extremely embarrassed by his physical appearance and lacks self confidence.

1. *During history taking it is most important to ask about:*
(a) Alcohol intake
(b) Allergies
(c) Occupation
(d) Personal and/or family history of autoimmune disease
(e) Smoking history

2. *During the consultation it is apparent that the man is depressed about his condition. You should:*
(a) Arrange for immediate section under the Mental Health Act
(b) Ignore the depression, you are only there to deal with his skin problem
(c) Approach this issue in a tactful manner. Suggest that he may benefit from a referral to a psychologist/psychiatrist
(d) Prescribe an antidepressant for him
(e) Suggest St John's Wort administration

3. *Therapeutic options for vitiligo include:*
(a) Topical steroids
(b) Phototherapy
(c) Tacrolimus
(d) Camouflage cosmetics
(e) All of the above

4. *In this patient an appropriate first-line agent may be:*
(a) Phototherapy
(b) Topical steroids
(c) Protopic (Tacrolimus) topical
(d) Dovonex (Calcipotriol) topical
(e) None of the above

Case 15: A patient with skin darkening on the face and hands

A 56-year-old Asian man with schizophrenia, diabetes and hypertension complains of progressive darkening of the skin of his face and hands.

1. *All but one of the following drugs might be responsible:*
(a) Chlorpromazine
(b) Oral contraceptive
(c) Amiodarone
(d) Furosemide
(e) Glibenclamide

A drug history confirms that the patient is on chlorpromazine, aspirin and amlodipine. He has diet-controlled diabetes.

2. *Hypermelanosis of drug origin occurs via the following mechanism(s):*
(a) Increased melanin synthesis
(b) Increased lipofuscin synthesis
(c) Cutaneous deposition of drug-related material
(d) None of the above
(e) All of the above

3. *The clinician suspects that the chlorpromazine is the likely cause of the patient's pigmentary changes. Other side effect(s) associated with chlorpromazine include:*
   (a) Cataracts
   (b) Increased conjunctival pigmentation
   (c) Increased nail bed pigmentation
   (d) None of the above
   (e) All of the above
4. *The physician should:*
   (a) Stop the culprit drug if feasible
   (b) Prescribe topical hydroquinone
   (c) Prescribe high potency topical steroids
   (d) Prescribe mercury containing de-pigmenting agents
   (e) None of the above

Case 16: An elderly patient with generalized skin blisters

An 88-year-old man, resident in a nursing home, presents with a 6-week history of generalized skin blisters. His past medical history includes a previous cerebrovascular accident (CVA). He is on aspirin. On examination, he is pyrexial (temperature 38°C), tachycardic (pulse of 100 beats/min, regular) and he is noted to have tense blisters (about 8) and scattered urticated plaques on his trunk and limbs. The blisters are on an erythematous base. On his thighs and back, he has ulcerated areas, the sites of previous intact blisters, now exuding pus. He has no mucosal blisters.

1. *The most likely diagnosis is:*
   (a) Linear IgA bullous disease
   (b) Bullous lupus erythematosus (LE)
   (c) Bullous pemphigoid (BP)
   (d) Paraneoplastic pemphigus
   (e) Bullous erythema multiforme
2. *In this man, no underlying drug aetiology is identified and the clinical suspicion is that of idiopathic BP. Which investigations should be performed to confirm this diagnosis?*
   (a) Lesional skin biopsy for H&E, with peri-lesional skin for direct immuno-fluorescence (DIF)
   (b) Wound swab
   (c) Blood glucose
   (d) Blood cultures
   (e) Chest X-ray
3. *His acute management should include all the following except:*
   (a) Involvement of the 'Care of the elderly' medical team
   (b) Intravenous antibiotics
   (c) Systemic steroids
   (d) Potassium permanganate soaks
   (e) Ciclosporin

Case 17: A patient with itching and diarrhoea

A 56-year-old Irish man is referred to outpatient clinic with a 2-year history of itching. He also complains of recent onset diarrhoea and is now awaiting gastroenterology review. Physical examination demonstrates the presence of small herpetiform blisters, distributed symmetrically on his elbows, knees and buttocks.

1. *The most likely diagnosis is:*
   (a) Scabies
   (b) Dermatitis herpertiformis (DH)
   (c) Drug-induced bullous pemphigoid
   (d) Linear IgA bullous disease
   (e) Porphyria cutanea tarda
2. *DH is suspected. Which simple non-invasive test should you do next?*
   (a) Skin scrapings for scabetic mites
   (b) Tissue transglutaminase levels
   (c) Serum, urine and faecal porphyrin levels
   (d) Full blood count
   (e) Serum iron, folate and vitamin B_{12} levels
3. *A lesional and peri-lesional skin biopsy is undertaken for both H&E and direct immunofluorescence (DIF) stains. Findings in keeping with DH on H&E is the:*
   (a) Presence of a sub-epidermal blister with eosinophils
   (b) Presence of a cell-poor sub-epidermal blister
   (c) Presence of a sub-epidermal blister with dermal papillary microabscesses
   (d) Festooning of the dermal papillae
   (e) Significant epidermal necrosis
4. *The patient is also reviewed by the gastroenterology team who confirm the presence of subtotal villous atrophy in keeping with coeliac disease. Your management approach should include:*
   (a) Institution of a gluten-free diet only
   (b) The use of antihistamines only
   (c) The use of dapsone only
   (d) Institute a gluten-free diet and commence dapsone
   (e) Topical steroids only

Case 18: A patient with targetoid lesions on the hands and feet

A 20-year-old woman presents with targetoid lesions on her hands and feet. She has no mucosal involvement. The clinical features are in keeping with erythema multiforme (EM).

1. *The following conditions all typically involve acral surfaces except:*
   (a) Erythema multiforme
   (b) Syphilis
   (c) Pityriasis rosea
   (d) Dermatomyositis
   (e) Perniosis
2. *Causes of EM include all the following except:*
   (a) Staphylococcus aureus
   (b) Herpes simplex virus
   (c) Streptococci
   (d) Drugs
   (e) Autoimmune diseases
3. *Further questioning reveals that the patient has been commenced on Septrin 3 days ago. What is your next approach?*
   (a) Start on empirical aciclovir
   (b) Perform an antistreptolysin (ASO) titre
   (c) Do an autoimmune screen
   (d) Stop the Septrin
   (e) None of the above

Dermatology: Answers

Case 1: A patient with an itchy skin eruption

1. (c) Phone the GP to find out the name of the new antihypertensive drug

All are indicated but (c) is the most important. The patient is ill with erythroderma with pustulosis. Blistering and tissue loss are suspected and high-output cardiac failure threatened. This is a dermatological emergency. The differential diagnosis is extensive and the management difficult. Although a dermatological opinion is needed the patient must be hospitalized, intravenous access obtained, fluid balance established, glucose monitored and the medical and dermatological differential diagnosis explored: all from a hospital bed.

2. (b) Skin biopsy

All are indicated but (b) is the most important, to address the dermatological differential diagnosis of erythrodermic pustular psoriasis, drug-induced exfoliative dermatitis, toxic epidermal necrolysis, staphylococcal scalded skin syndrome, cutaneous T cell lymphoma.

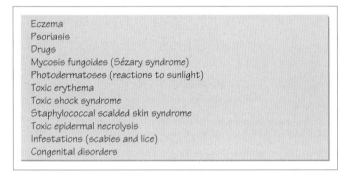

Eczema
Psoriasis
Drugs
Mycosis fungoides (Sézary syndrome)
Photodermatoses (reactions to sunlight)
Toxic erythema
Toxic shock syndrome
Staphylococcal scalded skin syndrome
Toxic epidermal necrolysis
Infestations (scabies and lice)
Congenital disorders

Figure 12.1.1 Causes of erythroderma.

3. (e) Cessation of all presenting medication

All *might* be considered but (e) is essential if TEN is suspected because this is usually drug induced. Intramuscular methotrexate might be indicated if the expert dermatological advice was that this is psoriasis (perhaps destabilized by intercurrent infection and the new antihypertensive (possibly a β-blocker) but an expectant policy would probably be followed for a day or two with bed rest, fluid balance and drug withdrawal. Potent topical steroids are contraindicated if unstable pustular psoriasis is suspected. Topical scabicides should only be given if scabies is unequivocally confirmed because they are highly irritant and would only worsen an already parlous cutaneous situation.

After five days in hospital the clinical presentation, results of investigations, course and response to treatment point to a diagnosis of *pustular psoriasis. Staphylococcus aureus* was grown from skin swabs at presentation. He is eventually discharged after 3 weeks on weekly methotrexate, daily folic acid, oral amlodipine glicazide and simvastatin: he was confirmed also to have diabetes mellitus and simple hyperlipidaemia.

4. (c) Regular haemoglobin, blood count, U&Es and liver function tests

All are important except (e) which is unlikely to be indicated. The patient has the metabolic syndrome where hyperlipidaemia, diabetes and atherosclerosis are associated with the chronic inflammatory state of psoriasis. Although alcohol and methotrexate are contraindications it is unlikely that this patient will need to be on methotrexate for more than a few months so monitoring for toxicity in the immediate to short term is the most important imperative, i.e. (c) is the answer.

Further reading: Chapter 69 in Medicine at a Glance.

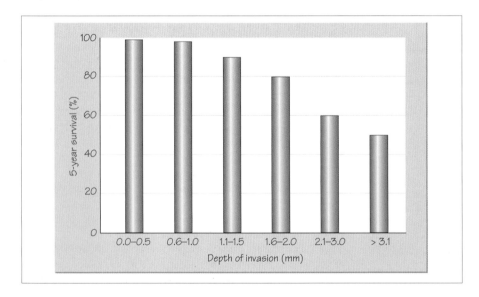

Figure 12.2.1 Outcome in malignant melanoma related to depth of skin invasion.

Case 2: A patient with a pigmented lesion on her arm

1. (a) Immediate excision of suspected melanoma

All are wrong save (a). Unless you can make an unequivocal diagnosis of a named benign lesion such as naevus, basal cell papilloma/seborrheic keratosis, histiocytoma/dermatofibroma, angioma, pyogenic granuloma, viral wart, molluscum, then new and changing skin lesions presenting in this way (often in real life less blatantly) *must* be excised and sent for histology.

2. (d) 1-cm wide re-excision of the forearm scar

Whilst (a), (b), and (c) *might* be done, both (d) and (e) are mandatory. Under the circumstances above the re-excision could predate the MDT whilst the others might be debated. Options (a) and (c) are probably unnecessary. Option (b) possibly could be omitted.

3. (b) 90% 5-year survival

This is the figure usually quoted for this Breslow thickness although the presence of ulceration is a indicator of worse prognosis. There is a 1/10 risk of a second melanoma.

4. (c) Superficial spreading melanoma/dysplastic nevus syndrome

Option (a) is not wrong but it is inadequate. Option (b) is a tautology: there is no such entity as a benign melanoma. Option (d) is wrong because all of the evidence from the history and signs point to (c). She and both parents were Scottish (celtic); the aunt was subsequently learnt to have died from cerebral metastasis of occult melanoma (5% of melanoma in oncological practice presents with no identifiable primary). Hutchinson's freckle (lentigo maligna melanoma) presents with a preceding history of a long-standing slowly changing freckle-like lesion in the elderly.

Further reading: Chapter 223.

Case 3: A patient with a pruritic rash

1. (d) Scabetic burrows

Generalized pruritus may be associated with iron deficiency anaemia, hyperthyroidism, systemic lymphomas and mastocytosis. However, in this clinical scenario, scabies is the most likely diagnosis for several reasons. First, the patient has a close personal contact that is also itchy. Second, he works in a nursing home and is likely to come into contact with people who may also have scabies. Finally, he has genital involvement, a site that is typically involved in scabetic infestations. Thus, it is important to search for scabetic burrows during his physical examination and a dermatoscope can aid in this quest.

2. (a) Isolation and visualization of a mite from infected sites

Isolation and visualization of a mite from infected sites is a simple bedside test that can be used to confirm the diagnosis of scabies. The mite is usually seen as a dark dot at one end of a burrow and various techniques can be used to extract this mite. Skin biopsies are time consuming and they do not always demonstrate the mite. There are no serological tests in humans for identification of the scabetic mite. PCR based testing is time consuming and not a first-line investigation.

3. (e) All of the above

All the above agents may be used for the treatment of scabies.

4. (e) All of the above

All the above are equally relevant and should be discussed with the patient prior to initiation of therapy. A simple information leaflet to re-enforce this information is desirable.

Further reading: Chapter 221.

Case 4: A child with hair loss

1. (c) Examination of scales from scalp by microscopy and culture

In children, tinea capitis can manifest as hair loss with/without cervical lymphadenopathy. Thus, the most likely diagnosis in this boy is tinea capitis and this should be confirmed with a simple non-invasive test, notably scalp scrapings for mycology.

2. (b) Oral terbinafine

Oral terbinafine. The *British National Formulary* (*BNF*) recommends using this agent over a 4-week interval. This oral therapy may be combined with 2% ketoconazole shampoo. It is important that repeat scalp scrapings are undertaken once the treatment is completed.

3. (b) The hair loss is usually reversible following adequate treatment of the child

This has significance in how one manages these children.

Further reading: Chapter 70.

Case 5: A patient with a chronic ulcer

1. (c) Venous ulcer

All the above are causes of leg ulceration, however chronic venous insufficiency is more likely to be a cause of her leg ulcer in view of the site of the ulcer and the history of a deep venous thrombosis involving that leg. It is worthwhile noting that venous ulcers account for 95% of ulcers above the medial malleolus.

2. (a) Concurrent cellulitis

All the above factors can cause problems with healing of leg ulcers. However, given the tenderness, erythema and warmth of the surrounding skin, the most likely cause for her current deterioration is the presence of cellulitis (a).

3. (e) Blood cultures

Although all the investigations above may be undertaken during this admission, it is imperative that blood cultures (e) are obtained prior to initiating antibiotic treatment.

4. (e) Topical steroids

All are relevant except for (e). A rectal examination is warranted on all patients with cellulitis to exclude obstruction of their lymphatic system due to an underlying malignant process. The initial source of the cellulitis may be from any untreated tinea pedis. It is important that the interdigital webs of the feet of all patients with cellulitis are examined thoroughly and appropriate treatment given for this. Intravenous antibiotics, such as benzylpenicillin and flucloxacillin are warranted in this setting. Potassium permanganate soaks can be applied to the infected venous ulcer. Topical steroids do not have a role in the acute management of this patient.

Further reading: Chapter 71.

Case 6: A patient with blisters on the backs of the hands

1. (a) Hypertrichosis

In this setting the most likely cause of the blisters is porphyria cutanea tarda (PCT), which is associated with hypertrichosis. All the other physical findings will be seen in the setting of chronic liver disease.

2. (c) Uroporphyrinogen decarboxylase

PCT occurs as a result of a deficiency of uroporphyrinogen decarboxylase. Protoporphyrinogen oxidase deficiency occurs in variegate porphyria, porphobilinogen deaminase deficiency in acute intermittent porphyria, uroporphyrinogen III synthase deficiency in congenital erythropoietic porphyria and coproporphyrinogen oxidase deficiency in hereditary coproporphyria.

3. (e) Uroporphyrin III in urine and faeces

PCT occurs as a result of a deficiency of uroporphyrinogen decarboxylase activity. The only conclusive test will be to demonstrate the presence of uroporphyrin III in urine and faeces.

4. (c) Systemic steroids

All the aforementioned suggestions are relevant in managing this patient with the exception of the use of systemic steroids (c). The latter does not have a role in the management of PCT.

Further reading: Chapter 72.

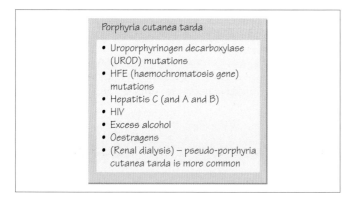

Figure 12.6.1 Causes of porphyria cutanea tarda.

Case 7: A patient with atopic dermatitis and worsening itch and rash

1. (a) Blood cultures

All are not without relevance but (a) is the most important because she is probably septic and requires intravenous antibiotics, so the blood cultures must be obtained straight away. The IgE estimation is not going to change the acute emergency management. All acute dermatological admissions should be HIV tested.

2. (a) Intravenous aciclovir

Intravenous aciclovir (or equivalent) i.e. (a) is indicated because eczema herpeticum is highly likely to be the diagnostic scenario. The other options *might* just possibly be indicated but are not mandatory.

3. (d) Long-term oral prednisolone

All are tenable save (d). Although there is a good case for short- to medium-term systemic steroids in unstable AD they are contraindicated for long-term use because of their well known dangerous side effects and the availability of safer more effective options. A single admission with eczema herpeticum having been acceptably stable for years is not an immediate indication for second-line treatment (e.g. azathioprine or ciclosporin).

Further reading: Chapter 216.

Case 8: A patient with recurrent hives

1. (a) Lesions lasting more than 24 hours and resolving with post-inflammatory hyperpigmentation

Urticated lesions lasting for more than 24 hours and resolving with post-inflammatory hyperpigmentation are cardinal features of urticarial vasculitis.

2. (a) Leukocytoclastic vasculitis

The histological features of urticaria are those of a 'dermal hypersensitivity reaction'. In this setting, a peri-vascular lymphocytic infiltrate, with scattered eosinophils and papillary dermal oedema is present. In contrast, urticarial vasculitis may show additional features of a leukocytoclastic vascuilitis. This is most likely if an early lesion is biopsied.

3. (e) Total IgE levels

All the investigations are warranted in the setting of urticarial vasculitis except for (e). The latter test is usually obtained for confirmation of atopic diathesis.

4. (e) Acitretin

All the drugs may be used for managing urticarial vasculitis except for acitretin, which has no pharmacological basis for use in this setting. In particular, given its teratogenicity, acitretin should generally be avoided in women of child-bearing age if possible. Systemic steroids have associated side effects and for this reason, steroid-sparing agents may be used instead.

Further reading: Chapter 216.

Case 9: A patient with hand eczema

1. (c) Irritant contact dermatitis occurring on a background of atopic diathesis

This is a common scenario that is seen in clinical practice. This young woman, following the birth of her child, is now undertaking more domestic duties. She has now developed irritant contact dermatitis in the setting of her atopic diathesis.

Physical examination shows lichenification on the dorsal aspects of both hands. In particular, she has eczema involving her interdigital webs and on sites under her wedding ring.

2. (d) Irritant contact dermatitis

These aforementioned sites are typically involved in cases of irritant contact dermatitis.

3. (d) Exclusion diet

Broadly speaking, dietary factors are not relevant in the pathogenesis of adult eczema. All the other aforementioned management strategies are relevant in this setting.

Further reading: Chapter 216.

Case 10: A patient with a psoriasiform rash

1. (e) Atopic eczema

All are relevant in this setting except for atopic eczema, which classically affects flexural sites, in the setting of an atopic diathesis.

2. (b) Antistreptolysin (ASO) titres

Given the history of a recent sore throat, ASO titres are warranted. This is relevant as streptococcal infections can trigger guttate psoriasis. Although not part of the patient's acute management, if there is strong clinical suspicion of HIV infection, repeating his serological tests after a 3-month interval is warranted. Current research indicates that patients with psoriasis are at a higher risk for cardiovascular disease. For this reason, it would be prudent to check this patient's serum glucose and cholesterol sometime in the near future.

3. (e) TLO1 phototherapy (narrow band UV-B)

All are treatment options for psoriasis. In guttate psoriasis spontaneous resolution occurs after a few months. However, TLO1 phototherapy may be used to help clear the cutaneous lesions.

4. (c) Advice to stop or reduce his alcohol intake and modify his cardiovascular risk factors

Alcohol can exacerbate psoriasis and he should be encouraged to stop or reduce his alcohol intake. Given the association between psoriasis and cardiovascular disease, his cardiovascular risk factors should be reviewed and modified appropriately. The use of phototherapy is associated with skin cancers. Thus, this treatment should be given under strict supervision to ensure cumulative ultraviolet light exposure is monitored.

Further reading: Chapter 217.

Case 11: A patient with acne

1. (e) No investigations

The uncomplicated scenario described requires no further investigations i.e. (e); these would only be required if prompted by specific gynaecological, endocrine, dermatological symptoms or signs or by other management choices.

2. (d) Augmentin

All would be reasonable except Augmentin (d).

3. (d) Start oral isotretinoin

Oral isotreinoin (d) is not indicated because maximal conventional medical therapy has not been exhibited and shown to have failed and she does not have nodulocystic acne or scarring.

4. (c) The patient must have a pregnancy test before treatment

The answer is (c) because isotretinoin is a teratogen. During treatment conception must not occur. Isotretinoin cannot be started immediately because it interacts with tetracyclines (benign intracranial hypertension) so there must be a 'wash out' period. Doing a clotting screen, e.g. for Factor V Leiden deficiency is not a bad idea but not mandatory.

Further reading: Chapter 218.

Case 12: A patient with facial redness

1. (e) All of the above

All the aforementioned entities are in the differential diagnosis as a cause of the red face in this setting.

2. (c) Improvement with topical steroids

The symptoms of rosacea can be precipitated or worsened with intake of alcohol, spicy food and coffee. Ophthalmological symptoms and signs are common in individuals with rosacea. Topical steroids worsen rosacea and are not a treatment option for this condition.

3. (b) An oral antibiotic such as doxycycline

Given the clinical description, this patient is likely to have papulo-pustular rosacea. In view of this, an oral antibiotic should be part of her first-line management strategy. Hydroxychloroquine has no role in managing rosacea but is of use in cutaneous lupus erythematosus. The pulse dye laser may be used as an adjunct for managing the patient's telangiectasia. Elidel and isotretinoin are not first-line agents in this patient.

4. (c) She has a chronic disease, and will likely have flares when her systemic therapy is discontinued

Like most patients with rosacea, this woman has a chronic disease, and will likely have flares upon discontinuation of her systemic therapy. Alcohol can exacerbate symptoms and signs of rosacea, however if the patient stops drinking her rosacea will not be permanently cured.

Further reading: Chapter 218.

Case 13: A patient with café-au-lait macules

1. (e) All the above

Café-au-lait macules are circumscribed melanotic macules. They may be seen in normal neonates at birth (up to 2% of all newborns have one or more of these pigmented lesions) but their occurrence may be a stigmata of an associated syndrome. A clinician should be alert to this possibility based on the number and size of the café-au-lait macules, and the presence of other stigmata of the syndrome. Most physicians are aware of the association of NF and café-au-lait macules, but these macules may be seen in

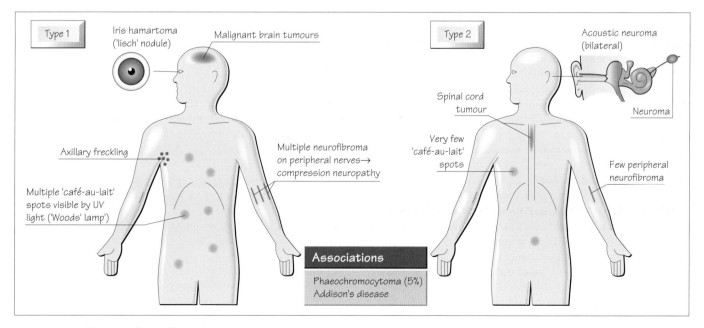

Figure 12.13.1 Features of neurofibromatosis.

other genodermatoses (e.g. McCune–Albright syndrome and tuberous sclerosis).

2. (a) Axillary freckling

The clinical information given on this young boy is in keeping with a diagnosis of neurofibromatosis (NF) type 1. Thus, another physical finding to look out for is the presence of axillary freckling. Mucocutaneous pigmented macules are seen in the setting of Peutz–Jeghers syndrome. Cutaneous myxomas may be seen in the setting of Carney's complex. There are many causes of hypomelanotic macules but ash-leaf macules are seen in the setting of tuberous sclerosis. Finally angiokeratoma corporis diffusum is seen in the setting of inherited metabolic disorders (e.g. Fabry's disease).

3. (b) Ophthalmological assessment

Ophthalmological assessment for the presence of Lisch nodules should be undertaken. In addition he should have his blood pressure monitored on a regular basis as hypertension is a feature of NF type 1. This can be essential hypertension or secondary to renal artery stenosis or the presence of phaeochromocytoma. The rest of the aforementioned investigations are not relevant in this setting.

4. (e) All the above

All the above are part of the clinical manifestation of NF type 1.

Further reading: Chapters 201 and 219.

Case 14: A patient with de-pigmented patches

1. (d) Personal and/or family history of autoimmune disease

All are relevant aspects of the history taking. However, given the association of vitiligo and other autoimmune diseases, it is important to clarify if there is a personal or family history of any autoimmune disorders.

2. (c) Approach this issue in a tactful manner and suggest to him that he may benefit from a referral to a psychologist/ psychiatrist

This is a difficult situation to manage in a general clinic. Nonetheless, it must be addressed, given that there is no cure for vitiligo. An approach in this situation is to encourage the patient to acknowledge that there is a mental health problem, although it is exogenous and in response to his physical condition. It could then be suggested to him that he would benefit from a referral to a psychologist or psychiatrist for their input. It is also worthwhile supplying him with written information about vitiligo and about patient support groups. It is also important to inform his GP of the situation and the outcome of your discussions with the patient.

3. (e) All of the above

All the above have been used for vitiligo with variable success.

4. (a) Phototherapy

In view of the wide area of distribution of his vitiligo, topical agents are not suitable. Furthermore, he has used high potency steroids already with minimal effect. If he is keen to have some sort of treatment, referral for phototherapy is indicated. It is important to inform the patient that re-pigmentation occurs initially around the follicles and for this reason it may look patchy. Furthermore, it is likely that he will need more than one course of phototherapy. Obviously the side effects of phototherapy should be discussed with him at length before initiating this treatment.

Further reading: Chapter 219.

Case 15: A patient with skin darkening on the face and hands

1. (b) Oral contraceptive

All these drugs can cause hyperpigmentaion possibly due to photosensitivity as hinted by the brief case history and it is not impossible that he might be taking all of them except (b). Other drugs that can cause dyspigmentation of the skin not listed above include phenytoin, anti-malarials and anti-tumour agents, such as busulfan and doxorubicin.

2. (e) All of the above

All the above mechanisms are relevant in drug-induced pigmentation of the skin.

3. (e) All of the above

All have been observed as side effects of chlorpromazine.

4. (a) Stop the culprit drug if feasible

If feasible it is important to stop the culprit drug, notably chlorpromazine. This must be done in conjunction with the patient's psychiatrists and an alternative drug instituted. Avoid prescribing de-pigmenting agents for symptomatic treatment of the hyperpigmentation since they can be associated with a range of side effects, e.g. exogenous ochronosis-induced topical hydroquinone.

Further reading: Chapter 219.

Case 16: An elderly patient with generalized skin blisters

1. (c) Bullous pemphigoid (BP)

Given the age of the patient and the presence of tense blisters and urticated plaques, the most likely diagnosis is BP. Prior to labelling a patient with idiopathic BP, a drug aetiology must be excluded.

2. (a) Lesional skin biopsy for H&E, with peri-lesional skin for direct immuno-fluorescence (DIF)

In BP, lesional skin biopsy shows a sub-epidermal blister with eosinophils. DIF demonstrates the presence of IgG and C3 at the dermal-epidermal junction. The rest of the aforementioned investigations are important as part of his overall management. In particular, chest X-ray is required to rule out a chest infection and/ or underlying malignant process. This is because there may be an association of BP and malignancy.

	Bullous pemphigoid	Pemphigus vulgaris	Dermatitis herpetiformis
Incidence	Common	Rare	Very rare
Age	Elderly	40–50 years	Young adults Elderly
Antibody attack target	Basement membrane hemidesmosome	Inter-epidermal cell desmosomal structure	Not characterized
Diagnosis	Biopsy	Biopsy Serum antibodies	Biopsy (skin and gut) Demonstration of villous atrophy
Treatment	Topical steroid Prednisolone 40–60 mg/day	Topical steroid Prednisolone 80–120 mg/day	Topical steroid Dapsone Gluten-free diet
Underlying malignancy	Possible	Rarely	GI Lymphoma risk
Prognosis	Excellent	Variable	Good

Figure 12.16.1 Features of common blistering skin diseases.

3. (e) Ciclosporin

It is important to involve a general/care of elderly physician in his management. While the pyrexia may be due to a superadded skin infection, this gentleman has had a previous CVA and is at risk for pneumonia, which should be excluded. In view of the ulcerated skin, he is at risk for fluid and electrolyte imbalance and he will need strict fluid balance charts. Systemic steroids should be started to control the blisters and appropriate antibiotics given to cover any potential cutaneous infections, while awaiting the swab results. Microbiological advice can be sought. The ulcerated areas may be treated with potassium permanganate soaks and the tense blisters can be carefully punctured using a sterile needle. The use of ciclosporin has no role in his acute management.

Further reading: Chapter 220.

Case 17: A patient with itching and diarrhoea

1. (b) Dermatitis herpertiformis (DH)

The clinical features are in keeping with DH.

2. (b) Tissue transglutaminase levels

Tissue transglutaminsae are the autoantigens of endomysial antibodies. Elevated serum tissue transglutaminase levels are seen in DH.

3. (c) Presence of a sub-epidermal blister with dermal papillary microabscesses

A collection of neutrophils in the dermal papilla may be seen in DH, in association with a sub-epidermal blister. Similar histo-logical findings are also seen in linear IgA disease and bullous LE. DIF in DH shows characteristic granular deposition of IgA at the dermal-epidermal junction.

4. (d) Institute a gluten-free diet and commence dapsone

Typically the patient starts a gluten-free diet and also com-mences on dapsone. Ensure glucose-6-phosphate dehydrogenase (G6PD) levels are checked before commencing on dapsone therapy to identify patients at risk of haemolytic anaemia.

Further reading: Chapters 124 and 220.

Case 18: A patient with targetoid lesions on the hands and feet

1. (c) Pityriasis rosea

This often involves the trunk and the individual lesions are distributed in a 'Christmas tree' pattern

2. (a) Staphylococcus aureus

It is important to be familiar with the associations of erythema multiforme (EM). Please do remember that in about 50% of cases no underlying cause is found.

3. (d) Stop the Septrin

The potential drug associated with EM should be stopped as soon as possible. The main concern is progression to EM major and/or toxic epidermal necrolysis (TEN) if the drug is continued. Topical steroids can be used on the rash, however there is no evidence that systemic steroids affect the overall prognosis.

Further reading: Chapter 224.

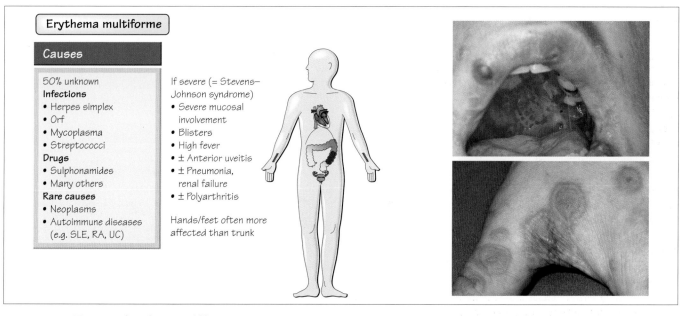

Figure 12.18.1 Features of erythema multiforme.

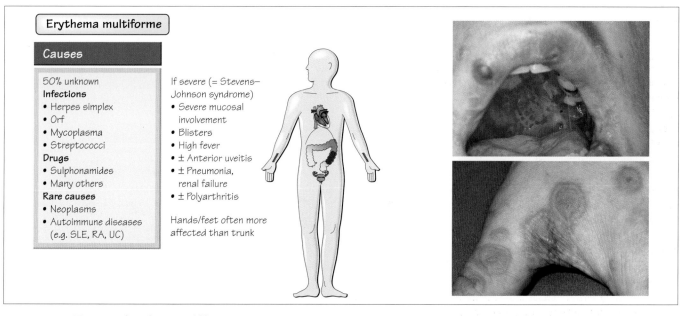

Other Emergencies: Cases and Questions

Case 1: A patient with dyspnoea and weight loss

A 58-year-old smoker presents to his GP with a 6-month history of progressive dyspnoea and weight loss. On talking to the patient it is noticed that he has a hoarse voice, which he says has been present for 3 months and he also admits to several episodes of haemoptysis. The GP is worried about the patient's appearance as he has lost 3 stone in weight since his last visit and is breathless at rest. He is referred to the acute medical take where a chest X-ray is performed. This demonstrates large bilateral effusions and nodules in both lung fields.

On examination the patient has a respiratory rate of 32 breaths/min, oxygen saturations of 88% on air and stony dullness at both bases. He is cachectic with a 4-finger breadth firm liver. The only other finding is that his right calf is warm and swollen with pitting oedema. The patient says that this has been present for approximately one week.

1. *What is the primary diagnosis?*
   (a) Tuberculosis
   (b) Community-acquired pneumonia
   (c) Carcinoma of the lung with metastasis
   (d) Wegener's granulomatosis
2. *How could the diagnosis be most easily confirmed?*

   (a) Computerized tomography (CT) scan
   (b) Bronchoscopy
   (c) Liver biopsy
   (d) Sending pleural fluid cytology or pleural biopsy
3. *Which of the following biochemical features are common in malignant pleural effusions?*
   (a) pH < 7.3
   (b) Blood
   (c) Exudate
   (d) Glucose <3.3 mmol/L
   (e) All of the above
4. *What are the MET teams' priorities in treating the patient?*
   (a) Immediate intubation and mechanical ventilation
   (b) Rapid infusion of intravenous fluid
   (c) Thrombolysis
   (d) Inform the patient's Consultant who should discuss palliation with the family

Case 2: A patient with abdominal pain and weight loss

A 72-year-old woman presents with a 2-month history of intermittent abdominal pain and weight loss of around half a stone which she attributes to poor appetite. She has noticed over this period of

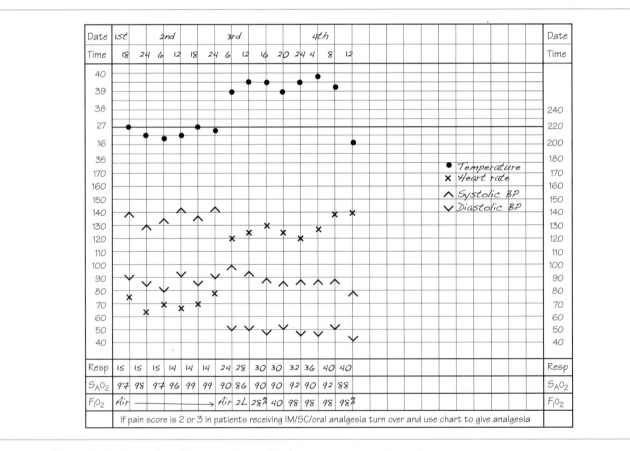

Figure 13.2.1 The patient's observation chart.

time that she has been more constipated, which she had put down to eating less. Her GP has referred her to A&E on Friday afternoon because the pain is worse in the last 24 hours and she is unable to keep anything down. She appears to be in pain and is vomiting. On examination her heart rate is 76 beats/min in sinus rhythm with a BP of 140/90 mmHg. Respiratory rate is recorded at 15 breaths/min and oxygen saturations are 99% on air. She is alert and orientated and able to give a good history of events. The abdomen appears distended and she is unsure when she last had her bowels open. Bowel sounds are present and there is no guarding or rebound. There is a suggestion of mass in the left iliac fossa. A nasogastric tube is inserted and the patient commenced on intravenous fluids. A CT scan is booked to investigate the abdominal findings further. The patient continues with fluid therapy over the weekend and analgesia in the form of morphine. She requires increasing amounts of analgesia as the pain is getting worse. You are called on the Monday morning by the ward staff as they are worried about her going down for her CT as she is 'unwell'. Her observation chart is shown in Fig. 13.2.1. On examining her abdomen there is evidence of guarding and rebound. She has become breathless and a chest X-ray is performed which shows air under the diaphragm.

1. *What is the diagnosis when you review the patient?*
   (a) Pancreatitis
   (b) Peritonitis
   (c) Cholecystitis
   (d) Leaking abdominal aneurysm
2. *When did the patient show signs that she was developing critical illness? (Fig. 13.2.1)*
   (a) 08.00 on the 4th (Monday)
   (b) Midnight on the 3rd
   (c) Midnight on the 2nd
   (d) 06.00 on the 3rd
3. *What are the priorities in managing the patient?*
   (a) Fluid resuscitate and transfer to CT
   (b) Fluid resuscitate, intubate and transfer to CT
   (c) Transfer to Intensive Care and start vasopressors for hypotension
   (d) Fluid resuscitate and transfer immediately to the operating theatre for a laparotomy
4. *Which of the following is most frequently abnormal in critical illness?*
   (a) Heart rate
   (b) Oxygen saturations

(c) Inspired oxygen concentration
(d) Respiratory rate

Case 3: A patient who has bumped his head getting out of the car

A 65-year-old man with a history of heavy alcohol consumption bumps his head getting out of the car. There is a small laceration on the left side of his head, which is bleeding profusely. He attends A&E for suturing of the cut. There was no history of loss of consciousness and the patient has no focal neurology. The patient complained that he had lost a lot of blood and so the casualty doctor performs a full blood count, which demonstrates a normal haemoglobin of 14.1 g/dL. The patient is discharged home with a head injury information sheet. He returns 2 weeks later in the company of his wife. He has not been feeling himself and complains of headache, nausea and vomiting. You are called to assess the patient. He is unsure of where he is and does not know which day of the week or year it is. He is sitting with his eyes open and his pupils appear normal. The patient will perform all the tasks you require of him to perform the examination. You notice some weakness on his right side, which is contralateral to the laceration, which is healing well. Oxygen saturations are 98% on air, respiratory rate is 16 breaths/minute, pulse 70 beats/min in sinus rhythm and BP 130/75 mmHg.

1. *Using the Glasgow Coma Score (GCS) work out the patient's score when he is examined (Fig. 13.3.1).*
   (a) 15
   (b) 14
   (c) 10
   (d) 2
2. *What blood test is mandatory to perform?*
   (a) Full blood count
   (b) Liver function tests
   (c) C-reactive protein (CRP)
   (d) Glucose

The patient suffers a generalized seizure lasting approximately 30 seconds. A nurse performs a blood glucose, which is 6.5 mmol/L. The patient is using inappropriate words, which make no sense. He will not open his eyes, even to a painful stimulus, but does flex his left arm to supra-orbital pressure. There is no motor response on the right. Pupils are midpoint and reactive to light.

3. *What is the patient's GCS now?*
   (a) 14
   (b) 7

Eyes open		Best verbal response		Best motor response	
Spontaneously	(4)	Orientated	(5)	Obeys commands	(6)
To speech	(3)	Confused	(4)	Localizes pain	(5)
To pain	(2)	Inappropriate words	(3)	Withdraws to pain	(4)
None	(1)	Incomprehensible sounds	(2)	Flexion (abnormal) to pain	(3)
		None	(1)	Extension to pain	(2)
				None	(1)
Glasgow coma scale = [ ]					

Figure 13.3.1 Glasgow coma scale.

(c) 8

(d) 10

4. *What are the priorities in assessing and treating the patient?*

 (a) Apply an ABCDE approach

 (b) Give an anti-epileptic drug immediately

 (c) Perform a CT immediately

 (d) Check a blood alcohol level

5. *What is the likely diagnosis?*

 (a) The patient is now an epileptic following the bump on his head

 (b) He is septic

 (c) Subdural haematoma

 (d) The patient has suffered a stroke (CVA)

Case 4: A patient who has taken a drug overdose

A 23-year-old woman is brought into A&E drowsy and appears confused. She had been found at home by her boyfriend with an empty bottle of vodka and some empty packets of medicines. He had only been out of the house for 1 hour and once he'd found her he'd brought her straight to A&E. He says she was feeling low after the death of her grandmother. Her BP is 90/60 mmHg, respiratory rate 10 breaths/min. Oxygen saturations are 94% on air. Her pupils are very small and non-reactive.

1. *What is the most likely cause of her pinpoint pupils?*

 (a) Alcohol intoxication

 (b) Opiate overdose

 (c) Tricyclic overdose

 (d) Benzodiazepine overdose

The patient's boyfriend does not know what the medicine packets were and did not bring them with him. He thinks she may have found them among her grandmother's things. He knows her grandmother had been taking painkillers for arthritis and had 'kidney problems'.

2. *What other blood tests should be done?*

 (a) Paracetamol levels

 (b) Opiate levels

 (c) Tricyclic levels

She is given a specific agent to reverse the poisoning intravenously, and 2 minutes later she sits up, sweaty and agitated, and seems to be hyperventilating, with large pupils. She asks to leave the department, and has to be restrained. Thirty minutes later she starts to become drowsy again.

3. *What was the agent she was given?*

 (a) Flumazenil

 (b) N-acetylcysteine

 (c) Glucagon

 (d) Naloxone

4. *What other immediate treatment may be indicated in this case?*

 (a) Activated charcoal with lactulose

 (b) Gastric lavage

 (c) Salt water emesis

 (d) Forced alkaline diuresis

Case 5: A patient who has taken a drug overdose

A 25-year-old man presents to A&E saying he has taken an overdose. He is well known to the department and to psychiatric services, as he often claims to have overdosed. In fact, he was here yesterday having taken a paracetamol overdose that did not require treatment. He is known to be a heavy drinker and is thought to have a personality disorder. He claims to have taken 20 paracetamol tablets. He lives alone, and brings his suicide note with him, saying he has now changed his mind.

1. *Which of the following factors are associated with a lower chance of completed suicide?*

 (a) Male gender

 (b) Personality disorder

 (c) Living alone

 (d) Previous attempts

 (e) Alcoholism

 (f) Age under 40

2. *The patient's paracetamol level now is 90 mg/L. He says he took the tablets 4 hours ago. This is below the high-risk treatment line found in the* British National Forumulary (BNF). *What factor might make you want to treat him anyway?*

 (a) He is alcoholic

 (b) He is malnourished

 (c) He has taken other paracetamol overdoses recently

 (d) He has been taking St John's Wort

3. *You ask for some blood tests prior to initiating treatment. Which of the following do you not need to request?*

 (a) 6-hour paracetamol levels

 (b) Liver function tests

 (c) International normalized ratio (INR)

 (d) Renal function tests

4. *He declines treatment and leaves the department without telling anyone. He cannot be found at home or work and is not contactable. His friend brings him to see his GP two days later complaining of abdominal pain and nausea. He looks jaundiced. What is the best course of action?*

 (a) Section him under Section 2 of the Mental Health Act, for treatment of his liver failure

 (b) Repeat the blood tests and ask him to come back the next day

 (c) Start an infusion of methionine in the surgery

 (d) Give an oral dose of acetylcysteine and transfer to A&E

 (e) Arrange immediate admission

5. *The following have all been proposed measures to reduce the death rate from poisoning. Which of the following has not been implemented, however?*

 (a) Restriction of maximal amount of paracetamol that can be bought at one time

 (b) Withdrawal of co-proxamol tablets (a combination of dextropropoxyphene, a weak opiate, and paracetamol)

 (c) Addition of the orally active paracetamol antidote methionine to all paracetamol-containing tablets

 (d) Encouraging doctors to prescribe selective serotonin reuptake inhibitors (SSRIs) rather than tricyclic antidepressants as first-line in depression in older adults

Case 6: A patient with acute confusional state

A 47-year-old construction worker was brought to hospital by his family. Five days previously he had begun to behave oddly, and his answers to questions had become increasingly muddled and confused. He had complained of a sore throat and a mild head-ache. He was taking no medication and had been previously well. He drinks around 70 units of alcohol a week.

1. *The least likely cause of his confusional state is:*
   (a) Severe hyponatraemia
   (b) Viral encephalitis
   (c) Infective endocarditis
   (d) Primary brain tumour

During examination the patient is alert but has confused speech. He is co-operative with the examination.

Vital signs are:

Pulse	68 beats/min
BP	150/88 mmHg
Respiratory rate	18 breaths/min
Oxygen saturation	96% on air
Temperature	37.7°C
Blood glucose	8.3 mmol/L

He has no jaundice, rash or lymphadenopathy; cardiovascular, respiratory and abdominal examination are all normal. There is no neck stiffness or focal neurological signs and fundi are normal. Urinalysis show 3+ protein and 2+ blood.

2. *The examination findings exclude:*
   (a) Viral encephalitis
   (b) Pneumonia
   (c) Infective endocarditis
   (d) Urinary tract infection

Blood tests showed:

Hb	14.3 g/dL
MCV	87 fL
WBC	21.3×10^9/L with neutrophilia
Platelets	298×10^9/L
CRP	281 mg/L
INR	1.2
APTT	34 sec (26–37)
Na	144 mmol/L
K	2.9 mmol/L
Creatinine	120 μmol/L
LFTs	normal

Blood and urine were sent for culture. Chest X-ray showed normal heart size and clear lungs.

3. *Which diagnosis is excluded by these results?*
   (a) Infective endocarditis
   (b) Cryptococcal meningitis
   (c) Viral encephalitis
   (d) Urinary tract infection
   (e) None of the above

4. *Which test should you do next?*
   (a) EEG
   (b) CT head
   (c) Echocardiography
   (d) Ultrasound of urinary tract

Case 7: A patient with acute confusional state

A 71-year-old woman was brought to hospital by her daughter with whom she lived. She had been increasingly unwell for 2 days, initially complaining of muscle aching, and then becoming agitated and confused. There was a background of type 2 diabetes, now treated with insulin, and chronic renal failure, for which she had started haemodialysis via a veno-venous catheter 3 months previously. She was taking over a dozen medications.

1. *The least likely cause of her confusional state is:*
   (a) Adverse effect of medications
   (b) Bacterial meningitis
   (c) Urinary tract infection
   (d) Severe hypothyroidism

Examination showed a restless elderly woman who was confused and poorly co-operative with examination.

Vital signs are:

Pulse	100 beats/min
BP	120/80 mmHg
Respiratory rate	28 breaths/min
Oxygen saturation	92% breathing air
Temperature	38.2°C
Blood glucose	22 mmol/L

Her score on the abbreviated mental test was 2/10. There was no neck stiffness or focal neurological signs. The fundi appeared normal on limited views. The entry site of the dialysis catheter was healthy, with no erythema or discharge. A soft mid-systolic murmur was heard. There were sparse crackles at the lung bases. She was not jaundiced, and the abdomen was soft and non-tender.

2. *The least likely diagnosis, based on history and examination findings, is:*
   (a) Bacterial meningitis
   (b) Ascending cholangitis
   (c) Infective endocarditis
   (d) Pneumonia

Blood tests showed:

Hb	8.3 g/dL
MCV	95 fL
WBC	17.5×10^9/L with neutrophilia
Platelets	180×10^9/L
CRP	190 mg/L
INR	1.3
APTT	33 sec (26–37)
Na	144 mmol/L
K	3.9 mmol/L
Urea	25 mmol/L
Creatinine	200 μmol/L
Albumin	25 g/L
Bilirubin	28 μmol/L

On chest X-ray the heart size is normal and the lungs clear. There is a dialysis catheter *in situ*. Blood was drawn for culture, via the dialysis catheter and from a peripheral vein.

3. *The priority in management is:*
   (a) To start empirical broad-spectrum antibiotic therapy
   (b) To arrange EEG to exclude non-convulsive status epilepticus
   (c) To perform immediate lumbar puncture to exclude bacterial meningitis
   (d) To arrange immediate echocardiography to exclude infective endocarditis.

Antibiotic therapy was started with vancomycin and gentamicin. CT of the head showed a right frontal cerebral infarction that was considered to be old. Lumbar puncture yielded normal CSF. Blood drawn from both dialysis catheter and peripheral vein grew *Staphylococcus aureus*, sensitive to flucloxacillin.

4. *Investigation of the source of her bacteraemia requires:*
  (a) CT of abdomen and pelvis
  (b) Transthoracic echocardiography
  (c) MRI of the spine
  (d) None of the above

Case 8: A patient with progressive confusion

A 52-year-old warehouseman was brought to A&E by his wife. He had been unwell for 10 days with difficulty concentrating, disturbed sleep and progressive confusion. He had also complained of feeling thirsty. He had lost around 5 kg in weight over the past month. His health had previously been good and he was taking no regular medications. He drank around 40 units of alcohol a week, although had drunk more heavily in the past, and had smoked 20 cigarettes daily for 30 years.

1. *Which is the least likely diagnosis?*
  (a) Diabetic ketoacidosis
  (b) Liver failure
  (c) Respiratory failure
  (d) Renal failure

Examination showed a well nourished man who was confused and mildly drowsy. His GCS score was 13/15 (E3 M6 V4).

Vital signs are:

Pulse	80 beats/min
BP	120/80 mmHg
Respiratory rate	28 breaths/min
Oxygen saturation	94% breathing air
Temperature	37.2°C
Blood glucose	8 mmol/L

There was no neck stiffness or focal neurological signs, and fundoscopy was normal. There was no jaundice, lymphadenopathy or clubbing. The rest of the general examination was normal.

2. *Which of the following diagnoses do these examination findings exclude?*
  (a) Cerebral metastases
  (b) Viral encephalitis
  (c) Liver failure
  (d) Renal failure
  (e) None of the above

Blood tests showed:

Hb	14.3 g/dL
MCV	87 fL
WBC	11.5×10^9/L
Platelets	320×10^9/L
INR	1.2
APTT	28 sec (26–37)
Na	146 mmol/L
K	5.1 mmol/L
Corrected Ca	3.94 mmol/L
Creatinine	230 µmol/L

Liver function tests are normal, and on chest X-ray heart size was normal and the lungs clear.

3. *What is the most likely cause of his hypercalcaemia?*
  (a) Myeloma
  (b) Primary hyperparathyroidism
  (c) Sarcoidosis
  (d) Malignancy

4. *What should be the initial treatment of his hypercalcaemia?*

  (a) Oral fluid intake of 3 L/day
  (b) Intravenous saline
  (c) Haemodialysis
  (d) High-dose steroid

Case 9: A patient with coma

A 49-year-old man was brought to hospital in coma following a major seizure. According to his wife, he had complained of feeling unwell 7 days before admission, and then developed an occipital headache. He had attended A&E 2 days before admission when fever (39°C) was noted, but no other abnormal signs. A diagnosis of influenza was made. He went home to bed. His headache persisted despite regular paracetamol. On the day of admission he had been confused and had vomited, and then had a tonic-clonic seizure lasting 10–15 minutes, without regaining consciousness after this. He had travelled to Spain two months previously. His health was good and he took no regular medication. He was a non-smoker. He drank around 30 units of alcohol a week. Other family members were well.

1. *Which is the least likely diagnosis?*
  (a) Infective endocarditis
  (b) Bacterial meningitis
  (c) Acute liver failure
  (d) Subarachnoid haemorrhage

Examination showed an unresponsive man with a Glasgow Coma Score score of 7/15. (E2, M4, V1). There was no rash or jaundice.

Vital signs are:

Pulse	90 beats/min
BP	110/90 mmHg
Respiratory rate	24 breaths/min
Oxygen saturation	94% breathing air
Temperature	38.7°C
Blood glucose	8 mmol/L

There was mild neck stiffness. Pupillary responses were normal. Fundoscopy showed normal discs and no retinal haemorrhages. Tendon reflexes were symmetrical. The plantar responses were extensor. There were no focal neurological signs. There was a soft mid-systolic murmur. The lungs were clear and the abdomen was normal.

2. *The finding of bilateral extensor plantar responses:*
  (a) Indicates a structural brain lesion involving both corticospinal tracts
  (b) Rules out bacterial meningitis
  (c) Is an absolute contraindication to lumbar puncture
  (d) Is a transient finding after tonic-clonic seizure

Blood tests showed:

Hb	13.8 g/dL
MCV	92 fL
WBC	14.2×10^9/L, 82% neutrophils
Platelets	267×10^9/L
INR	1.2
APTT	34 sec (26–37)
Na	144 mmol/L
K	4.1 mmol/L
Creatinine	92 µmol/L
LFTs	Normal

Blood was sent for culture. On chest X-ray the heart size is normal and lungs are clear. CT head (without contrast) is normal, with no evidence of intracranial bleeding.

3. *The normal findings on CT exclude:*
   (a) Subarachnoid haemorrhage
   (b) Bacterial meningitis
   (c) Cerebellar infarction
   (d) Infective endocarditis
   (e) None of the above
4. *The next investigation should be:*
   (a) EEG
   (b) Lumbar puncture
   (c) Echocardiography
   (d) Toxicology screen

Case 10: A patient with coma

A 38-year-old man was found unconscious on a bench in a local park and given intravenous glucose by a paramedic, with no improvement in his conscious level. He was brought to hospital. Contact with his GP's surgery established that he was taking no prescribed medications and had not been seen there for 2 years. He was separated from his wife, and lived alone. He was a car mechanic and had been at work the previous day.

1. *The least likely cause of his coma is:*
   (a) Bacterial meningitis
   (b) Subarachnoid haemorrhage
   (c) Viral encephalitis
   (d) Acute liver failure

Examination showed no external signs of injury. He was unconscious with a Glasgow Coma Score score of 8 (E2, M4, V2).

Vital signs are:

Pulse	90 beats/min
BP	85/50 mmHg
Respiratory rate	36 breaths/min
Oxygen saturation	99% breathing 60% oxygen
Temperature	36.4°C
Blood glucose	12 mmol/L

There was no neck stiffness. Pupillary responses were normal and there were no focal neurological signs. Fundoscopy showed normal discs and no retinal haemorrhages. General examination was normal. There was no jaundice or rash. A bladder catheter was placed and drained clear urine.

2. *Which is the least likely diagnosis?*
   (a) Bacterial meningitis
   (b) Subarachnoid haemorrhage
   (c) Acute renal failure
   (d) Alcohol intoxication

Investigations showed:

Arterial blood gases/pH, breathing 60% oxygen

PO_2	17.5 kPa
PCO_2	3.1 kPa
pH	7.15

Blood tests showed:

Hb	16.3 g/dL
MCV	97 fL
WBC	22.5×10^9/L, 95% neutrophils
Platelets	320×10^9/L
INR	1.2
APTT	28 sec (26–37)
Na	146 mmol/L
K	5.1 mmol/L
Corrected Ca	2.20 mmol/L

Creatinine	230 µmol/L
LFTs	Normal
Glucose	9.5 mmol/L

ECG showed sinus rhythm with normal conduction, with normal QRS duration and QT interval. Chest X-ray showed heart size normal, and lungs clear.

3. *Which is the least likely cause of his metabolic acidosis?*
   (a) Tonic-clonic seizure prior to admission
   (b) Alcoholic ketoacidosis
   (c) Bacterial meningitis
   (d) Poisoning
4. *Which investigation is not needed as a priority?*
   (a) CT head, to exclude intracranial haemorrhage
   (b) Measurement of blood alcohol, paracetamol and salicylate levels
   (c) EEG, to exclude non-convulsive status epilepticus
   (d) Toxicological screen of urine

Case 11: A patient with bloody diarrhoea and pain

A 64-year-old man with ulcerative colitis (UC) is admitted to hospital with bloody diarrhoea and abdominal pain. He has been getting progressively more unwell over the previous 2 years with frequent episodes of severe colitis, which are becoming increasingly difficult to treat. He has been on ciclosporin for the last 12 months and has been taking 4 mg of prednisolone a day for the last week. Stool frequency is more than 10 per day, he has a high fever of 39°C. He is flushed and looks unwell. Capillary refill is prolonged at 5 seconds and jugular venous pressure is not visible. A tachycardia of 120 beats/min in sinus rhythm is recorded with a BP of 90/60 mmHg. Respiratory rate is 28 breaths/min with oxygen saturations of 94% on air, the lungs are clear. His abdomen is tender and he has guarding but no rebound. He appears unwell and a catheter is introduced; he passes 20 mL of urine for each of the following 2 hours. Routine blood tests show that he is: anaemic with a haemoglobin of 8 g/dL, Urea is raised at 18 mmol/L, creatinine is normal and CRP >200 mg/L.

He is given high-flow oxygen and an arterial blood gas performed:

pH	7.29
PaO_2	48 kPa
$PaCO_2$	3.2 kPa
HCO_3	15 mmol/L
Base excess	−8
SaO_2	100%
Lactate	4.1 mmol/L

1. *Which of the following are true?*
   (a) The patient has hypovolaemic shock
   (b) The patient has a respiratory acidosis
   (c) The patient has metabolic acidosis with respiratory compensation
   (d) The anaemia and raised urea are indications for upper GI endoscopy
2. *Which of the following should be given?*
   (a) 5% dextrose 1000 mL over 6 hours
   (b) Normal saline 1000 mL over 1 hour
   (c) 500 mL HAES-Steril over 10 minutes
   (d) 500 mL Hartmann's over 10 minutes

3. *The patient is given 4 L of fluid, his pulse is then 90 beats/min, BP 120/70 mmHg, respiratory rate 24 breaths/min and urine output increases to 50 mL/hour. A plain abdominal film shows a pancolitis, which is dilated to 12 cm. What treatment is indicated next?*

(a) Urgent total colectomy
(b) Pulsed methylprednisolone
(c) Broad-spectrum antibiotics
(d) Urgent cyclosporin levels

4. *The patient makes a full recovery and is seen 4 months later in the outpatient clinic. He is well and his only complaint is that he has developed intense itching. What might be the cause?*

(a) Extra-intestinal manifestation of UC
(b) Side effect of multiple steroid doses
(c) The patient was resuscitated with HAES-Steril
(d) The patient has developed a bowel cancer related to UC

Case 12: A patient with mild haematemesis

A 24-year-old woman with severe alcoholic liver disease and varices is admitted with mild haematemesis of about 100 mL of blood. She has a BP of 110/65 mmHg, but is otherwise haemodynamically stable. Her blood test results are as follows:

Hb	11.1 g/dL
WBC	8.1×10^9/L
Platelets	90×10^9/L
PT	20 (12–14 sec)
APTT	Normal

1. *Which of the following explain the thrombocytopenia and the prolonged prothrombin time (PT)?*

(a) GI blood loss
(b) Patient has taken aspirin
(c) Alcohol effects
(d) Disseminated intravascular coagulation (DIC)

2. *A further 500 mL of fresh blood is vomited and the BP drops to 95 mmHg systolic. She is given 500 mL of gelofusin by rapid infusion. A few minutes later she complains of itching and abdominal pain. She is dyspnoeic and wheezy with a respiratory rate of 40 breaths/min. She becomes tachycardic, 110 beats/min and more hypotensive, 80/50 mmHg. What has happened?*

(a) Acute alcohol withdrawal
(b) Anaphylactoid reaction
(c) Oesophageal perforation
(d) Massive GI bleeding

Case 13: A patient with recurrent tongue swelling

A 69-year-old woman presents to you with recurrent angioedema, affecting the tongue for the last 3 months, and waking her at night; she has also had attacks at various times during the day. She has never had this before. She lives by herself and is quite anxious about this. She believes that she is allergic to potatoes, as she has always eaten these the evening before the attacks happen. She has previously been fit and well, apart from moderate hypertension for which she has been taking lisinopril for the last five years. Ultrasound of the abdomen shows normal liver, spleen and kidneys.

1. *The most likely diagnosis is:*

(a) Hereditary angioedema
(b) Angiotensin-converting enzyme (ACE) inhibitor induced angioedema
(c) Splenic villous lymphoma
(d) Allergy to potatoes

Case 14: A patient who has collapsed after eating a take-away

A 19-year-old student is brought into A&E having collapsed at home after eating a Chinese take-away with some friends. They have driven him straight to A&E. He had been to the pub first and had had 6 pints of lager. He has itchy hives on his arms and face, and his lips are swollen. He says his chest feels tight. He normally has mild exercise-induced asthma and has used his salbutamol inhaler without effect. He feels dizzy and has stomach cramps. When he was younger, he had had lip and tongue swelling when he ate peanuts, so has avoided them since. On arrival in A&E his oxygen saturation is 92%, BP 85/50 mmHg, heart rate 116 beats/min. There is widespread wheeze in the chest.

1. *The most likely diagnosis is:*

(a) Anaphylaxis to nuts in the Chinese meal
(b) Asthma triggered by additives in the lager and take-away
(c) Alcohol intolerance due to deficiency of the enzyme alcohol dehydrogenase
(d) Food poisoning from fried rice contaminated with *Bacillus cereus*

Case 15: An asthmatic patient with breathlessness

A 26-year-old woman with known asthma has become suddenly breathless. She has seen her dentist earlier in the day for toothache and been given a course of amoxicillin which she has previously tolerated without any problems. Twenty minutes after taking a single dose of amoxicillin she developed a rash, and become suddenly short of breath. She had difficulty swallowing because of the sensation of a lump in her throat. She called 999 as she felt so unwell and on arrival at A&E was found to have a widespread urticarial rash. Her heart rate was 132 beats/min and her BP was 88/56 mmHg.

1. *What is the most likely cause of her symptoms?*

(a) Exacerbation of asthma
(b) Acute urticaria and angioedema
(c) Anaphylaxis
(d) Vasovagal episode

2. *Which of the following medications should be given first in established anaphylaxis?*

(a) Salbutamol nebulizer
(b) Intravenous adrenaline
(c) Intramuscular adrenalin
(d) Intravenous chlorphenamine

3. *Which of the following investigations would be useful to identify the cause of her symptoms?*

(a) Pulmonary function tests
(b) Mast cell tryptase
(c) Total IgE
(d) Specific IgE to penicillins

Case 16: A patient with light-headedness and faintness

A 34-year-old woman attends for a routine cervical smear. She has a history of seasonal hayfever and eczema for which she takes antihistamines and nasal spray. Thirty minutes after the smear she begins to feel light headed and faint. Examination reveals diffuse erythema, wheezy chest and hypotension. A diagnosis of anaphylaxis is made and her symptoms improve after a dose of adrenalin.

1. *What is the correct dose of adrenaline?*
   (a) 0.5 mL subcutaneous adrenaline 1:1000
   (b) 0.5 mL intramuscular adrenaline 1:10000
   (c) 0.5 mL intramuscular adrenaline 1:1000
   (d) 0.5 mL intravenous adrenaline 1:10000
2. *What other treatments should be considered?*
   (a) Intravenous antihistamine
   (b) Oral antihistamine
   (c) Intravenous steroid
   (d) Oral steroid
   (e) All of the above
3. *What is the most likely cause for her anaphylaxis?*
   (a) Pollen allergy
   (b) Food allergy
   (c) Latex allergy
   (d) Idiopathic anaphylaxis

Case 17: A patient with a peanut allergy

A 15-year-old boy attends his GP clinic to discuss his peanut allergy. As a child he was diagnosed with a nut allergy after several episodes of urticaria, angioedema, vomiting and wheezing after the ingestion of nuts. He has been avoiding them for many years but recently whilst out with his friends ate a curry and within a few minutes began to feel unwell. He vomited and had diarrhoea, and had to leave the restaurant. On his walk home he became increasingly wheezy and required his salbutamol inhaler. His friend gave him some antihistamines at his house. Gradually his symptoms eased. He has a history of asthma but has not attended your asthma clinic for many years despite numerous appointments.

1. *What type of hypersensitivity reaction is he describing?*
   (a) Type 1
   (b) Type II
   (c) Type III
   (d) Type IV
2. *What would be your management?*
   (a) Issue him with epipens and train him in the use of these
   (b) Advise him that it is important that his asthma is optimally controlled
   (c) Get him to see the dietician with regard to avoiding traces of nuts
   (d) Advise him to carry salbultamol and antihistamines at all times
   (e) All of the above
3. *When should he be advised to use his epipens?*
   (a) When he develops an urticarial rash
   (b) If he develops peripheral swelling
   (c) If he feels nauseous
   (d) If he eats a peanut
   (e) None of the above

Case 18: A patient with a widespread itchy rash

A 56-year-old woman presents to her GP with a 6-week history of widespread itchy rash. On the day the rash began she awoke with the rash which covered her abdomen. Since then she has had intermittent rashes which can appear anywhere on her body. She describes the rash as itchy, raised wheals similar in appearance to nettle rash. Each wheal lasts less than 24 hours in duration and fades leaving no residual lesion. She has been taking some chlorphenamine tablets intermittently but over the past few days her symptoms have become worse. The rash has now spread to affect her back, arms, legs and face. Today she has had some facial swelling affecting her left eye and upper lip which was present when she awoke. She is concerned that she has developed a food allergy but has not been able to identify any particular triggers; she is now avoiding milk, wheat and colourings.

1. *What investigations are appropriate?*
   (a) Skin prick tests to foods
   (b) Blood tests for specific IgE to foods
   (c) Food intolerance tests available at health food shops
   (d) C1 inhibitor level
   (e) None of the above
2. *What is the most likely diagnosis?*
   (a) Wheat allergy
   (b) Food colouring allergy
   (c) Urticarial vasculitis
   (d) Hereditary angioedema
   (e) Idiopathic urticaria and angioedema
3. *What would be the next step in the management of this patient?*
   (a) Regular antihistamine medication
   (b) A 5-day course of oral steroids
   (c) Long-term low-dose steroids
   (d) All of the above

Case 19: A patient with hayfever

A 28-year-old policeman attends for problems with hayfever. He describes symptoms of nasal blockage, running of the nose, sinus pain and itching of the eyes starting in May of each year and lasting through to the end of August. His symptoms are worst outside and he finds he sometimes has difficulty driving due to itching and watering of the eyes. He has had his seasonal hayfever symptoms since the age of 17 years. He has a history of eczema as a child.

1. *What is the most likely allergen responsible?*
   (a) Tree
   (b) Weeds
   (c) House dust mite
   (d) Animal dander
   (e) Grass
2. *What treatments would you recommend?*
   (a) Nasal steroid spray
   (b) Intramuscular Kenalog injection
   (c) Oral corticosteroids
   (d) Montelukast
3. *The patient wants to take an antihistamine but because of driving needs one which is non drowsy. Which would you recommend?*
   (a) Chlorpheniramine
   (b) Hydroxyzine

(c) Dothiepin
(d) Cetirizine

Case 20: A baby with severe pneumonia

A boy was admitted to his local hospital at the age of 9 months with severe pneumonia. *Haemophilus influenzae* was isolated. He was treated with antibiotics and made a gradual recovery. During his admission he was noted to have loose stools and his weight had fallen from 75% at 3 months to 0.2nd centile on admission. *Cryptosporidium* was isolated from his stools. His immunoglobulin results were measured as follows:

		Normal range
IgG	2.0 g/L	3.0–10.9 g/L
IgA	<0.1 g/L	0.20–0.7 g/L
IgM	2.3 g/L	0.60–2.10 g/L

1. *What is the likely diagnosis?*
   (a) Chronic granulomatous disease
   (b) Common variable immunodeficiency
   (c) Specific antibody deficiency
   (d) Wiskott–Aldrich syndrome
   (e) CD40L deficiency
2. *What advice should be given to this patient's parents?*
   (a) Avoid live vaccines
   (b) Boil drinking water
   (c) Commence immunoglobulin replacement therapy
   (d) All of the above
   (e) None of the above

Case 21: A child with fever, irritability and vomiting

A 4-year-old boy presents to A&E with a 2-week history of fever, irritability, vomiting and right upper quadrant (RUQ) pain. He had a past medical history of intermittent loose stools and failure to thrive, as well as two previous superficial skin abscesses which were treated by incision and drainage. He had also had one episode of lymphadenitis and biopsy showed the presence of granulomas. He has one sister who is well and one brother who has also had a superficial abscess. On examination he was noted to have a temperature of 38°C, was tachycardic with mild hypotension. His oxygen saturations were reduced on room air. He was found to have an enlarged liver and ultrasound demonstrated the presence of two liver abscesses.

1. *What is the most likely diagnosis?*
   (a) Complement deficiency
   (b) Primary antibody deficiency
   (c) Tuberculosis
   (d) Severe combined immunodeficiency
   (e) Chronic granulomatous disease (CGD)
2. *Which investigation would be most useful to confirm the diagnosis of CGD?*
   (a) Blood film
   (b) Bone marrow examination
   (c) Liver biopsy
   (d) Neutrophil oxidative burst
   (e) Lymphocyte counts

Case 22: A patient with bronchiectasis

A 56-year-old woman attends the chest clinic with a diagnosis of bronchiectasis. She gives a history of infections dating back to childhood which affected her chest and ears. As well as bronchiectasis, she has chronic sinusitis. *Haemophilus influenzae* and *Streptococcus pneumoniae* are pathogens frequently isolated from her sputum. At her last clinic visit blood test revealed an iron deficiency anaemia, low platelet count, abnormal liver function tests (LFTs) with raised alkaline phosphatase, alanine transaminase and bilirubin. Her total protein level was noted to be low although her albumin level was normal. A possible diagnosis of antibody deficiency was considered.

1. *Which of the following investigations would be the most appropriate in establishing whether this patient has an antibody deficiency?*
   (a) IgG subclasses
   (b) Specific antibody levels
   (c) Immunoglobulin (Ig) levels
   (d) Lymphocyte surface markers
   (e) All of the above
2. *Which of the following is incorrect?*
   (a) Patients who have not responded to immunoglobulin therapy within 6 months of starting should have their therapy discontinued as it is unlikely that it will be of any further benefit
   (b) Ig replacement therapy can be given at home
   (c) Ig replacement therapy can be administered intravenously
   (d) Ig replacement therapy can be administered subcutaneously
   (e) Ig is manufactured from pooled plasma with multiple purification and viral inactivation steps in the manufacturing process

Case 23: A patient with severe headache, vomiting and photophobia

A 24-year-old student presents with a 24-hour history of severe headache, vomiting and photophobia. Neurological examination was normal. His temperature was 38°C. He was noted to have neck stiffness and a petechial rash. A CT scan showed no evidence of raised intracranial pressure. A lumbar puncture was undertaken which showed increased protein, reduced glucose and increased white cell count (predominantly neutrophils) in the CSF. Gram stain revealed Gram-negative diplococci. On reviewing his history he had previously been treated for an episode of Neisserial meningitis at the age of 14 but there is no other history of infections. His younger brother also had an episode of meningitis aged 10 years.

1. *What is the most likely underlying cause for his recurrent meningitis?*
   (a) Anatomical defect
   (b) Chronic granulomatous disease
   (c) T-cell disorder
   (d) Complement deficiency
   (e) Antibody deficiency
2. *How should this patient be managed to try to prevent further infection?*
   (a) Immunoglobulin replacement
   (b) Complement replacement with fresh frozen plasma
   (c) Vaccination and prophylactic antibiotics
   (d) Avoidance of international travel
   (e) Long-term high-dose antibiotics

Case 24: A patient with lip swelling

A 56-year-old man with hypertension presents to his GP two months after starting on an ACE inhibitor. He has had several episodes of recurrent lip swelling, most of which have occurred overnight. On this occasion his upper lip, left side of his tongue and left jaw were swollen. He was afraid that the swelling might affect his throat, although he had had no difficulty swallowing or breathing with his attacks.

1. *What is the most likely cause of his swelling?*
   (a) Food allergy
   (b) Idiopathic angioedema
   (c) Angiotensin-converting enzyme (ACE) inhibitor induced angioedema
   (d) ACE inhibitor allergy
   (e) Contact dermatitis
2. *What would be the next stage in his management?*
   (a) Stop his ACE inhibitor, advise that all ACE inhibitor medication should be avoided in the future and consider alternative antihypertensive medication
   (b) Stop his current ACE inhibitor and recommence an alternative ACE inhibitor.
   (c) Stop his ACE inhibitor and advise that all antihypertensive medication should be avoided

(d) Continue his ACE inhibitor medication, add regular antihistamines to his medications and issue him with a supply of prednisolone should he have further episodes of swelling
(e) None of the above

Case 25: A patient with a persistent dry cough

A 52-year-old woman complains of a persistent dry cough. She has had this for several months but has not experienced any chest pain, shortness of breath or wheeze. She has had no sputum production. Her current medication is aspirin, lisinopril and atenolol which she commenced 6 months ago for hypertension. She also takes thyroxine which was commenced 2 years ago for hypothyroidism.

1. *What is the most likely cause of her cough?*
   (a) β-Blocker-induced asthma
   (b) Thyrotoxicosis
   (c) Hypothyroidism
   (d) Angiotensin-converting enzyme (ACE) inhibitor induced cough
   (e) Aspirin allergy

Other Emergencies: Answers

Case 1: A patient with dyspnoea and weight loss

1. (c) Carcinoma of the lung with metastasis

The combination of hoarse voice, haemoptysis, dyspnoea and severe weight loss along with the clinical findings of bilateral pleural effusions, pulmonary nodules and hepatomegaly in a smoker imply a diagnosis of metastatic lung cancer.

Wegener's granulomatosis is a rare vasculitic disorder, which occurs with predominance in the fourth or fifth decade. Dyspnoea, haemoptysis and weight loss all occur and rarely there is hoarseness of the voice. Pleural effusions and pulmonary nodules are also a feature, however firm hepatomegaly is not. Patients with Wegener's also have fever, lethargy and often involvement of eyes, nose, kidneys, heart, joints, skin and nerve. Tuberculosis may also lead to many of the same symptoms and signs, however fever and night sweats are usually prominent in the history. Large hepatomegaly and hoarse voice would be rare findings.

2. (d) Sending pleural fluid cytology or pleural biopsy

A CT scan will show the extent of disease and may well be suggestive of lung cancer but it does not give a histological diagnosis. Each of the other three answers (b–d) will give a histological diagnosis, however pleural aspiration is the simplest, least invasive procedure, which is least likely to distress the patient. Bronchoscopy may worsen the patient's hypoxia (despite oxygen therapy) and cause bleeding in the airway following biopsy, cytological brushings or washings. Liver biopsy can be complicated by haemorrhage.

3. (e) All of the above

Malignant pleural effusions are exudates. An effusion that is grossly bloody is suggestive of malignancy; other common causes include pulmonary embolus with infarction and trauma. A low pH in malignant pleural effusions increases the likelihood of positive cytology, more extensive disease and failed pleurodesis. It is also associated with a reduced median survival.

Pleural sampling shows an exudate with a pH of 7.1 and cytological analysis confirms that the patient has squamous cell carcinoma of the lung. A decision is made to drain the pleural fluid to improve the patient's dyspnoea. Four days later the patient develops severe pleuritic chest pain, increasing hypoxia with oxygen saturations of 70% on high-flow oxygen, tachycardia of 130 beats/min and hypotension with a BP of 80/40 mmHg. The patient is identified as being critically ill and peri-arrest by a severity scoring system and the hospital Medical Emergency Team (MET) is called.

4. (d) Inform the patient's Consultant who should discuss palliation with the family

The patient has almost certainly suffered a massive pulmonary embolism (he had evidence of a deep venous thrombosis (DVT) on admission) and he is shocked, cardiac arrest is imminent. Answers (a)–(c) are appropriate treatments for a pulmonary embolus in other circumstances, however this patient has incurable disseminated malignancy for which the only therapeutic options are symptom control. He has suffered a terminal event in this context and is in the process of dying. Institution of aggressive treatment is likely to be distressing for the patient and to prolong his death.

Further reading: Chapter 76 in Medicine at a Glance.

Case 2: A patient with abdominal pain and weight loss

1. (b) Peritonitis

The patient presented with symptoms of bowel obstruction (pain, distension, vomiting and constipation). She now has signs of peritonitis (guarding rebound and air under the diaphragm) due to intestinal perforation.

2. (d) 06.00 on the 3rd

The patient develops tachypnoea (respiratory rate 24 breaths/min), hypoxia (oxygen saturation falls), tachycardia (120 beats/min), hypotension (MAP 100/60 mmHg) and fever 39°C.

3. (d) Fluid resuscitate and transfer immediately to the operating theatre for a laparotomy

The patient is shocked as a consequence of peritonitis. A CT scan adds nothing to the diagnosis and delays definitive management, which is a laparotomy and wash out with defunctioning of the bowel (source control). The history is suggestive of a malignancy but the patient could easily have diverticular or inflammatory bowel disease. Transfer to Intensive Care is also inappropriate because this again delays definitive treatment. The Consultant Surgeon should be informed and an experienced surgeon should

Example of an early warning scoring system for critically ill patients. Scores >5 can be used for triggering an emergency medical team

Score	3	2	1	0	1	2	3
HR		<40	40–50	51–100	101–110	111–129	>130
BP	<45%	<30%	<15%	Normal for patient	>15%	>30%	>45%
RR		<8		9–14	15–20	21–29	>30
TEMP		<35		35–38.4		<38.4	
CNS				A	V	P	U
URINE	Nil	<0.5mL/kg/h	<1mL/kg/h		>1.5mL/kg/h		

Figure 13.2.2 Early warning score to detect critical illness at an early stage.

undertake the procedure. The patient should be transferred to Intensive Care following surgery as a level 3 case (patient mechanically ventilated) because she already shows signs of respiratory and cardiovascular failure. It is likely that she will develop multi-organ failure as a consequence of septic shock. Admission to Intensive Care should be discussed between the consultant surgeon and consultant intensivist.

4. (d) Respiratory rate

Although, non-specific, respiratory rate is the commonest abnormality in critical illness, and it is vitally important to record it accurately.

Further reading: Chapter 12.

Case 3: A patient who has bumped his head getting out of the car

1. (b) 14

The patient is disorientated in time and place, in other words confused (4). He obeys commands (6) and has his eyes spontaneously open (4). This may also be written as E4 V5 M6. A score of two is not possible even when dead!

2. (d) Glucose

The patient is confused with focal neurological signs. This may occur with hypoglycaemia (focal signs are not common, however) and forms part of the assessment of patients with altered neurological status. There is a higher incidence of hypoglycaemia in individuals with heavy alcohol consumption.

3. (b) 7

E1 V3 M3.

4. (a) Apply an ABCDE approach

The ABCDE assessment and treatment may be life-saving in this patient. The airway is not obstructed because the patient can speak. One of the presenting symptoms was vomiting, the patient has a GCS of <8 and is therefore unable to protect his airway. He should be put in the recovery position immediately and given high-flow oxygen to prevent secondary brain injury.

5. (c) Subdural haematoma

Subdural haematomas are commoner in the elderly and in alcoholics. There is often a history of minor head trauma. Typically there is a slow progression of neurology over days or weeks. They behave like space-occupying lesions (nausea, vomiting, headaches, focal neurology). This patient had an abnormal GCS and focal neurology. A CT scan should be performed and then the clot removed surgically. This patient is unable to protect his airway and may deteriorate further. He will require intubation and mechanical ventilation to: protect the airway (he has been vomiting and may aspirate gastric contents into the lung), facilitate oxygenation and avoid secondary brain injury, control carbon dioxide and avoid further rises in intracranial pressure.

Further reading: Chapter 12.

Case 4: A patient who has taken a drug overdose

1. (b) Opiate overdose

Opiate overdose will make the pupils constrict, tricyclics may cause them to dilate, alcohol and benzodiazepines should not affect the pupils, so the correct answer is an opiate overdose. Opiates include morphine, heroin, pethidine; codeine is metabolized to morphine.

2. (a) Paracetamol levels

Paracetamol levels may be key here, as the painkiller is likely to have been paracetamol-based. Opiate and tricyclic levels are not normally measured.

3. (d) Naloxone

This is a classical response to naloxone given intravenously at a reasonably large dose to someone who has taken an opiate overdose. Flumazenil is a benzodiazepam antagonist, given intravenously, which also acts within a minute or so; N-acetylcysteine is used to prevent hepatic toxicity in paracetamol overdose, and glucagon is a physiological hormone, used pharmaceutically to reverse severe hypoglycaemia. It is given IV, IM or subcutaneously.

4. (a) Activated charcoal with lactulose

Activated charcoal is useful to delay absorption of drugs if given within 2 hours of their ingestion (or longer in the case of some modified release drugs) It causes constipation so should be given with some form of laxative. Gastric lavage is almost never used, nor is salt water emesis, which can cause hypernatraemia. Forced alkaline diuresis is a treatment that has been used for salicylate poisoning.

Further reading: Chapter 73.

Case 5: A patient who has taken a drug overdose

1. (f) Age under 40

Young age is the only factor associated with a reduced chance of completed suicide; all the others are associated with a higher risk of completed suicide.

2. (c) He has taken other paracetamol overdoses recently

Alcohol, malnourishment and St John's Wort are all factors that would make you use the high-risk treatment line rather than the low-risk one. However, the recent paracetamol overdose is much more worrying, as his glutathione stores will not have recovered by now. The graph is designed for a single overdose, not a cumulative one.

3. (a) 6-hour paracetamol levels

Liver function tests and clotting are essential, and severe paracetamol poisoning may cause renal failure. He has already had 4-hour paracetamol concentrations and you have decided to treat, so 6-hour ones are not necessary.

4. (e) Arrange immediate admission

Section 2 of the Mental Health Act can only be used for treatment of psychiatric illnesses, not physical ones. He is showing symptoms of liver failure and needs urgent admission and treatment. Methionine is an oral drug, acetylcysteine is given intravenously, and neither is likely to be readily available in the community.

5. (c) Addition of the orally active paracetamol antidote methionine to all paracetamol-containing tablets

Paracetamol can only be sold in packs of no more than 16 tablets, and only two packs can be sold to one person in one transaction. Co-proxamol was withdrawn as it was a common drug of overdose, and dextropropoxyphene may be less safe in overdose than other opiates. Methionine has not been added to paracetamol tablets due to cost, but could in theory be very helpful. SSRIs are safer in overdose than tricyclics, but may increase suicidal ideation in adolescents.

Further reading: Chapter 73.

Case 6: A patient with acute confusional state

1. (b) Viral encephalitis

Primary brain tumours typically present with fits, focal neurological symptoms or symptoms of raised intracranial pressure (e.g. headache). The presentation in this case, with systemic symptoms and confusional state, is against a diagnosis of primary brain tumour.

2. (b) Pneumonia

Pneumonia is effectively excluded by the absence of tachypnoea, hypoxaemia or focal chest signs.

3. (e) None of the above

None of these diagnoses is excluded by these results. They all remain possible, although urinary tract infection is unlikely to cause an acute confusional state in a man of this age.

4. (b) CT head

CT head should be done to exclude a contraindication to lumbar puncture.

The working diagnosis was viral encephalitis, and treatment with aciclovir was started pending CT of the head (which was normal) and lumbar puncture. Surprisingly, lumbar puncture disclosed purulent CSF, with group B meningococcus identified on polymerase-chain-reaction analysis. Blood culture also yielded meningococcus. Urine microscopy and culture were normal. His confusion rapidly resolved on treatment with ceftriaxone, and he was discharged home 14 days after admission.

This was an unusual presentation of meningococcal infection with meningitis, in which meningeal features were not prominent. The case exemplifies the importance of lumbar puncture in patients with acute confusional state and fever, to exclude meningitis/ encephalitis, if no other source of infection is apparent.

Further reading: Chapter 200.

Case 7: A patient with acute confusional state

1. (d) Severe hypothyroidism

While severe hypothyroidism can cause myalgia and confusional state, the rapid time course of this patient's illness is against this diagnosis.

2. (b) Ascending cholangitis

While not impossible, ascending cholangitis is the least likely diagnosis. Ascending cholangitis typically causes fever with rigors, right upper quadrant pain and jaundice.

3. (a) To start empirical broad-spectrum antibiotic therapy

The clinical picture is of severe sepsis, and prompt antibiotic therapy is needed for a good outcome. In the absence of an obvious focus of infection on clinical examination and chest X-ray, infective endocarditis and line-related sepsis are strong possibilities. Choice of antibiotic therapy should be discussed with a microbiologist. Possibilities would include vancomycin or teicoplanin (to cover gram-positive bacteria including MRSA) plus gentamicin (to cover Gram-negative organisms).

4. (b) Transthoracic echocardiography

It is a useful aphorism that every patient with a bacteraemia has infective endocarditis until proven otherwise. She should have transthoracic echocardiography to look for vegetations and/or valve destruction. Transthoracic echocardiography was normal. Transoesophageal echocardiography showed vegetations on the dialysis catheter. Antibiotic therapy was continued with flucloxacillin, and the catheter changed. She made a slow recovery.

Patients with chronic renal failure are at increased risk of sepsis, particularly if they have an indwelling vascular catheter. Coagulase-negative staphylococci and *Staphylococcus aureus* account for around 50% of cases of line-related sepsis.

Further reading: Chapter 161.

Case 8: A patient with progressive confusion

1. (c) Respiratory failure

While respiratory failure can cause a confusional state, it is an unlikely diagnosis in a patient with no past history of respiratory disease or current respiratory symptoms.

2. (e) None of the above

None of these diagnoses is excluded by the examination findings.

3. (d) Malignancy

The tempo of his illness, the marked weight loss, the absence of anaemia (which would be expected in myeloma) and the absence of clinical or radiological evidence of sarcoidosis, make malignancy the most likely cause.

4. (b) Intravenous saline

Patients with severe hypercalcaemia should be treated with IV saline, with monitoring of central venous pressure and urine output. If malignancy is the likely cause, a bisphosphonate should then be given.

The patient's confusional state resolved with correction of hypercalcaemia. CT thorax revealed a right upper lobe pulmonary nodule and mediastinal lymphadenopathy. Biopsy showed small-cell carcinoma of the bronchus, for which he received chemotherapy.

When plasma calcium concentration rises above 3 mmol/L, patients may develop polyuria (from hypercalciuria-induced nephrogenic diabetes insipidus), vomiting, constipation and abdominal pain. Confusional state and coma are seen when plasma calcium is over 3.5 mmol/L. Malignancy may cause hypercalcaemia by bone metastases or by synthesis of parathyroid-hormone-related protein. A clear chest X-ray does not exclude carcinoma of the bronchus.

Further reading: Chapter 157.

Case 9: A patient with coma

1. (c) Acute liver failure

All these diagnoses are possible, on the history presented. However, no cause for acute liver failure is apparent (paracetamol poisoning is a remote possibility but would not account for the onset of his illness), and jaundice is not a feature.

2. (d) Is a transient finding after tonic-clonic seizure

Extensor plantar responses are seen transiently after 50% of tonic-clonic seizures.

3. (e) None of the above

It is critically important in medicine to be fully aware of the false negative rate of any investigation; all investigations will occasionally fail to diagnose an illness when it is actually present. The issue is, how frequently does this occur and what are the consequences of a failed diagnosis. A CT scan will miss 2–5% of subarachnoid bleeds and is normal in nearly all cases of meningitis. Likewise, the CT is normal in 98% of cases of infective endocarditis and in 10–20% of cases of encephalitis. If the consequences of a missed diagnosis are serious, then in the face of a negative test a more sensible one is often ordered.

4. (b) Lumbar puncture

Lumbar puncture is needed to confirm or exclude bacterial meningitis, viral encephalitis and subarachnoid haemorrhage.

Empirical treatment for bacterial meningitis (ceftriaxone) and herpes simplex viral encephalitis (aciclovir) were started. Lumbar puncture was done, and yielded CSF with a high lymphocyte count and increased protein concentration. Herpes simplex DNA was detected by polymerase-chain-reaction analysis. Aciclovir was continued. He required hospital care for 4 weeks and eventually made a good recovery, although was left with some impairment of memory and concentration.

Encephalitis should be considered in any patient with fever and an abnormal mental state (which may range from abnormal behaviour to coma). Herpes simplex infection is an important – because treatable – cause of encephalitis, and if suspected, aciclovir should be started pending investigation results.

Further reading: Chapter 78.

Case 10: A patient with coma

1. (c) Viral encephalitis

The rapid tempo of his illness is against a diagnosis of viral encephalitis causing coma.

2. (d) Alcohol intoxication

Alcohol intoxication sufficient to cause coma would be expected to result in respiratory depression, while this patient is tachypnoeic.

3. (a) Tonic-clonic seizure prior to admission

Transient metabolic acidosis is seen after tonic-clonic seizure. In this case, no seizure was reported, and the patient has a severe metabolic acidosis. Another cause for the metabolic acidosis is therefore more likely.

4. (c) EEG, to exclude non-convulsive status epilepticus

All these investigations may be helpful in diagnosing the cause of coma. However, given the clinical features, and the finding of metabolic acidosis, EEG is not needed as a priority.

The patient was electively intubated and ventilated, and given IV fluids. Ceftriaxone was started as empirical therapy for possible bacterial meningitis. Blood alcohol, paracetamol and salicylate levels were negative. Urinary microscopy showed needle-shaped crystals of calcium oxalate monohydrate, a metabolite of ethylene glycol. A diagnosis of poisoning with ethylene glycol (a component of anti-freeze) was made. He was treated with fomepizole and supportive care, and made a full recovery.

The combination of metabolic acidosis and coma may be seen in several settings, including post-cardiac arrest, severe sepsis and poisoning. The clinical features in this case made poisoning the most likely cause. Poisons associated with metabolic acidosis include carbon monoxide, ethylene glycol and tricyclics.

Further reading: Chapter 138.

Case 11: A patient with bloody diarrhoea and pain

1. (a) The patient has hypovolaemic shock

(c) The patient has metabolic acidosis with respiratory compensation

The patient has evidence of shock: hypotension, tachycardia, tachypnoea, oliguria and lactic acidosis. The patient is acidotic which is metabolic (pH 7.29, HCO_3 15 mmol/L, base excess –8, lactate 4.1 mmol/L). The lungs are attempting to compensate by eliminating CO_2. The primary aetiology of the shock state is GI fluid loss from the diarrhoea. The anaemia and raised urea do not indicate upper GI bleeding, the urea is raised as a consequence of dehydration. The patient is anaemic because of the chronic inflammation and lower GI blood loss.

2. (c) 500 mL HAES-Steril over 10 minutes

(d) 500 mL Hartmann's over 10 minutes

The patient requires rapid infusion of fluid via a large-bore cannula; it is less important whether this is colloid or crystalloid than it is administered as a 'fluid challenge' (bolus of 250-500 mL over 10-15 minutes). Physiological parameters should be monitored to assess the effects of the fluid challenge.

3. (a) Urgent total colectomy

The patient has had severe colitis for many months which is difficult to control with aggressive immunosupression. He presents to hospital with shock and a toxic megacolon; urgent surgery is indicated.

4. (c) The patient was resuscitated with HAES-Steril

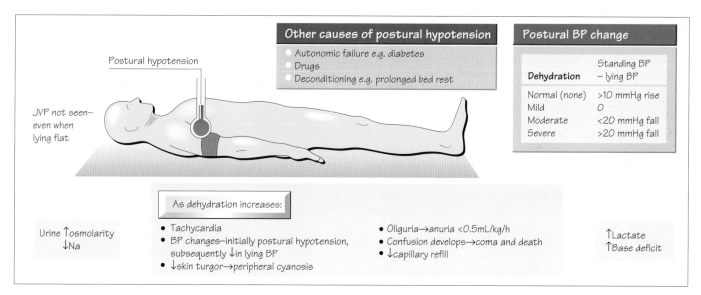

Figure 13.11.1 Assessment of hypovolaemia.

Itching can last many months and even up to 2 years following administration of starch solutions. Itching is not a feature of UC. Malignancy may be associated with itching and UC carries a 20% malignancy risk after 30 years. However the patient had a pancolectomy and UC does not extend outside the large bowel.
Further reading: Chapter 225.

Case 12: A patient with mild haematemesis

1. (c) Alcohol effects

Megakaryocytes are particularly sensitive to the toxic effects of alcohol and thrombocytopenia is not uncommon. Some coagulation factors are made in the liver and PT is often prolonged in severe liver disease.

2. (b) Anaphylactoid reaction

These are features of an anaphylactoid reaction to gelofusin. Treatments include: steroids, antihistamines, fluids, bronchodilators; adrenaline is required in severe reactions (which includes hypoxia and haemodynamic instability). Mast cell tryptase becomes elevated and should be measured after the reaction to confirm the diagnosis.
Further reading: Chapter 74.

Case 13: A patient with recurrent tongue swelling

1. (b) Angiotensin-converting enzyme (ACE) inhibitor induced angioedema

Even though she has been on this for 5 years, this is still the most likely cause. Angioedema may occur at any time and up to 5% of patients on ACE inhibitors may develop angioedema at some point. The drug should be stopped; it may take up to 3 months for the effect to wear off. Hereditary angioedema is very unlikely to present *de novo* at this age, as it is a genetic disease; splenic villous lymphoma is rare, but is a cause of acquired angioedema. The spleen is invariably enlarged. Foods taken the day before an attack are not going to be the cause of angioedema. Allergy is immediate.
Further reading: Chapter 75.

Case 14: A patient who has collapsed after eating a take-away

1. (a) Anaphylaxis to nuts in the Chinese meal

He has the typical features of anaphylaxis with breathing difficulty, reduced oxygen saturation, hypotension, tachycardia, bowel symptoms and rash (only 50% have rash); allergy to peanuts has been previously documented. Treat immediately with adrenaline intramuscularly, followed by antihistamine and hydrocortisone. (b) Is very unlikely and he has more than just asthma; (c) this deficiency causes flushing on alcohol consumption, it does not cause the other features that this man has; (d) while this is a recognized problem from Chinese take-aways where the rice has been pre-cooked and then kept warm, it does not cause immediate reactions, and the symptoms are gastrointestinal rather than respiratory.
Further reading: Chapter 75.

Case 15: An asthmatic patient with breathlessness

1. (c) Anaphylaxis

The patient has evidence of low blood pressure and breathlessness as well as rash and swelling.

2. (c) Intramuscular adrenalin

Intramuscular adrenalin is the first-line treatment of anaphylaxis. Intravenous adrenalin should not be given as first-line treatment.

3. (d) Specific IgE to penicillins

Specific IgE to penicillins may be positive in patients with penicillin allergy which can occur after previously tolerating penicillin-based drugs without any problems. A negative test does not exclude the diagnosis and patients may need further investigations in an allergy clinic.
Further reading: Chapter 75.

Case 16: A patient with light-headedness and faintness

1. (c) 0.5 mL intramuscular adrenaline 1 : 1000

2. (e) All of the above

The route of administration of antihistamine and steroids will be determined by the clinical status of the patient.

3. (c) Latex allergy

Latex should be considered as a potential cause of any allergic reaction occurring in a healthcare setting.
Further reading: Chapter 74.

Case 17: A patient with a peanut allergy

1. (a) Type 1

2. (e) All of the above

Adolescent patients with asthma and nut allergy are at high risk of severe allergic reactions after accidental exposure. If epipens are issued patients need to be trained in their use and advised when to use them. Dietary advice is important so that foods containing traces of nuts can be avoided. Asthma control should be optimized.

3. (e) None of the above

An epipen should be administered if he has symptoms of anaphylaxis, i.e. difficulty breathing or symptoms of low blood pressure (dizziness or feeling faint) in the setting of an allergic reaction.
Further reading: Chapter 75.

Case 18: A patient with a widespread itchy rash

1. (e) None of the above

For an explanation see the answer to Que~~stion 2~~ (below).

2. (e) Idiopathic urticaria and angioedema

Food allergy does not cause urticaria and angioedema symptoms that last for days, and does not cause swellings/rash with onset several hours after ingestion (e.g. overnight, first thing in the morning). Tests to confirm type 1 allergy to foods are therefore inappropriate. Food intolerance tests including vega testing, impedance testing, hair analysis and IgG measurement to foods have no evidence to support their use in any clinical setting. Patients with hereditary angioedema present with angioedema but not urticaria and therefore testing for C1 esterase is inappropriate. Lesions of urticarial vasculitis generally last more than 24 hours, are painful rather than itchy and may leave residual bruising or pigmentation; patients may have other clinical features such as arthralgia, fatigue, weight loss, raised inflammatory markers and low complement levels. Most cases of chronic urticaria and angioedema are idiopathic in nature and may have a physical component to it (i.e. exacerbation of symptoms by physical factors such as heat, pressure, stress).

3. (a) Regular antihistamine medication

Regular antihistamine medication would be most appropriate. Steroids should not generally be used in the treatment of urticaria and angioedema.

Further reading: Chapter 216.

Case 19: A patient with hayfever

1. (e) Grass

House dust mite and animal dander allergies cause perennial symptoms. Tree pollen allergy causes symptoms in spring and weeds in late summer/early autumn. Grass pollen allergy causes symptoms generally from May through to August.

2. (a) Nasal steroid spray

Nasal steroid spray is the first-line treatment of allergic rhino-conjunctivitis; oral antihistamines may also be used. Intramuscular kenalog should never be given for hayfever and oral corticosteroids should be avoided.

3. (d) Cetirizine

Chlorpheniramine is a relatively weak antihistamine which can be sedating so should generally be avoided. Hydoxyzine and dothiepin are both sedating and are prescribed at night. Cetirizine, along with, e.g. loratidine and fexofendine, is a second-generation antihistamine which is non-sedating and has a long half life so can be given once daily.

Further reading: Chapter 75.

Case 20: A baby with severe pneumonia

1. (e) CD40L deficiency

Severe infections (pneumonia) and unusual infections (*Cryptosporidium*) should raise the possibility of immunodeficicency, as well as persistent infections and recurrent infections (SPUR). Low IgG results would raise the possibility of an antibody deficiency; this patient had a low IgG level but a raised IgM level suggesting a HyperIgM syndrome. The commonest cause of this is CD40L deficiency; absence of CD40L on T cells can be detected by flow cytometry. *Cryptospoidium* in stools is found in patients with CD40L deficiency but not in most antibody deficiency conditions.

2. (d) All of the above

Live vaccines should be avoided in all patients with possible or confirmed immunodeficiency. Patients should be advised to boil all drinking water as *Cryptosporidium* may be present in mains water supply. Treatment of the condition, which is lifelong and progressive, includes immunoglobulin replacement therapy, which can be given intravenously or subcutaneously, and prompt treatment of infection. Immunologists should be involved in the diagnosis of and management of patients with suspected and confirmed immunodeficiency.

Further reading: Chapter 170.

Case 21: A child with fever, irritability and vomiting

1. (e) Chronic granulomatous disease (CGD)

This patient also has a history strongly suggestive of immunodeficiency with a history of recurrent infection and failure to thrive. Abscesses are commonly seen in CGD which is a condition resulting from impaired neutrophil function. Liver abscesses in children are almost exclusively seen in patients with CGD. Infections are generally with catalase positive organisms. Fungal infection is common and can affect the lungs, bone and brain. *Aspergillus* is one of the most common causes of mortality in patients with CGD. Two-thirds of cases of CGD are x-linked; female family members may therefore be carriers. Autosomal recessive forms can occur.

2. (d) Neutrophil oxidative burst

CGD is a condition caused by defects in the reduced nicotinamide adenine dinucleotide phosphate (NADPH) oxidase, the enzyme responsible for the generation of superoxide in neutrophils. Superoxide is then further converted into enzymes, including hydrogen peroxide, that activate neutrophil granule proteins which are essential in microbial killing. The neutrophil oxidative burst is a flow cytometric assay designed to detect hydrogen peroxide production within neutrophils.

Further reading: Chapter 170.

Case 22: A patient with bronchiectasis

1. (c) Immunoglobulin levels

The most appropriate test at this stage would be immunoglobulin measurement. Hypogammaglobulinaemia is likely as she had a low protein level but normal albumin levels. Patients with common variable immunodeficiency have low IgG levels and, as well as recurrent bacterial infections, often affecting chest, ears and sinuses, may develop granulomatous hepatosplemegaly (abnormal LFTs) and lymphadenopathy; autoimmune disease can also be a feature (e.g. autoimmune thrombocytopenia). Lymphocyte numbers may also be altered in this condition with abnormalities in T and B cell numbers. IgG subclass measurement can be helpful particularly in patients with normal IgG levels who have features of immunodeficiency. IgG2 subclass deficiency in association with IgA deficiency is associated with immunodeficiency in some patients. Specific antibody levels are used to assess a patient's immune response to a previous vaccine. If specific antibody levels are low, immunization with appropriate killed vaccines may be appropriate and levels checked after 4–6 weeks to establish that the patient has responded to these vaccines. Failure to respond is associated with significant bacterial infections especially in combination with low/ borderline IgG levels, absent IgA levels or low/ absent IgG2 levels. Therefore, although immunoglobulin measurement is the most appropriate next step, all these tests are useful in confirming the diagnosis of antibody deficiency syndromes.

2. (a) Patients who have not responded to immunoglobulin therapy within 6 months of starting should have their therapy discontinued as it is unlikely that it will be of any further benefit

Immunoglobulin is a highly purified plasma product with multiple steps in the processing to remove and inactivate viral particles. Different products are available for both intravenous and subcutaneous use. Intravenous therapy is given at 3-weekly intervals and subcutaneous therapy is given weekly. The dose recommended is 400–600 mg/kg/month. Patients can be trained to administer both these products at home. When commenced in patients with antibody deficiency (e.g. common variable immunodeficiency, specific antibody deficiency, X-linked agammaglobulinaemia, secondary antibody deficiency) patients may have a marked improvement in symptoms quite quickly; in others however, particularly in those with evidence of end-organ damage from previous infection, e.g. bronchiectasis, improvement in symptoms may be more gradual. Treatment should be continued to prevent further progression.

Further reading: Chapter 170.

Case 23: A patient with severe headache, vomiting and photophobia

1. (d) Complement deficiency

While bacterial meningitis is relatively common, recurrent meningitis is definitely uncommon. Cases of recurrent bacterial meningitis require a search for an underlying abnormality. The abnormality may be anatomical or immunological. Immunological problems are suggested by recurrent episodes of infections in multiple sites or a family history of similar problems. Anatomical abnormalities where there is an abnormal connection exists between the CNS and a mucosal surface or the skin predisposes to meningitis. In this case the family history is suggestive of an immune defect. The lack of other infections makes a T cell disorder, antibody deficiency or chronic granulomatous disease much less likely. Complement deficiencies are associated with increased susceptibility to Neisserial infections.

2. (c) Vaccination and prophylactic antibiotics

Definitive treatment of complement deficiencies requires replacing the missing component of the cascade, either through direct infusion of the protein or through gene therapy. Because neither of these options is currently available, treatment of these patients focuses on managing the sequelae of the particular complement

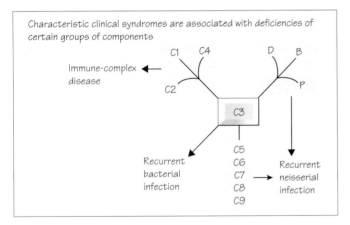

Figure 13.23.1 Consequences of complement deficiency.

deficiencies. Administration of the multivalent meningococcal vaccine is recommended in patients with known complement deficiency, especially those patients deficient in the terminal complement components. Similarly, administration of the pneumococcal vaccine and the *Haemophilus influenzae* vaccine provides protection against these encapsulated organisms. Long-term antibiotic prophylaxis should be given, although compliance is often poor. Patients with an identified complement deficiency should be counselled regarding possible complications and risks associated with this deficiency so they can take steps for early diagnosis and treatment should infections occur. Family members should be screened.

Further reading: Chapter 169.

Case 24: A patient with lip swelling

1. (c) Angiotensin-converting enzyme (ACE) inhibitor induced angioedema

The swelling described is suggestive of angioedema, swelling of the deep layers of the skin. ACE inhibitor medication can be associated with angioedema in patients taking these medications. Onset of symptoms may be shortly after commencing the drug or after many years for therapy. Attacks of angioedema may, however, occur up to 6 months after treatment is stopped. Attacks can be severe and may result in laryngeal obstruction. The angioedema resulting from ACE inhibitor medication is due to the pharmacological action of the drug resulting in increased bradykinin, which in turn results in angioedema. The history is not suggestive of food allergy which usually has symptoms onset shortly after the ingestion of foods, or contact dermatitis.

2. (a) Stop his ACE inhibitor, advise that all ACE inhibitor medication should be avoided in the future and consider alternative antihypertensive medication

ACE inhibitors are contraindicated in patients with a history of angioedema; it is a class effect rather than being drug specific. Other antihypertensive medication should be considered; there are case reports of angioedema occurring in patients treated with angiotensin receptor blockers.

Further reading: Chapter 75.

Case 25: A patient with a persistent dry cough

1. (d) Angiotensin-converting enzyme (ACE) inhibitor induced cough

ACE inhibitors may cause a persistent dry, tickly cough without sputum production or chest pain in patients taking them. Cessation of the drug is necessary to alleviate symptoms.

Further reading: Chapter 19.

Case 1: A patient with chest pain following a fall

A 32-year-old male decorator presents to the A&E department following a fall off a ladder. The only past medical history is of mild asthma for which he takes salbutamol occasionally. Although he fell from a height of only 1.5 m he caught his left side on a cabinet lying below and now is in considerable pain. The patient was conscious throughout and there was no suggestion of a head injury. He is obviously in pain and is unable to take a deep breath. Respiratory rate is recorded as 30 breaths/min with oxygen saturations of 99% on air. Chest expansion is limited, but symmetrical. He has vesicular breath sounds. Bruising is noted over the lower thoracic cage on the left and it is painful to touch. Heart rate is 120 beats/min with a BP of 150/95 mmHg. Examination is otherwise unremarkable. The patient is given morphine 5 mg with an antiemetic, paracetamol and 400 mg of ibuprofen. A chest radiograph is performed and fractures of the 8th to 10th ribs are visible. You return to the patient to discuss the radiograph findings and his observations are now: respiratory rate 14 breaths/min, oxygen saturations 100%, BP 110/70 mmHg, heart rate 60 beats/min.

1. *Why has there been a change in the physiological variables?*
   (a) These parameters can vary widely
   (b) Patient had an asthma attack following his fall (precipitated by the stress)
   (c) He was seeking attention
   (d) He was in pain, which was adequately treated

2. *The patient suddenly complains that he is feeling breathless and becomes tachypnoeic with a respiratory rate of 35 breaths/min. Oxygen saturations fall to 90%, he is tachycardic (120 beats/min) but BP is unaltered at 110/70 mmHg. Which of the following might have occurred?*
   (a) Asthma attack
   (b) Pneumothorax
   (c) Haemothorax
   (d) Pulmonary embolism (PE)

3. *The chest radiograph shows a 5 cm pneumothorax on the left side with no significant pleural fluid. Following the administration of high-flow oxygen how should this be treated?*
   (a) Observation
   (b) Aspiration
   (c) Surgery
   (d) Intercostal tube drainage with underwater seal

4. *The patient's physiology improves rapidly following the insertion of a chest drain. The following day the lung has re-expanded and the underwater seal is swinging with respiration. Suddenly the patient feels unwell. BP drops to 90/50 mmHg, pulse increases to 130 beats/min, respiratory rate to 30 breaths/min, and oxygen saturations are not recordable. The patient is now confused. High-flow oxygen is administered and a rapid infusion of colloid administered. A blood gas is taken; which parameter is of most concern?*
   (a) PaO_2 40 kPa on high-flow oxygen
   (b) $PaCO_2$ 3.5 kPa
   (c) pH 7.40
   (d) Lactate 8 mmol/L

5. *A chest radiograph is also performed and shows the drain in the correct position, the lung is fully expanded and there is no pleural fluid. What diagnosis must be excluded?*
   (a) Septic shock
   (b) Tension pneumothorax
   (c) Ruptured spleen (haemorrhagic shock)
   (d) Myocardial infarct

Case 2: A hospitalized patient who develops neutropenia and a temperature

A 45-year-old woman with acute myeloid leukaemia is in hospital receiving chemotherapy. Four days after this treatment is completed she becomes neutropenic and develops a fever of 39°C. An examination is performed of the patient, which is unremarkable. She is given paracetamol and venous blood cultures are taken. The following day the microbiologist phones to say that the blood cultures have Gram-positive cocci in both bottles. You go to review the patient. The temperature is now 34.5°C and the patient is confused with a Glasgow Coma Score (GCS) of 12. There is no focal neurology, neck stiffness or rash. Glucose is 5.5 mmol/L. The respiratory rate is 30 breaths/min, oxygen saturations are 90% on air and the chest has vesicular breath sounds only. BP has fallen from 120/70 to 84/50 mmHg and the pulse has risen to 128 from 90 beats/min in sinus rhythm. She is cold and clammy to touch, and capillary refill is 5 seconds. The patient is not catheterized but has not passed urine for 12 hours. Abdominal examination is unremarkable. The patient has a Hickman line (long-term central venous catheter), which was inserted 3 weeks previously for the administration of chemotherapy. The Hickman line has some erythema at the site of insertion. A chest radiograph is normal. The patient is catheterized, there is a residual volume of 200 mL and the patient passes 15 mL in the first hour. A dipstick is negative for nitrites and leukocytes.

1. *What is the diagnosis?*
   (a) Pulmonary embolism (PE)
   (b) Cardiogenic shock
   (c) Septic shock
   (d) Dehydration

2. *Which of the following would be useful treatments whilst the patient is still on the ward?*
   (a) Rapid infusion of fluids
   (b) Antibiotics
   (c) 28% oxygen
   (d) Noradrenaline (norepinephrine)

3. *The patient is transferred to intensive care; what important procedure must be performed without delay?*
   (a) Remove the Hickman line
   (b) Repeat blood cultures
   (c) Perform a lumbar puncture
   (d) Insert a central line

Case 3: A patient with septic shock

An obese 40-year-old woman is referred by her GP with right upper quadrant abdominal pain. She has noticed that her urine has been dark for the last few days and her stools pale. She complains of feeling hot and cold with involuntary shaking for the last 12 hours. On examination she appears jaundiced and has a fever of 39.4°C. BP is recorded as 100/60 mmHg (she is normally hypertensive) and a pulse of 120 beats/min in sinus rhythm. Respiratory rate is 24 breaths/min with oxygen saturations of 92% on air. The Glasgow Coma Score (GCS) is 15 with no focal neurology. Examination of the abdomen reveals some tenderness in the right upper quadrant. An arterial blood gas is performed which shows a base excess of −8 and a lactate of 5 mmol/L. The patient is given high-flow oxygen and rapid boluses of fluid up to a total of 4 L, with little change in BP. A diagnosis of septic shock is made and the patient transferred to critical care.

1. *What is the likely cause of this patient's septic shock?*
   (a) Diverticular disease
   (b) Cholangitis caused by gallstones
   (c) Pancreatitis
   (d) Peritonitis due to a perforated duodenal ulcer
2. *What non-invasive investigation should be performed?*
   (a) Plain abdominal radiograph
   (b) Ultrasound of the biliary tract
   (c) Magnetic resonance cholangiopancreatography (MRCP)
   (d) An erect chest radiograph
3. *The ultrasound demonstrates a normal pancreas (amylase is also normal) but the common bile duct is grossly dilated with a stone sitting in the duct. There is little dilatation of the intrahepatic ducts. Which of the following should be undertaken?*
   (a) Endoscopic retrograde cholangiopancreatography (ERCP)
   (b) Intravenous antibiotics
   (c) Cholecystectomy
   (d) Percutaneous transhepatic cholangiography (PTC)

Case 4: A feverish patient with a productive cough

A 34-year-old woman is referred by her GP to the medical admissions unit. She has had a cough productive of purulent sputum for 4 days and has become increasingly short of breath and more unwell. She also describes being feverish. She has no history of foreign travel nor does she keep any pets.

On examination, she looks pale, unwell and is confused. Her BP is 85/30 mmHg, and her pulse 120 beats/min sinus. She has cool peripheries and a capillary refill time of 5 seconds. Her urine output in the last hour was just 10 mL. Her respiratory rate is 32 breaths/min, and SpO_2 is 94% on 15 L/min oxygen. Auscultation reveals quiet breath sounds at the right base with a dull percussion note. There are some coarse crepitations in this area and you note some bronchial breath sounds in the right mid zone.

Arterial blood gas (ABG) levels are as follows:

pH	7.42
PO_2	9.6 kPa
PCO_2	3.8 kPa
Base excess	−7
HCO_3	19 mmol/L
Lactate	4.8 mmol/L

Blood tests showed:

Na	33 mmol/L
K	4.1 mmol/L
Urea	12.6 mmol/L

Creatinine	165 μmol/L
WCC	17.9×10^9/L
CRP	386 mg/L

Chest X-ray is consistent with a right lower and middle lobe pneumonia.

1. *What is the significance of the lactate level on the ABG?*
   (a) It shows that hypoxia is causing poor oxygen delivery to the tissues
   (b) There is poor peripheral perfusion due to a shock state
   (c) Probable liver dysfunction meaning the lactate is not being removed
   (d) It is slightly high, but requires no treatment currently. Monitor carefully.
2. *What is the first-line treatment for her low urine output?*
   (a) Fluid bolus
   (b) Noradrenaline infusion
   (c) Renal dose dopamine infusion
   (d) Frusemide
3. *What is this patient's CURB-65 score?*
   (a) 2
   (b) 3
   (c) 4
   (d) 5
4. *What are the recommendations regarding the timing of antibiotic therapy in this woman with septic shock?*
   (a) When a positive culture is yielded from either blood or sputum
   (b) Within 6 hours
   (c) Immediately once the radiological the diagnosis is confirmed
   (d) Within an hour

Case 5: A patient with haematemesis

A 61-year-old male is admitted to hospital with massive haematemesis. He had slipped and fallen a week earlier at work, hurting his knee in the process. To help with the pain the patient has been taking ibuprofen three times a day. There is no other past medical history. Following initial resuscitation the patient undergoes an emergency endoscopy, which shows a large ulcer in the first part of the duodenum with a bleeding vessel. The endoscopist is uncertain whether the bleeding has stopped because of the large amount of blood present in the gastrointestinal tract. The ulcer is injected and the patient returned to the high dependency unit for observation. The patient is kept nil-by-mouth and given fluid via a central venous catheter. However, the patient continues to vomit blood and pass melaena. Thirty minutes later he remains tachycardic at 120 beats/min and his systolic blood pressure cannot be sustained above 90 mmHg. Respiratory rate is 32 beats/min, but oxygen saturations are well maintained at 100% on high-flow oxygen. His lactate is persistently raised at 4.5 mmol/L.

1. *What should be done next?*
   (a) Repeat endoscopy
   (b) Check full blood count and coagulation urgently
   (c) Give more blood
   (d) Urgent laparotomy
   (e) Omeprazole infusion
2. *In total the patient receives 18 units of blood and 8 units of fresh frozen plasma (FFP). A laparotomy with oversewing of the ulcer is performed; the patient is extubated and returned to*

the high dependency unit. The patient is now haemodynamically stable and his lactate has returned to normal. He is orientated and passing good volumes of urine. However, he remains tachypnoeic and his oxygen saturations are 92% on high-flow oxygen. A chest radiograph is performed and shows a normal cardiac silhouette but airspace shadowing in all four quadrants of the lung. Which of the following may have occurred?

(a) The patient has sustained a myocardial infarct
(b) The patient is fluid overloaded
(c) The patient has transfusion-related acute lung injury (TRALI)
(d) The patient has an aspiration pneumonitis
(e) All of the above

3. *An ECG is performed, which is normal, and an echocardiogram shows vigorous left ventricular function with no regional wall abnormality. The patient is commenced on non-invasive ventilation but quickly deteriorates so that he is on 100% oxygen with an inspiratory positive airway pressure (IPAP) of 20 cmH₂O and expiratory positive airway pressure (EPAP) of 10 cmH₂O. The patient's respiratory rate is 40 breaths/min, SaO₂ 84% and pH 7.21. The patient is intubated and mechanically ventilated. The patient's body mass index is 22 (normal) and he weighs 70 kg. Which of the following are appropriate initial ventilator settings?*

(a) Synchronized intermittent mandatory ventilation (SIMV), tidal volume 700 mL, rate 12/min, positive end-expiratory pressure (PEEP) 2 cmH₂O
(b) SIMV, tidal volume 700 mL, rate 12/min, PEEP 12 cmH₂O
(c) SIMV, tidal volume 420 ml, rate 12/min, PEEP 2 cmH₂O
(d) SIMV, tidal volume 420 ml, rate 12/min, PEEP 12 cmH₂O

4. *The patient is sedated and ventilated with SIMV. The following are set: tidal volume 420 ml, PEEP 5 cmH₂O, rate 15/min, inspired oxygen 100%, inspiratory time 1 sec; plateau pressure is 24 cmH₂O on these settings. The pH is 7.35, PaO₂ 6 kPa, PaCO₂ 5.5 kPa and SaO₂ 80%. What is the inspiration to expiration (I : E) ratio?*

(a) 1 : 2
(b) 1 : 1
(c) 1 : 4
(d) 1 : 3

5. *What could be done to improve oxygenation?*

(a) Turn patient from supine to prone
(b) Give inhaled nitric oxide
(c) Increase PEEP
(d) Decrease PEEP
(e) Increase inspiratory time and reduce the I : E ratio

Case 6: A patient with a severe asthma attack

A 25-year-old female with asthma is admitted with dyspnoea, cough, wheeze and green sputum. She has been unwell for the last 3 days and has been unable to sleep at night because of cough and wheeze. She has used her salbutamol so many times that it has now run out. On examination she is unable to speak and has a respiratory rate of 50 breaths/min but there is no audible wheeze. Oxygen saturations are 88% on high-flow oxygen and she is being given continuous salbutamol nebulizers on oxygen. She is recognized as having a severe asthma attack and in danger of a cardiorespiratory arrest and the critical care consultant is called to see her in the emergency department. As he enters the room the patient stops breathing and is immediately intubated. There is no loss of cardiac output at any stage.

1. *Which of the following drugs are indicated?*
(a) Magnesium sulphate intravenously
(b) Salbutamol
(c) Corticosteroids
(d) Antibiotics

2. *Following intubation the blood pressure drops from 100 mmHg systolic to 60 mmHg. An arterial blood gas shows: pH 7.1, PaO₂ 12 kPa, PaCO₂ 10 kPa and SaO₂ 100%. Which of the following may explain the hypotension after intubation?*
(a) The patient is dehydrated/hypovolaemic
(b) A pneumothorax has developed
(c) The patient has been given magnesium sulphate too rapidly
(d) It is related to hypercapnia
(e) The patient is being hand ventilated too quickly
(f) All of the above

3. *There is no evidence of a pneumothorax and following 2000 mL of Hartmann's solution the systolic pressure returns to 110 mmHg systolic. The patient is transferred to intensive care and is commenced on synchronized intermittent mandatory ventilation (SIMV), with tidal volume 320 mL, inspiratory time 1 sec, respiratory rate 10 breaths/min, inspired oxygen 40% and PEEP 5 cmH₂O. Plateau pressure is 30 cmH₂O. An arterial blood gas shows: pH 7.15, PaO₂ 14 kPa, PaCO₂ 10.3 and SaO₂ 100%. A doctor comes along and increases the respiratory rate to 20 breaths/min to reduce the PaCO₂ and improve pH. The systolic pressure again falls to 70 mmHg. What has happened?*
(a) The patient is having a pulmonary embolism
(b) Auto-PEEP has increased
(c) PaCO₂ has been reduced to quickly
(d) The patient has plugged off and collapsed a segment of lung

4. *Five days later the patient is much better and has weaned to a pressure support mode of 15 cmH₂O and a PEEP of 5 cmH₂O. There is little wheeze audible. The patient now develops a fever of 39°C and her respiratory rate has increased from 14 to 28 breaths/min. Oxygen requirements have also increased from 28 to 45%. What might have happened?*
(a) The patient is developing ventilator-associated pneumonia (VAP)
(b) Asthma is getting worse again
(c) The patient has plugged off and collapsed a lobe
(d) She patient has a pneumothorax

The Acutely Unwell Patient: Answers

Case 1: A patient with chest pain following a fall

1. (d) He was in pain, which was adequately treated

Physiological variables are an important way to define severity of illness and deviation from the 'normal' must be carefully appraised. Variation in a single parameter may be sensitive for severity of illness but has low specificity. In this case the patient's physiological response was in relation to pain. He could have had an asthma attack but there was no audible wheeze and it would not have got better without specific treatment.

2. (a) Asthma attack (b) Pneumothorax
(c) Haemothorax

The patient received the non-steroidal drug (NSAID) ibuprofen. Approximately 3–4% of individuals with asthma have attacks following aspirin or NSAIDs. However, patients usually know if they are aspirin sensitive because this drug is freely available over the counter. Rib fractures are difficult to visualize on chest radiographs and there are usually as many unseen as seen ones. Bleeding from the fractures (haemothorax) or laceration of the pleura (pneumothorax) are both highly likely. In a young patient significant bleeding may occur whilst BP is preserved in the early stages of haemorrhage. Pulmonary embolus would occur at no greater incidence than any other 32-year-old at this early stage.

3. (d) Intercostal tube drainage with underwater seal

Chest radiographs are two-dimensional representations of the thorax and so under-represent the size of pneumothoraces. Indeed, a 1 cm rim of air round the lung corresponds to a 27% pneumothorax, whilst 2 cm rim of air is equivalent to 50%. The patient has marked physiological abnormality and is critically ill, observation is not appropriate, and he may die if this is left untreated. Aspiration is only indicated in spontaneous pneumothoraces or small secondary pneumothoraces (<2 cm) where there is minimal breathlessness and the patient is <50 years of age. Surgery is only indicated when intercostal tube drainage has failed.

4. (d) Lactate 8 mmol/L

The patient's oxygenation is not normal; as a very rough rule PaO_2 should be about 10 kPa less than the inspired oxygen percentage. The inability of the saturation probe to record in this instance is related to an inadequate peripheral circulation. The $PaCO_2$ is low, which in the context of a normal pH implies respiratory compensation for a metabolic acidosis. The lactate is very high. This patient has shock: hypotension, tachycardia, tachypnoea, compensated metabolic acidosis, poor peripheral circulation, confusion and hyperlactaemia. This patient is extremely ill.

5. (c) Ruptured spleen (haemorrhagic shock)

The patient is not immunocompromised. The drain could provide a potential portal of infection but providing this is inserted using a sterile technique infection is very uncommon (particularly after only 1 day). Tension pneumothorax has been excluded by the chest radiograph and the drain swinging with respiration. Myocardial infarct would be unlikely in a young man in the absence of risk factors. The site of trauma was the 8th to 10th ribs and the spleen lies immediately below. Delayed haemorrhage of the spleen can occur days after blunt trauma.

Further reading: Chapter 12 in Medicine at a Glance.

Case 2: A hospitalized patient who develops neutropenia and a temperature

1. (c) Septic shock

The patient is shocked: hypoxia, tachypnoea, altered mental state, hypotension, tachycardia and oliguria. This shock state is associated with positive blood cultures. Septic shock may be associated with fever or hypothermia.

2. (a) Rapid infusion of fluids
(b) Antibiotics

Appropriate antibiotics are life saving and should be given immediately. Survival decreases by 7.6% for each hour delay in administration of antibiotics after the onset of hypotension in septic shock. Rapid infusion of fluid is a requisite, as is oxygen therapy, but this must be high flow through a non-rebreath bag (not 28%). Noradrenaline is often used in septic shock but this should be done in a critical care area with arterial pressure monitoring.

3. (a) Remove the Hickman line

There is no focus of sepsis other than the Hickman line, which is showing signs of erythema. Line infections are typically associated with Gram-positive infections with organisms such as *Staphylococcus aureus*. An essential part of treating septic shock is source control , i.e. if there is an abscess, drain it; if there is peritonitis, wash out the abdomen and repair the perforated viscus. The patient will not get better unless the Hickman line is removed; this can be replaced, the patient cannot!

Further reading: Chapter 18.

Case 3: A patient with septic shock

1. (b) Cholangitis caused by gallstones
(c) Pancreatitis

The patient has symptoms of obstructive jaundice. She is in the typical demographic group for gallstones. Septic shock could also be the result of pancreatitis, which is often caused by gallstones. In other words the gallstone has caused obstructive jaundice in the absence of cholangitis and pancreatitis.

2. (b) Ultrasound of the biliary tract

About 20% of gallstones are present on plain radiographs, but this does not add to the diagnostic process. MRCP will adequately image the biliary tree; however the patient is in septic shock. Magnetic resonance imaging is often situated a long way from acute service areas of the hospital, monitoring is technically more difficult (because of the magnetic field) and the imaging itself is not quick to perform. MRCP is not appropriate in this patient. An ultrasound will show whether the biliary tree is dilated and may demonstrate a gallstone. It can be undertaken at the patient's bedside. Ultrasound can also examine the pancreas if pancreatitis is suspected.

3. (a) Endoscopic retrograde cholangiopancreatography (ERCP)
(b) Intravenous antibiotics

Antibiotics are life saving in septic shock. Source control must be achieved, which means draining the biliary tree. This can be achieved with ERCP, where the stone can be retrieved using a basket and a sphincterotomy performed to achieve adequate drainage; alternatively a stent can be inserted if the stone can not be removed. Cholecystectomy alone does not affect biliary drainage. PTC carries the risk of trauma and bleeding to the liver and should only be performed if ERCP fails; it is only feasible when there is intrahepatic duct dilatation.

Further reading: Chapter 161.

Case 4: A feverish patient with a productive cough

1. (b) There is poor peripheral perfusion due to a shock state

The patient is not currently hypoxic so there is sufficient oxygen content in the blood. The problem is that there is poor delivery of the oxygen to the peripheral tissues. This is evidenced by the cool peripheries and delayed capillary refill time. The raised lactate is a worrying feature and needs prompt treatment.

2. (a) Fluid bolus

This patient has septic shock and will be intravascularly fluid deplete. Frusemide and renal dose dopamine have no role in treating oliguria. The mainstay of initial treatment is aggressive fluid challenges of either crystalloid (0.9% saline or Hartmann's) or colloid solutions. If these fail vasopressor agents such as noradrenaline can be instituted. Early, aggressive resuscitation saves lives and prevents the development of further organ dysfunction.

3. (c) 4

The CURB-65 is a mortality prediction tool for severe community-acquired pneumonia. One point is given for each parameter present:

C – confusion
U – Urea >7 mmol/L
R – Respiratory rate >30 beats/min
B – BP <90 mmHg systolic or <60 mmHg diastolic
65 – age 65 or older

Her mortality, with a score of 4, is actually 41.5% which helps to highlight just how unwell she is.

4. (d) Within an hour

This is the maximum time recommended by the comprehensive Surviving Sepsis Campaign guidelines, which are important

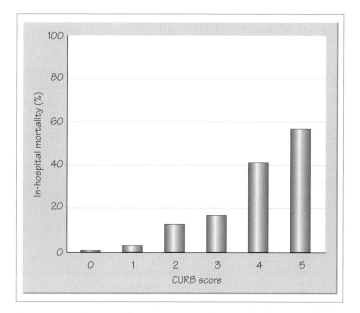

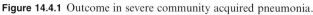

Figure 14.4.1 Outcome in severe community acquired pneumonia.

reading (*Crit Care Med* 2008 36(1); 296–327). You should ensure that appropriate cultures are taken prior to starting antibiotics. In hypotensive patients with septic shock the mortality rate increases by 7.6% for each hour delay in antibiotic administration.

Further reading: Chapter 161.

Case 5: A patient with haematemesis

1. (d) Urgent laparotomy

The patient is shocked (hypotension, tachycardia, tachypnoea, hyperlactaemia) due to continued bleeding. In other words the patient has had a failed therapeutic endoscopy. Giving blood or proton pump inhibitors will not stop the bleeding and the patient requires definitive surgery. Had the patient initially stopped bleeding following the procedure and then re-bled, a repeat therapeutic endoscopy might have been indicated, followed by surgery if this second procedure failed. Mortality increases with age, co-morbidities, shock and endoscopic stigmata of major haemorrhage. These indices are included in the Rockall scoring system, which defines the risk of re-bleeding and death following admission to hospital with non-variceal acute gastrointestinal haemorrhage.

2. (e) All of the above

All of the answers are possibilities in this patient. Although the patient has no co-morbid history, severe haemorrhagic shock may precipitate an ischaemic event in a patient with subclinical coronary artery disease (the patient is 61 years). There has been vigorous fluid replacement and fluid overload is possible if the patient has abnormal LV function. Aspiration pneumonitis is a possibility but is less likely if the patient has remained conscious and therefore able to protect his airway. One may also expect to see soiling of the airway at intubation or suction gastric contents from the endotracheal tube. TRALI is the leading cause of mortality in transfusion-related reactions. It is probably due to the presence of antibodies to human leukocyte antigen (HLA) molecules in the recipient; it is therefore commoner with FFP but can occur with packed red cells. Essentially, this is a form of non-cardiogenic pulmonary oedema caused by microvascular inflammation and capillary leak. Treatment is supportive. If this diagnosis is suspected then the blood bank should be informed so that this can be investigated further.

3. (d) SIMV, tidal volume 420 ml, rate 12/min, PEEP 12 cmH$_2$O

The patient has lung injury and ventilating at 10 mL/kg ideal body weight will cause further damage and increase mortality. The PEEP should be set so that the lung is optimally recruited; this is a somewhat complex topic and beyond the scope of this text. However a PEEP of 2 cmH$_2$O is too low and mechanical ventilation at this level will cause repeated opening and closing of lung units (alectotrauma), again contributing to lung injury.

Lung injury is characterized as acute lung injury (ALI) or adult respiratory distress syndrome (ARDS) and is defined by a measure called the P/F ratio. This refers to the partial pressure of arterial oxygen (in mmHg) divided by the inspired oxygen fraction: ALI 200–300, ARDS <200. Thus if PaO_2 is 10 kPa (76 mmHg) and the inspired oxygen is 100%, then the P/F ratio is 76 ÷ 1.0 = 76. The definition of ALI/ARDS takes no account of PEEP, which may radically alter this value. The definition also requires an acute onset, bilateral infiltrates on chest X-ray and the absence of LV failure.

4. (d) 1:3

Each breath has an inspiratory time of 1s and there are 15 breaths/min. In total inspiration lasts 15sec, thus expiration lasts 45sec (60–15). The ratio of I:E is therefore 15:45 = 1:3.

5. (a) Turn patient from supine to prone
   (b) Give inhaled nitric oxide
   (c) Increase PEEP
   (e) Increase inspiratory time and reduce the I:E ratio

Prone positioning and inhaled nitric oxide can improve oxygenation in some patients with ALI/ARDS by improving $\dot{V}/\dot{Q}$ relationships. Oxygenation is a function of mean airway pressure, which is increased by elevating PEEP or increasing inspiratory time. The increase in mean airway pressure recruits more lung, improving $\dot{V}/\dot{Q}$ relationships. Rarely an inspiratory time longer than expiration is required; this so-called inverse ratio ventilation is uncomfortable for patients, who need to be deeply sedated (and sometimes paralysed with neuromuscular blocking drugs), and may also adversely effect haemodynamics if the patient is dehydrated.

Further reading: Chapter 101.

Case 6: A patient with a severe asthma attack

1. (a) Magnesium sulphate intravenously
   (b) Salbutamol
   (c) Corticosteroids

Steroids, β_2-agonists and magnesium sulphate are all useful drugs in the treatment of bronchospasm. Antibiotics are only indicated if there is evidence of pneumonia. The presence of green sputum alone in asthma in the absence of other indicators of infection is not an indication for antibiotics as this may reflect inflammatory cells in the airways.

2. (f) All of the above

Patients with severe asthma tend to have had little to drink and have increased insensible losses, particularly if they have been unwell for several days. The introduction of positive pressure ventilation reduces venous return and cardiac output and blood pressure drops. This responds to fluid replacement. A pneumothorax may be a life-threatening complication and may cause cardiac tamponade; indeed this could have been the cause of the cardiac arrest. Whilst a chest X-ray will show a pneumothorax, it should be possible to diagnose and treat this clinically. Magnesium sulphate dilates smooth muscle, hence its use in bronchospasm; however, it can cause vasodilatation and a drop in blood pressure, especially if administered rapidly. Hypercapnia causes pulmonary vasoconstriction and dilatation of the systemic vasculature and can therefore contribute to hypotension. Overvigorous ventilation causes air trapping and increases intrinsic or auto positive end-expiratory pressure (PEEP). The high intrathoracic pressures reduce venous return and thus blood pressure.

3. (b) Auto-PEEP has increased

The probability of pulmonary embolism is low but higher than in a well individual. In the context of severe bronchospasm, this probability will not change greatly with this ventilator change. 'Plugging off' by tenacious sputum plugs is common in severe asthma, but this would tend to cause hypoxia. Hypoxia would have to be extremely severe for hypotension to occur in a young adult. The I:E ratio has changed from 1:5 (10:50sec) to 1:2 (20:40sec). Asthma is a disease of the small airways, which tend to collapse on expiration; different lung units empty at different rates. If expiration is not prolonged, gas is still emptying from the lung when the next breath is delivered. This leads to progressive breath stacking and the lungs become increasingly hyperinflated, also known as auto-PEEP. The high intrathoracic pressures reduce venous return. This hypotension will respond to fluid and lengthening the inspiration to expiration (I:E) ratio.

4. (a) The patient is developing ventilator-associated pneumonia (VAP)

There is nothing to suggest the patient's asthma has got worse. The primary problem is that the patient has a deterioration in oxygenation which could be caused by a pneumothorax or plugging; however, the new high fever should initiate the search for a new infection. VAP can be difficult to diagnose; it is associated with new or abundant secretions, chest X-ray changes, fever, increased white blood cell count and positive microbiology on lung lavage.

Further reading: Chapter 101.

Keep up with critical fields

Would you like to receive up-to-date information on our books, journals and databases in the areas that interest you, direct to your mailbox?

Join the **Wiley e-mail service** - a convenient way to receive updates and exclusive discount offers on products from us.

Simply visit www.wiley.com/email and register online

We won't bombard you with emails and we'll only email you with information that's relevant to you. We will ALWAYS respect your e-mail privacy and NEVER sell, rent, or exchange your e-mail address to any outside company. Full details on our privacy policy can be found online.

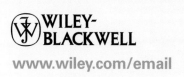

WILEY-BLACKWELL

www.wiley.com/email

17841

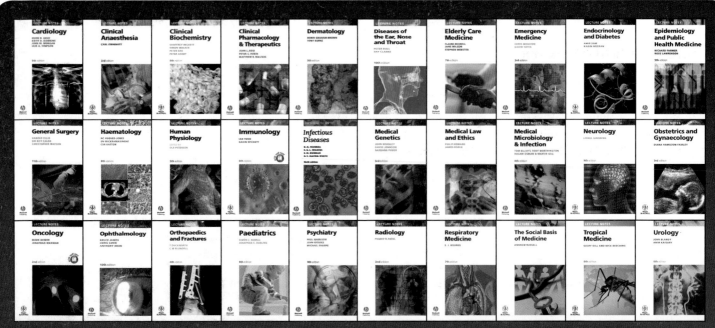
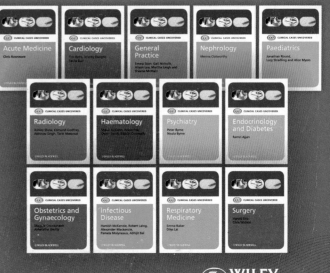
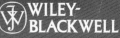